KETO
QUICKSTART

A Beginner's Guide to a Whole–Foods Ketogenic Diet

New York Times bestselling author
DIANE SANFILIPPO

VICTORY BELT PUBLISHING Inc.
Las Vegas

First Published in 2019 by Victory Belt Publishing Inc.

Copyright © 2019 by Diane Sanfilippo

ISBN-13: 978-1-628603-47-7

Cover photography by Diane Sanfilippo
Food photography by Diane Sanfilippo
Cover design by Charisse Reyes
Interior design by Yordan Terziev and Boryana Yordanova

Printed in Canada
TC 0118

CONTENTS

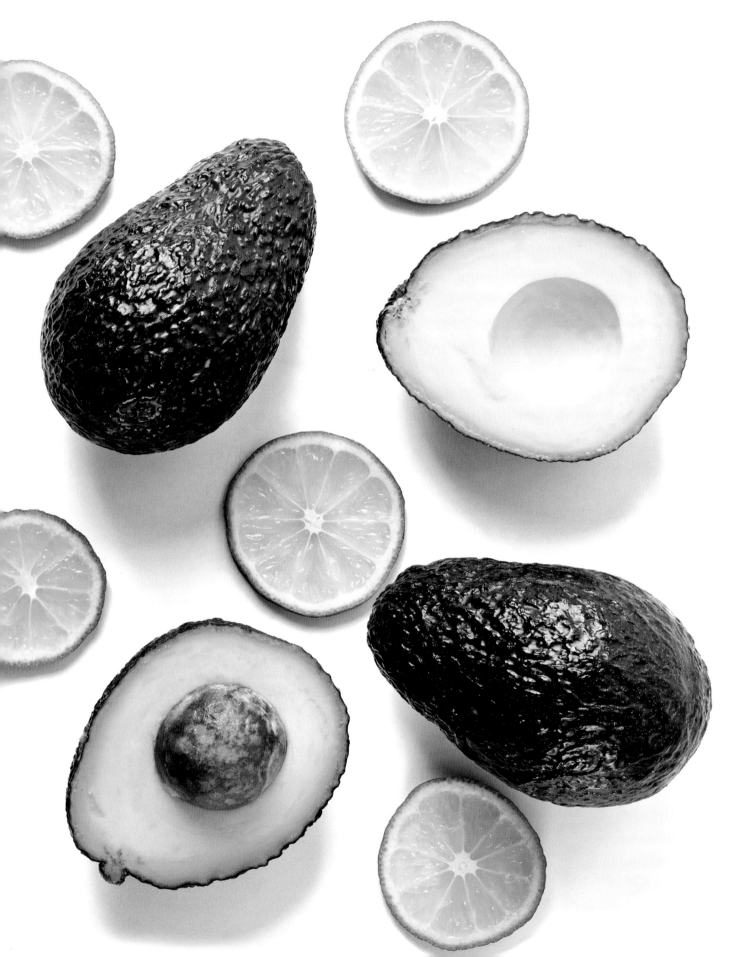

Introduction

Welcome to a new way of looking at your plate!

We all want to eat what's best for ourselves and our health, but at some point, figuring out what that means can become overwhelming, and when the media is full of conflicting information, it's enough to make even the savviest of eaters throw up their hands and ask, "What gives?!"

Allow me to set your mind at ease. This book will give you a new way of approaching how you eat. You may choose to use this approach solely for a short-term reset to get yourself off of a blood sugar roller coaster, lose some body fat, or kick some bad habits that have crept in over a stressful period of time—or you may find that this becomes your new lifestyle going forward. Either way, there are amazing benefits to experience by filling your plate with nutrient-dense, satiating foods, focusing on quality protein, healthy fats, and plenty of vegetables while cutting out processed foods and excess carbs—which is exactly what you'll learn how to do in this book.

A NATIONAL HEALTH CRISIS

In the last forty years or so, we've gone all too far to the opposite extreme of what healthy eating can and should look like. Starting with the invention of hydrogenated oils (in the early 1900s), continuing with the introduction of high-fructose corn syrup (in the 1970s) and canola oil (in 1978) into the marketplace, and finally coming to a largely grain-based (nay, *sugar*-based) diet today, our health has gotten progressively worse.

According to the Centers for Disease Control and Prevention, as of 2017, diabetes is the seventh-leading cause of death in the United States and affects nearly one in ten Americans. (This refers primarily to type 2 diabetes, a condition brought on by diet and lifestyle, not type 1 diabetes, an autoimmune disease. Of all diabetes patients in the US, 90 to 95 percent have type 2.) Worldwide, this number is even more staggering: in 2011, over 366 million people had diabetes, half of which were undiagnosed, and this number will reportedly rise to well over 500 million by the year 2030. In 2000, this number was just 150 million—so by 2030, the number of cases of diabetes worldwide will have *tripled* over the course of three decades.

It's hard to know for sure how many cases of heart disease—the number one cause of death—type 2 diabetes contributes to, but I'd venture to guess it's a large percentage. The National Heart, Lung, and Blood Institute states that "type 2 diabetes raises your risk of having 'silent' heart disease—that is, heart disease with no signs or symptoms. You can even have a heart attack without feeling symptoms. Diabetes-related nerve damage that blunts heart pain may explain why symptoms aren't noticed."* So we see that even though it's the number seven cause of death in the United States, type 2 diabetes is likely contributing significantly to the number one cause of death.

I believe there's a strong connection between our national health and our national diet.

Today people are also being diagnosed with autoimmune conditions at higher rates than ever. The various incarnations of autoimmune disease—celiac disease, colitis, Crohn's disease, lupus, psoriasis, rheumatoid arthritis, Hashimoto's thyroiditis, and many more—impact over twenty-three million Americans, according to the National Institute of Environmental Health. I believe there's a strong connection between our national health and our national diet.

---

* *"Diabetic Heart Disease," National Heart, Lung, and Blood Institute, n.d., www.nhlbi.nih.gov/health-topics/ diabetic-heart-disease.*

FINDING A SOLUTION IN FOOD

We can't expect our health-care system to fix what's broken. Problems rooted in diet and lifestyle simply cannot be solved in a medical setting. For example: your doctor cannot possibly reverse type 2 diabetes with medication—period. It won't happen. Diabetes medication can improve *numbers*, but it cannot *heal your body*.

But I've heard from countless people who, after just a week on my 21-Day Sugar Detox program, which is similar in many ways to a keto diet, stopped needing multiple prescription medications. Within seven days of changing the food on their plates, people's bodies are righting themselves. This isn't wizardry; it's nature. Our bodies work optimally when given a better set of inputs—that is, *real food*, not processed, carb-loaded junk. Of course these folks all consult with their doctors before ceasing any medications (as should you!), but this is staggering. Doctors aren't typically giving nutritional advice to cut back on refined carbs and sugar, but they're quick to say "Keep doing what you're doing" when they see the results.

> **Our bodies work optimally when given a better set of inputs—that is, *real food*, not processed, carb-loaded junk.**

Naysayers will argue that keto is just another fad diet. To that I say: not the case. There's a reason why various diets or ways of eating gain traction and begin to fill up bookstore shelves: *they work for and help a lot of people!* And science backs up the experiences so many people have had on keto. In the coming chapters, I'll explain why eating few carbs, more fat, and a good amount of protein will stabilize blood sugar, promote weight loss, and improve the symptoms of many health conditions, including type 2 diabetes, epilepsy, heart disease, and more. And besides, to me, trying something new isn't following a fad; it's being open-minded and experimenting to find what works best for you.

WHY A KETO BOOK?

Many of you may know me as the author of *Practical Paleo*, and you may be wondering why I've written a book about keto. Well, as you'll read in the next chapter, I've eaten a Paleo-style keto diet on and off for years—consistently for about a year and a half and as a reset diet many times since. I know and love the merits of this way of eating, but I think that many approaches to keto go to extremes or don't focus on how to easily eat keto with a real-foods focus, and that can make it not only difficult to sustain but also less beneficial in the longer term for overall health.

So I decided to write this book to explain how to come up with a truly healthy keto diet that you can live with for the long term—or use as a short-term reset diet if you find yourself feeling off or what you've been doing stops working, or use to launch a low-carb diet that works for you but may not be strictly keto. My focus is on the practical: what to expect when you start eating keto; how to ease into keto in a doable way; how to determine if you need more carbs than is standard on keto and how to incorporate those carbs in a healthy way; how to customize keto for particular goals, especially weight loss; and things to be aware of if you're concerned about a particular health issue, such as type 2 diabetes, cancer, heart disease, or liver health.

WHO THIS BOOK IS FOR

Understandably, many folks are worn out on dietary advice. If you feel like rebelling entirely against the diet industry, you're not alone! For some people, simply moderating what they eat feels comfortable; they can have a bite of something here or there and don't feel out of control, and it even works to keep them healthy. If you're feeling perfectly happy with where you're at with your food and your health, then keep doing what's working for you.

But chances are, that isn't you. If it were you, you probably wouldn't be reading a book on keto! For many, improving health through different food choices, whether they're major or minor changes, is always going to be relevant. And as humans, we need to turn to one another, to those who are experts on various topics, for advice and guidance in making changes in our lives. That's my goal with this book: to support you as you seek a way of eating that will help you feel better.

That's my goal with this book: to support you as you seek a way of eating that will help you feel better.

I find there are two camps of people who are interested in learning about and implementing a ketogenic diet, and this book is for both.

THE FIRST CAMP: You're generally healthy, but you want to optimize or tweak your nutrition and see if keto could be a way to feel better. You're not feeling worn out on dietary advice—in fact, that's why you've picked up this book. You want to read my take on how keto can help you, how to do it, what to eat, and what to look out for in terms of pitfalls and tweaking. Perfect. Welcome! You'll find plenty here about ways to truly nourish your body and how keto can help you level up in many areas of health.

THE SECOND CAMP: You've heard that eating keto can help you to heal. Maybe you are dealing with unstable blood sugar or metabolic issues (type 2 diabetes, for example), have an autoimmune condition, suffer with inflammatory issues, need to lose body fat to improve your health, or currently experience general fatigue. Or maybe you want to eat preventatively to ward off neurological or metabolic problems. For any and all of these concerns, you've probably heard that keto can help.

I want you to know that I've written this book with both camps in mind. For those looking to optimize your health, I see you and hear you! I will always offer my best, most balanced and thoughtful advice, and I believe there's so much here that you'll find valuable and helpful.

In my heart, however, I most want to reach those of you who are desperately seeking to *transform* your health. I'm talking to those of you who are on medications and seeking to get off of them (with the help of a medical professional, of course!), those of you who are struggling with autoimmune flares, and those of you who feel at a total loss for how to get your health back on track when you don't want to be deprived of good food. Your stories move me, and the desire to help you is what gets me out of bed in the morning and keeps me writing. If I help one person to reverse disease or get off a medication that had previously been a lifetime prescription, I'll have done my job.

The Limits of Weight Loss

I'd like to note here that when I present information in this book that may help you to lose weight or body fat, I am in no way expressing that I think that losing weight is ever the key to health or wellness, and certainly not happiness. If you've picked up this book presuming that "once I lose that last five or ten pounds, I'll be happy," allow me to stop you right here—it doesn't work that way.

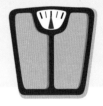

WHO THIS BOOK IS NOT FOR

Even if you want or need to make nutritional changes in your life, a keto diet may not be right for you.

First, if you have a diagnosed medical condition, talk to a qualified, keto-knowledgeable health professional about your specific condition and any medications you may be taking.

Some populations I'd say are not best suited to eating keto are:

- **Children of rapid growth and developmental ages (generally under age 18),** except in the cases of neurological or behavioral conditions that a medical professional and parents have agreed to address nutritionally (in combination with other therapeutic interventions). Keto won't necessarily inhibit growth or development, but if calories are not carefully maintained or some nutrients are missing from the diet, it may not be ideal. That said, if a child is provided with a variety of real, whole foods and tends to eat more fat and protein and fewer carbs naturally, I would not consider it cause for concern.

- **The elderly.** A keto diet is very satiating, and many people experience a drop in appetite as they age, so on keto, they may not eat enough to get adequate calories.

- **"Hardgainers"**—folks who consistently have trouble gaining weight and fall below a healthy weight when not working diligently to maintain it.

- **Those with disordered eating patterns.** If this is you, I recommend you work with an expert on disordered eating or a medical professional and avoid keto. Any way of eating that becomes restrictive or triggering can cause problems, and it's best not to put yourself in that situation.

- **Those with diagnosed hypoglycemia.** I'm not referring to someone who feels like they have low blood sugar now and then; I'm talking about hypoglycemia that's been diagnosed by a medical doctor. You cannot diagnose this by feel; it requires blood glucose testing.

- **Pregnant or breastfeeding women who were not eating keto before becoming pregnant.** Keto isn't contraindicated during pregnancy, but because changing your diet brings a set of lifestyle changes and new potential stressors—using new criteria to decide what to eat, cooking more often and with new ingredients, investing the emotional energy to commit to something new, and other changes that can wear on a pregnant woman—I think it's not worth experimenting with your eating habits during this time. It's also very common to have an aversion to protein, at least in the first trimester, which would make your keto-friendly options much more limited. I think trusting what your body is telling you during this time is really important, and I wouldn't force any one way of eating (other than to say avoiding poor-quality and refined foods is always a good idea). I suggest you consult a keto-educated health practitioner for a recommendation here. All this applies to breastfeeding women, too, especially those with a newborn; with all the changes that a new baby brings, it may not be a good time to try out another lifestyle change.

- **Those struggling with adrenal fatigue or extreme exhaustion.** Transitioning to a keto diet can add physical and emotional stress that exacerbate this condition. However, if part of what caused the adrenal stress was a high-carb diet or blood sugar dysregulation, then using keto to regulate blood sugar and appetite may be helpful. Work with the practitioner who diagnosed you with adrenal fatigue or exhaustion to determine the best diet for you.

Finally, this book may not be right for you if:

- you are looking for a quick fix and are unwilling to put in the time it will take to reap the benefits. While four weeks is a great amount of time to reboot healthy habits, seeing the effects in your physical appearance and in your blood work will likely require at least eight to twelve weeks.

- you eat (or want to eat) a mostly plant-based diet (see page 20)

HOW TO USE THIS BOOK

While there are certainly some folks for whom eating keto is a permanent lifestyle, there are many more for whom it's a way to quick-start an overall lower-carb lifestyle. Regardless of how you decide to use keto, here's how I suggest you approach your first experience with it: commit to keto for at least three months. This initial three-month period is your Keto Quick Start.

For the first month, follow it strictly, without adding any extra carbs. The idea here is that you jump-start your body's transition to burning fat for fuel and prime your metabolism to be in a fat-burning state. From there, you can develop a keto (or mostly keto) lifestyle, or you can learn what you need to learn from how you feel in the initial three months, and adjust and move away from it.

In this book, you'll find the tools and resources to discover what to eat, how much, and how to move through life for those first three months. Should you choose to continue with keto after those three months, I'll suggest ways to balance eating more carbs now and then according to your activity and energy levels. In fact, after the first month, if you're not working to heal a specific health condition, I recommend tinkering with these levels to find what works best for you in terms of (1) how you feel—your energy, moods, sleep, etc., (2) how your body is responding, especially in terms of fat loss if that's a primary goal, and (3) how manageable or maintainable it feels to eat keto 100 percent of the time, or if maybe 90 percent would work better for you.

The therapeutic benefits of a ketogenic diet are many, and I'll discuss them in the following chapters, but if the diet weren't sustainable, that wouldn't matter. I strongly believe that the absolute best way of eating for the longer term is one that you can maintain without feeling like you're imprisoned by rules or someone else's plan.

It's imperative that we all find what works best for each of us, whether that's eating strictly keto all of the time or most of the time, or eating low-carb, or even eating more carbs. As a nutritionist, it's my job to help you find what works to support your body in naturally achieving optimal health. With this book, I propose that you see how keto works for you and your body, with a "quick start" approach that you can customize for your needs.

There isn't a right or wrong way to utilize keto as a nutritional tool. You're not "wrong" if you eat keto for three months of the year and incorporate more carbs for the other nine months. In fact, some would argue it's very seasonally appropriate to eat lower-carb for three to six months of the year—generally late fall into spring, when fruit isn't in season—and then eat more carbs when seasonally appropriate—when nutrient-dense whole foods rich in carbs, like fruit, are abundant.

The tools are all here for you to use in whatever way works best for you. Listen to your body, and enjoy the many benefits of a low-carb, high-fat diet!

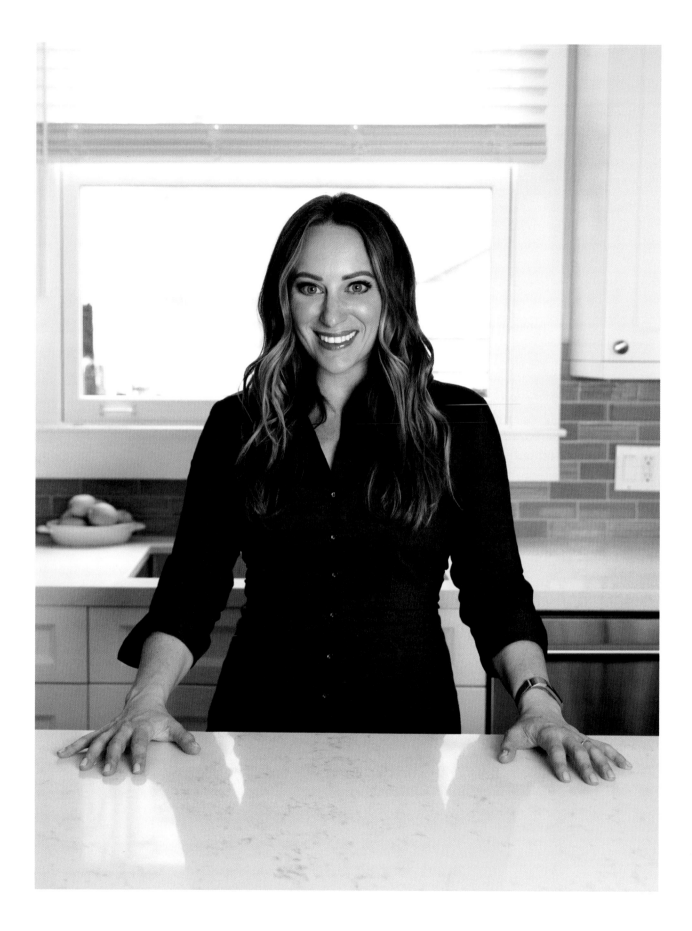

My Keto Story

Like most kids, I never thought about nutrition when I was growing up. I ate whatever I liked, I was always in pretty good shape, and I considered myself to be healthy and strong.

Then, during high school, I began to have disruptive bouts of digestive distress, to the extent that I took Imodium A-D several times a week. I also suffered from repeated sinus infections, which became so old hat that I simply demanded antibiotics when I visited the doctor. After all, I had been taught that pills were the best way to handle symptoms.

My close friends struggled with the same health issues. All of us had a range of chronic ailments, such as acne, pharyngitis, heartburn, headaches, dental cavities, and deteriorating vision, in addition to sinus and digestive discomfort. It never occurred to any of us that we had the power to prevent these problems.

After eighteen years as an active youth, I became much less active in college, and my weight started to rise. My late nights with pizza and Buffalo wings meant that the "freshman fifteen" didn't go away after freshman year. I continued to eat like an athlete even though I had all but abandoned that aspect of my life. By the time I finished college, I had put on thirty pounds. There is a photo from my graduation dinner that shows my bloated midsection—it's one I use as a "before" picture when I tell my story at seminars. At the time, I had no idea my body had fallen completely apart.

Like many people who gain weight during their college years, I thought, "This is just what happens when people get older." I learned later, of course, that it's what happens when people stop exercising and eat foods that do not support a healthy body. My symptoms may have been common, but what I didn't realize until later is that "common" doesn't necessarily mean "normal."

In the year after college, I gained yet another ten pounds, and a nurse practitioner brought up my weight during a routine checkup. She talked to me about food portion sizes, and I suddenly realized how out of control my eating had become. Even though everyone around me ate the same way, I couldn't deny that I didn't feel or look good.

That winter, I joined a gym and tried to watch what I ate, but I had no clue what that meant. I dined out on burgers and fries (on large seedy buns, of course) and washed it all down with Coke. I did know that soda wasn't healthy, so I sometimes substituted water instead. At home, I made dinners of pasta with red sauce and analyzed the meal in my head. "Well, that's just some pasta and tomatoes," I'd think, "so it's healthy." I gave myself a bit less than I served my boyfriend, and I sweated away on the cardio machines at the gym. You probably aren't surprised to hear that my weight did not budge.

Months later, I started a new job and found myself surrounded by women on Weight Watchers. "Okay," I thought, "if they can do it, I can do it." So I started the diet and stayed on it . . . until the end of each workday, when I found myself still hungry and with no points left. I knew that going home and not eating anything for the rest of the evening wasn't an option, so I bent the rules on the points system. But I had started to work out, and in spite of my rule-bending, the diet began to work. I was losing weight.

What Weight Watchers taught me more than anything was to read food labels. Granted, I now teach people to read labels more for ingredients, which reveal the quality of the item in their hand, but paying attention to calories, fat, and fiber was a start for me. I lost twelve pounds simply by watching my diet and working out on the elliptical machine for thirty minutes several times a week. The initial weight loss gave me the confidence to exercise at the gym more often, and I started lifting weights again for the first time in four years.

Days turned into weeks and months, and before I knew it, I had lost thirty pounds. In many ways, I felt amazing—my body was finally getting back to a size that was more comfortable for me. But the rest of my system was the same as it had always been: riddled with digestive distress, chronic sinus infections, and deteriorating vision.

But the rest of my system was the same as it had always been: riddled with digestive distress, chronic sinus infections, and deteriorating vision.

I even had a new ailment to add to the mix: bouts of low blood sugar, which caused me to nearly pass out at times. When I became shaky, sweaty, and light-headed, a friend usually said, "Get her a granola bar!" Of course, it turned out that was the last thing I needed.

FIRST CAME PALEO

It wasn't until several years later that I discovered the root cause of my chronic symptoms of low blood sugar was my high carb intake. I was eating close to 300 grams of carbohydrates a day, reaching for bread with olive oil if my dinner wasn't filling enough, but I thought it was crazy that bread—innocent old bread— could be the source of such hefty problems.

When I finally came to terms with the long list of conditions associated with not only gluten intolerance but also a high-carb diet, it still took me more time to finally make the switch to a lower-carb, gluten-free diet—not quite Paleo yet, but in that direction. It took reading books on the topic, attending seminars for health-care practitioners on gluten sensitivity, and tuning in to how my body was truly reacting when I ate pasta (indigestion), whole-wheat bread (digestive distress), and more carbs than I really needed (bloating, weight gain, and overall lethargy).

It wasn't until several years later that I discovered the root cause of my chronic symptoms of low blood sugar was my high carb intake.

Then there were was a big turning point for me. Not long after converting to a 90 percent gluten-free and lower-carb way of eating, I attended Robb Wolf's Paleo Solution seminar. By then I had already studied nutrition for many years, but one of the biggest takeaways for me that day was that managing blood sugar, insulin levels, and systemic inflammation is critical for health and can be done fairly easily by avoiding certain foods we've come to rely on as staples in our diet: grains, legumes, poor-quality dairy, and sugar-laden foods. (Shocker, right?)

I went home and gutted my pantry, cleaning it of every grain—quinoa, buckwheat, rice, millet, gluten-free oats, and more. I stopped eating gluten-free grains and legumes entirely, shifted my meals away from carbs, and focused on protein and healthy fats, along with more vegetables. For dinner, I started preparing meat and vegetables with some fat and spices, and I cooked eggs and bacon in the mornings, packing them in a glass container to take to work so I could eat at my desk.

My coworkers were jealous as they chowed on bagels and granola bars and downed bowls of cereal, all of which were always well stocked in the office kitchen. When it was time for our lunch orders, I designed mine to provide me with as much protein and as many veggies as possible. When a last-minute work meeting over breakfast offered only pastries and fruit, I took a short walk to the corner deli for hard-boiled eggs to eat alongside the fruit for a much more satisfying meal. When I couldn't get enough healthy fare from a restaurant or deli, I brought extra food with me. That took a bit of planning, of course, but it was easier than you'd think.

The results were dramatic. I stopped suffering from the chronic ailments that had plagued me for most of my life. My digestion started working predictably well, I rarely got sinus infections, and the hypoglycemia disappeared. I no longer worried that I might pass out without a snack or that I might have to run to the bathroom when it wasn't convenient. The vision deterioration I had experienced for years halted, and I have not had a cavity in a long time.

Changing my diet resolved all of the ailments that had haunted me for years. It was a matter of healing my gut—which, in turn, healed my entire body—and balancing my blood sugar levels.

After these two main issues were addressed, I took the next step and fine-tuned my diet to optimize my health with keto.

THEN CAME KETO

I first started eating a ketogenic diet in 2010, long before I wrote the book I'm best known for, *Practical Paleo*—in fact, I was eating keto-Paleo when I wrote it!

A personal trainer friend of mine, Steve, heard me say that Paleo had been great for me, but I still wanted to find a better way to manage my blood sugar levels and appetite, and I wanted to see if I could also lose some body fat by tweaking my diet. Steve told me about the basic tenets of keto: that it's a low-carb, high-fat diet and causes your body to switch from primarily burning sugar to primarily burning fat. He suggested that I aim for about 30 grams of total carbs per day, and he also warned me that I would not likely see much in the way of results for around four to six weeks. But if I stuck with it, he said, I'd definitely see my body fat drop and feel improvements in my blood sugar control, my appetite wouldn't be so crazy (I'd be less hungry in general), and my overall energy would be much more even throughout the day.

Knowing that I needed to hang in there for a month helped me get through those first weeks, when I was fumbling and figuring out this new way of eating through trial and error. There weren't books on keto, and no one was really talking about it outside of bodybuilder communities and medical circles (where it was primarily seen as a treatment for epilepsy).

My "keto-Paleo" diet was still focused on whole, unprocessed foods; it just had more healthy fats and fewer carbs, and it was dairy-free.

So I started out simply paying attention to the carbs I ate, without trying too hard to cut them way back. I counted the carbs I ate each day, aiming for 30 grams but going over it now and then and not stressing about it. (I'd later come to learn that I was essentially eating the 30 grams of net carbs—total carbs minus fiber—on the days when I ate closer to 40 or 45 grams total carbs.) I also omitted starchy and sugary foods. Since I was already eating Paleo, this wasn't difficult, but it did require that I pay more attention to my food than I was accustomed to. My "keto-Paleo" diet was still focused on whole, unprocessed foods; it just had more healthy fats and fewer carbs, and it was dairy-free.

I got really lucky: I felt fine. Most people experience the "keto flu" for a couple of weeks when starting out on keto as their bodies adapt to the new diet. I didn't experience any of those ill effects, most likely because I was eating fairly low-carb beforehand. And sure enough, over time, I started to feel pretty darned awesome.

For the first time in my life, I was able to fast for twelve to sixteen hours without feeling so hungry and shaky that I thought I'd pass out. At this point, I was working full-time as a nutritionist: leading small-group talks, consulting one-on-one with clients, and teaching half- and full-day seminars all over the country. It was on weekends when I was traveling for these seminars that I felt the most direct positive effects of my keto-Paleo diet. There weren't as many healthy snack options then as there are now. I carried some almonds and 100% dark chocolate as well as homemade jerky with me, and that was about it. Eating keto allowed me to make long trips with just these small snacks, without feeling shaky, light-headed, or hungry. This was one of the biggest breakthroughs for me about this way of eating. Going far longer than three or four hours between meals felt like the ultimate freedom!

FitDay Journal for dianesanfilippo (Sep 11, 2010)

Food Eaten

Food Name	Amount	Unit	Cals	Carb	Fat	Prot
		Total	1,569	27.0	109.4	116.2
---BREAKFAST---	1	oz	0	0.0	0.0	0.0
Egg, whole, cooked	2	medium	147	1.1	10.7	10.8
Chicken, thigh, skin not eaten	1	oz	59	0.0	3.1	7.3
Chorizos	1	oz	129	0.5	10.8	6.8
Sauerkraut, 1/2 cup (Bubbie's, Fresh)	0.5	serving	3	1.5	0.0	0.0
Nuts, coconut milk, canned (liquid expressed from grated mea...	60	grams	118	1.7	12.8	1.2
Coffee	12	fl oz	4	0.2	0.1	0.4
---LUNCH---	1	serving	0	0.0	0.0	0.0
Lamb, roast, cooked	8	oz, boneless, cooked	603	0.0	41.2	54.3
Squash, spaghetti, cooked	100	grams	47	6.3	2.6	0.6
Onions, mature, cooked	25	grams	15	2.5	0.5	0.3
Tomatoes, cooked	25	grams	4	1.0	0.0	0.2
---DINNER---	1	serving	0	0.0	0.0	0.0
Lamb, roast, cooked	4	oz, boneless, cooked	302	0.0	20.6	27.1
Carrots, cooked	50	grams	27	4.0	1.2	0.4
Tomatoes, cooked	25	grams	4	1.0	0.0	0.2
Onions, mature, cooked	25	grams	15	2.5	0.5	0.3
---SNACK---	1	serving	0	0.0	0.0	0.0
Fig, raw	0.5	medium (2-1/4" dia)	18	4.8	0.1	0.2
Salami (Applegate: Organic Genoa, 1oz)	0.75	serving	75	0.0	5.2	6.0
		Total	1,569	27.0	109.4	116.2

Calories Eaten

	Grams	Calories	%-Cals
Calories		1,569	
Fat	109.4	977	62 %
Saturated	48.6	431	27 %
Polyunsaturated	9.8	88	6 %
Monounsaturated	39.0	351	22 %
Carbohydrate	27.0	101	6 %
Dietary Fiber	5.7		
Protein	116.2	489	31 %
Alcohol	0.0	0	0 %

Fat (62%) Carbs (6%)
Protein (31%) Alcohol (0%)

Here's an example of a FitDay.com record I kept in my early days of eating keto.

Over the last nearly decade or so, I've dabbled with various approaches to healthy eating—partially for the sake of self-experimentation and partially to offer insight to others on what may work for them. And time and time again, the way of eating I come back to for my own best-bet nutritional reset and overall lifestyle, the one that I can maintain for the longest amount of time, is based on keto. True, I don't always stick to a strict 30 grams of carbs per day. I don't think it's necessary for everyone to live in that space for prolonged durations of time. But getting most of my fuel from healthy fats and quality proteins while limiting my carb intake has proven to be the most sustainable and healthiest diet and lifestyle choice for me.

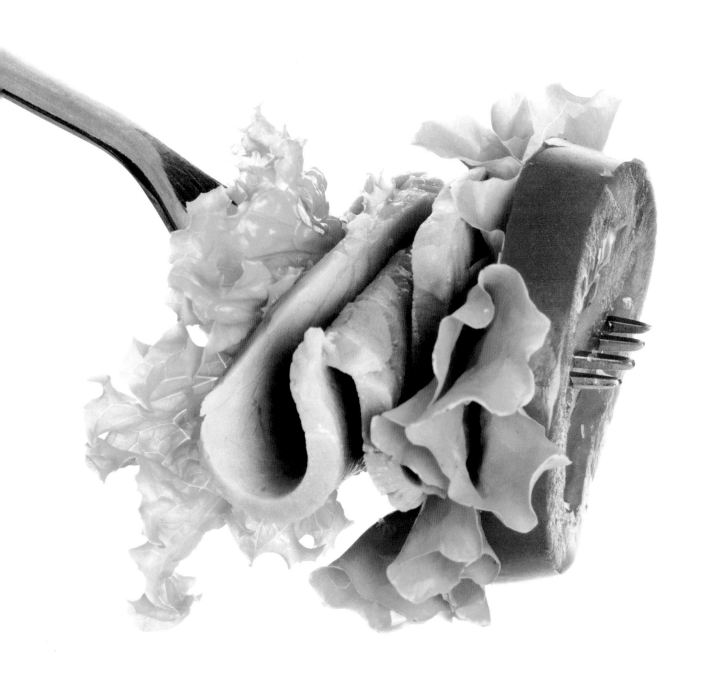

CHAPTER 1

Fueling Your Body

Before we dive headfirst into the details and nuances of eating keto, it's important to understand foundational aspects of nutrition and how foods work in the body. We're also going to look at how the body responds to different nutrients and how adjusting how much you eat of each one, and the balance of them on your plate, can hugely impact how you feel every day.

THE FUNDAMENTALS

Can Vegans Eat Keto?

While, technically speaking, eating keto without animal foods is certainly *possible*, in terms of fueling for optimal health, it's not something I recommend. There are vital nutrients that we all need to maintain our health that will be absent in a diet without animal foods (see page 49).

Furthermore, the specific aim of keto is to keep carbohydrate intake extremely low, and this becomes increasingly difficult if you're avoiding animal protein due to the carbohydrate content in vegan protein sources. For example, let's say you turn to lentils as a source of plant protein. To get 20 grams of protein from lentils, you'd also be consuming about 25 grams of net carbohydrates.

To make eating keto as easy and nutritious as possible, including animal foods is ideal because it allows you to obtain protein from sources that do not also include carbohydrates. This leaves a lot more room on your plate for colorful, nutrient-dense vegetables.

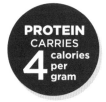

First, let's define the basics. There are three macronutrients that make up every food: fat, protein, and carbohydrate. Everything that goes onto your plate and into your body can be categorized as one of these or, more likely, some combination of the three. While some foods are called "proteins," for example, they typically also contain some fat. Likewise, foods that are called "fats" usually contain some protein. For our purposes, calling a food a "fat," "protein," or "carb" simply means that that's the primary macronutrient in the food.

Protein

Proteins are the building blocks of our bodies. We need to eat adequate protein in order to feel satiated from meals, to build and maintain muscle mass (critical for a healthy metabolism and fat-burning), to regulate our immune and endocrine systems, and to provide the foundation for balanced mental health.

Proteins are made of amino acids. There are nine essential amino acids—our bodies can't manufacture them, so we must eat them in our foods. These essential amino acids are histidine, isoleucine, leucine, methionine, phenylalanine, threonine, tryptophan, valine, and lysine. But as long as you're getting protein from animal foods, you don't need to know all that! If you aren't eating animal foods, then you'll need to make sure your foods are providing all of those essential amino acids to keep your body in good working order.

While we can get some trivial amounts of protein from plant-based foods, especially legumes, they're not a solid source of protein—in fact, the primary macronutrient in those foods is carbohydrate.

Fat

Fats allow us to store energy and regulate its use, insulate us, and serve as protection for our vital organs. Fats also work as messengers and help control essential functions like growth, immunity, reproduction, and basic metabolism. Fats also help us to absorb nutrients that are not water-soluble, namely vitamins

A, D, E, and K—also known as fat-soluble vitamins. We need dietary fats for proper vision, neurological health, immune health, healthy skin, hair, and nails, and just about every major body function.

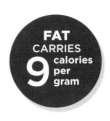

There are two classes of essential fatty acids (meaning our bodies can't make them, we must eat them): omega-6 and omega-3. We tend to get plenty of omega-6 fatty acids from foods such as nuts, seeds, meat, eggs, and vegetable oils (you'll avoid vegetable oils on your Keto Quick Start—more on this later), but most of us need to make an effort to include more omega-3-rich foods in our diets.

Omega-6 fatty acids are known to be pro-inflammatory and are therefore often demonized. But when they're consumed in whole foods (that is, not in vegetable oils and other refined foods), there is likely not a great cause for concern. Mild, short-term inflammation—what's called acute inflammation, the kind that you get when you cut your finger—helps us heal from whatever ails us, and supporting that isn't a bad thing! Just as long as we are also supporting our bodies' anti-inflammatory processes.

Omega-3 fatty acids are known to be anti-inflammatory. But although they're present in many foods—such as salmon, mackerel, sardines, and other cold-water fatty fish, as well as walnuts, chia seeds, and flax seeds—most people don't consume as much omega-3 as they should. Since, by default, we typically eat *way* more omega-6, we need to make a conscious, deliberate effort to include as many omega-3-rich foods in our diet as possible in order to balance pro- and anti-inflammatory effects of these fatty acids.

Of course, we eat other fats, too: saturated, monounsaturated, and polyunsaturated fats. You'll take a deep dive into tons of details on fats we should eat and avoid in chapter 5.

Carbohydrate

Often referred to as *saccharides* (not to be confused with sacchar*in*, which is an artificial sweetener), carbohydrates include sugars, starches, and cellulose (fiber). These are often categorized based on their molecule structure as monosaccharides, disaccharides, oligosaccharides, or polysaccharides. What's important to know about the variety of types of carbohydrates is that, while they do offer health benefits, none are essential to human life (unlike proteins and fats).

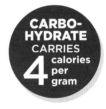

All carbohydrates break down in our bodies into glucose—sugar—whether those carbs come from pizza or a sweet potato. But foods that are good sources of healthy carbohydrates also provide vitamins and minerals, phytonutrients (compounds that give plants their variety of colors and have important health benefits, like lycopene and chlorophyll), antioxidants (which are known for their anti-inflammatory effects), fiber, and fuel for our beneficial gut bacteria. While your carbohydrate intake will be initially very low on keto, over time you'll learn how to include a variety of healthy carbohydrates in a balanced low-carb diet.

THE EFFECTS OF THE STANDARD AMERICAN DIET

The body doesn't respond to protein, fat, and carbs the same way. The amount of insulin released in response to each is different, they're stored in the body differently, and they affect satiety differently. The balance of macronutrients in your diet ends up literally changing how your body works.

The average American today eats a diet that's 10 to 15 percent protein, 40 to 50 percent carbohydrate, and 30 to 50 percent fat. This makes most of us sugar-burners—our bodies are primarily fueled by carbohydrates.

This balance of macronutrients often causes two common problems that can lead to many other issues (including insulin resistance, type 2 diabetes, heart disease, and cancer): unstable blood sugar and excess body fat. Both problems have their roots in the high amount of refined carbs in the standard American diet.

> **The average American today eats a diet that's 10 to 15 percent protein, 40 to 50 percent carbohydrate, and 30 to 50 percent fat.**

The Blood Sugar Roller Coaster

You know that feeling when you need a "second breakfast" around 10 a.m. or a snack around 3 p.m.? You know that feeling you get when you started out as simply hungry but then you had to wait another 30 or 40 minutes before eating and now you're ready to bite someone's head off? Yeah, that's "hangry," and it's a sign that what you're eating just plain isn't working for you.

What's happening is that your blood sugar is spiking after a meal and then crashing back down. To understand why, you have to understand the role of insulin, a hormone produced by the beta cells of the pancreas. It is insulin's job to move nutrients—including glucose—from your bloodstream, where they land after you digest your food, into your cells, where they can be utilized. This is why people with type 1 diabetes, who do not produce insulin, can experience rapid and extreme weight loss despite eating well. Without insulin, the nutrients from the food they eat never make it into their cells. In fact, before the discovery of insulin, type 1 diabetes was a death sentence: patients slowly starved to death, no matter how much they ate. Insulin moves nutrients from the bloodstream to cells over a period of one to two hours after you eat. It's especially important for insulin to clear excess glucose from the bloodstream, since high blood sugar is dangerous and is a key sign of the development of diabetes, both type 1 and type 2.

Carbs trigger the release of more insulin than fat and protein (especially in those of us for whom a high-carb diet simply doesn't work well or feel good). So a meal or snack heavy in carbs sends insulin into overdrive to put away all that glucose—

exactly as it should. But the spike in insulin, in response to the spike in blood glucose, can actually end up moving too much glucose out of your bloodstream. That's when the crash happens: your blood sugar drops below normal and you feel tired, irritable, foggy, and hungry.

Those are just the immediate symptoms. Frequently sending your blood sugar too high by eating a diet rich in refined carbs, as most of us do, also leads to poor sleep quality; hormonal imbalances; skin problems like acne, eczema, and psoriasis; digestive upset; and other inflammatory conditions. In the long term, it can lead to serious blood sugar problems like insulin resistance and type 2 diabetes.

So if you're dealing with any of those symptoms, it's a great sign that trying a keto way of eating for a period of time may help you feel a lot better, as it will kick off a new, healthy way of looking at food and building your meals from day to day. Or you may find that you want to carry it forward into a lifestyle shift for good!

The Post-Workout Window

For about thirty minutes to two hours after a workout, your muscles have first dibs on the carbs you eat by a process known as non-insulin-mediated glucose transport. This post-workout process allows your muscles to be replenished and restored for your next workout without a release of insulin. Just one of the many benefits of exercise!

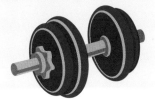

Body Fat and Visceral Fat

Even when you eat more glucose than your cells can use, it still has to be moved out of the bloodstream. So whatever glucose can't be used right away is stored in your body as one of two things: glycogen (the technical term for "stored glucose") or fat. Yes, fat.

Your body can only store glycogen in your liver and your muscles. When you eat carbohydrates, your body checks to see how much glycogen is already stored in those two places before deciding how to handle what you've just eaten. If you have been active and used up some of those glycogen stores, your body will replenish them with glycogen from the new food.

So what happens when there's no more room in your liver or muscles for glycogen? While your body has only limited places to store glycogen, it has *un*limited storage sites for fat. So your liver converts the extra glucose into one of three types of fat: triglycerides, which circulate in the blood; visceral fat, which is stored closely around your organs; or adipose fat, which is stored *on* the body and is generally unsightly but not as dangerous as visceral fat.

Visceral fat is more dangerous than that extra weight around your hips and thighs because it has the capacity to impede organ function. And this fat is responsible for more than just disturbing your appearance: research has shown that visceral fat acts like an additional organ, interacting with your endocrine

Can You Measure Visceral Fat?

Yes! There are body fat-measuring methods that can test both adipose (body fat) and visceral fat (organ fat) with a noninvasive procedure such as bioelectrical impedance or even CT scans. However, there's a very simple, practical way to get a baseline reading on whether or not you have a high amount of visceral fat, and we can call it the "belly from the floor test." Lie down on the floor and see if your stomach pretty much flattens out or if it remains rounded. If it remains quite rounded or protruding when lying down, visceral fat is responsible for the shape! If it sort of falls off to the sides, that's adipose, and while you may want to lose it, it isn't as harmful as visceral fat.

and immune systems and stimulating inflammation.* This builds the case for not only a lower-sugar diet but also one that promotes lowering inflammation in the body overall, so that we reduce visceral fat as well as adipose. Visceral fat may be to blame for "pot bellies" or "beer bellies," where there may not be much "pinchable" fat but the abdomen is distended.

Blame It on the Carbs?

Now, let's not get this twisted—simply eating carbs isn't automatically going to lead to weight gain! Eating to a calorie surplus of *any* food can lead to weight gain. But our bodies are very efficient at converting the excess carbohydrates we consume into body fat. And since carbohydrate-rich foods tend to set off the reward centers in our brain, it's easy to reach for more and more. Eating carbs in moderate amounts also doesn't necessarily cause a blood sugar roller coaster—but it does trigger the release of more insulin than either fat or protein, which are not connected to unstable blood sugar.

Protein and fat also don't have the same connection to weight gain. Protein is highly satiating and doesn't stimulate that same feeling of reward, so we don't tend to overeat protein-rich foods. And since fat on its own, without carbs, protein, salt, or sugar, is not extremely palatable (anyone try spooning straight coconut oil into your mouth? You won't get too far!), we don't tend to overeat it, either.

In the end, it's pretty simple: unstable blood sugar and excess body fat are closely related to the overconsumption of carbohydrates, particularly refined carbs.

But let's be clear: carbs aren't all bad or all good. There are carbohydrate-rich foods that are nutrient-dense, and there are ones that are nutrient-poor. When eating a keto diet, a lot of folks demonize carbohydrates, saying that they're flat-out unhealthy or don't deserve a place in your diet. But we stand to gain a lot of amazing nutrients from carbohydrate-rich foods like vegetables and fruits! Whole-food carbohydrates are not inherently bad or unhealthy, nor are foods like sweet potatoes or cherries to blame for the development of diseases like type 2 diabetes. Refined and processed carbohydrates, however, are disease promoting for a variety of reasons, not least of which is their impact on insulin and blood sugar levels and their lack of vitamins and minerals found in whole foods.

---

* *Stephen B. Hanauer, "Obesity and Visceral Fat: A Growing Inflammatory Disease,"* Nature Clinical Practice Gastroenterology & Hepatology 2, no. 6 (June 2005): 245; M. Alvehus et al., "The Human Visceral Fat Depot Has a Unique Inflammatory Profile," Obesity 18, no. 5 (May 2010): 879–883.

THE FLIP SIDE: BURNING FAT

If insulin is the key to how the body uses carbs, the key to how the body uses stored body fat is insulin's counterpart, glucagon. Glucagon is produced by the alpha cells of the pancreas, and its job is the opposite of insulin's: it signals your cells to *release* stored energy to make sure your blood sugar levels remain even. Remember, high blood sugar is toxic, but so is low blood sugar! When it's healthy and working optimally, your body is a well-oiled machine at prioritizing that steady blood sugar level through balancing the signals from insulin and glucagon: put glucose away when blood sugar is high; get some from storage—body fat and glycogen—when blood sugar drops.

And *this* is exactly what we're looking for to solve the problems of unstable blood sugar and excess body fat. Burning body fat for fuel means that instead of getting hangry, you just feel hungry, and then an hour later you're still at a low level of hunger because your body is being fueled by stored body fat—so blood sugar stays steady. And body fat is being burned, rather than created! Now, this doesn't mean you don't have to eat when you're hungry, but it does mean that you're able to wait longer from that first twinge until you eat, and in that time, you're happily burning body fat to hold you over.

Here's the catch, though (and you knew there was one, right?): if your body is not adapted to using fat as its primary fuel, it struggles to pull energy from fat stores. Instead of staying stable, blood sugar drops, the hangry feeling intensifies, and you can't wait too long before you—*must*—*eat*.

This is where keto comes in. The most important tenet of a ketogenic diet is that your body is encouraged to burn primarily fat for fuel rather than carbohydrates, and over time, it makes the body more efficient at burning fat—what's called "fat-adapted." In other words, we become everyday fat-burners.

My Friend Eats Donuts Every Morning and Is Still a Stick. WHY?

Frankly, some of us simply process or tolerate carbs better than others, both in terms of weight gain and blood sugar regulation. There are a variety of reasons for this, some of which may be genetic and some of which may have to do with our own unique metabolism based on our muscle mass and activity level.

But it's not always a matter of processing carbs *well*—people just process them *differently*. Your genes have some say in where your body stores fat. You may know people, for example, who seem to be able to eat lots of carbs, never work out, and remain thin. Their bodies are likely converting more of their excess carbohydrate intake into triglycerides and visceral fat than into visible body fat that would make their clothes tighter. They *seem* lucky because their clothing size remains the same, but they're actually in more trouble because visceral fat and high triglycerides are more dangerous than a little extra body fat. Unfortunately, the absence of any visible cue leaves people in the dark about their inner state of health. Remember that someone who isn't visibly overweight isn't necessarily healthy, particularly if they're eating more carbs than they are able to burn (which is typical of those eating lots of refined carbs day in and day out). And while genetics are a factor in where you store fat, you can certainly improve your health by refusing to add to visceral fat and avoiding excess carbs.

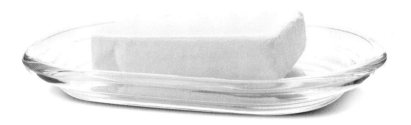

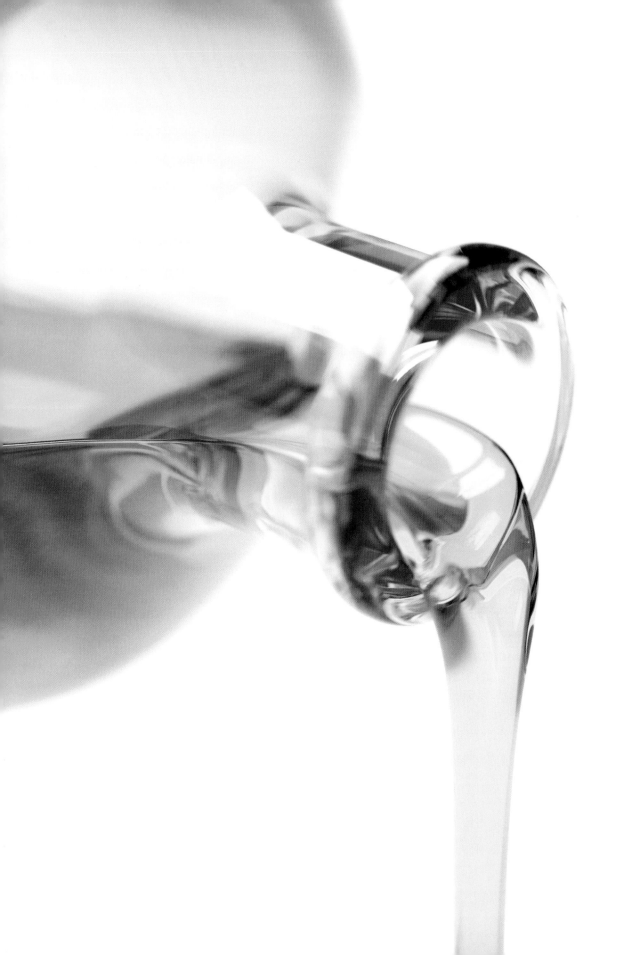

CHAPTER 2

Burning Fat for Fuel

Fat is a perfect long-lasting fuel source for your body, but your body can't efficiently burn fat (from your food or from your stored body fat) if you are constantly eating a steady stream of carbohydrates.

In order to become fat-adapted, meaning your body knows how to effectively use fat for fuel, you have to stop giving it carbs all day, every day. When you stop eating so many carbs and fearing natural, healthy fats, your body burns not only the fat you eat but also body fat—the same fat you've been trying to burn off for years by cranking away on the elliptical machine.

So what's a good guide for balancing protein, fat, and carbs in your meals? I've got all the details in later chapters, but here's the basic formula:

PROTEIN: In each meal, serve yourself *at least* 20 grams of protein for women, 30 grams for men.

FAT: Make sure there is adequate healthy fat in the meal—anywhere from 30 to 75 grams.

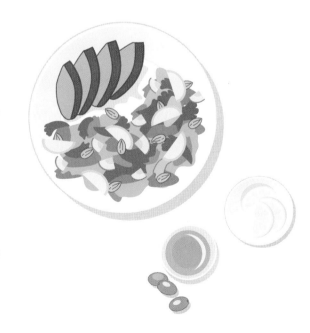

CARBS: In each meal, add nonstarchy vegetables from the very-low-carb veggies section in the Keto Foods List (pages 56 to 57) for a total of not more than about 10 grams net carbs (total carbs minus fiber, which doesn't get absorbed and therefore doesn't affect blood sugar). This amount of carbs per meal will set you up to hit 30 grams per day, but of course you are welcome to vary that and eat, for example, zero carbs at breakfast, then 10 grams or so at lunch and 20 or so at dinner.

These are just general basics, provided here to give you an idea of what a balanced keto plate looks like. I'll talk much more about what to eat on keto in chapters 4 and 5 and how to customize your keto diet for your needs in chapter 7.

The process of becoming fat-adapted can take anywhere from three to eight weeks, depending on your health, metabolism, and overall inflammation. I'm sorry to be the bearer of bad news, but that's just how it works—your body needs time to ramp up its fat-burning capabilities and fully switch to being a fat-burner. I'll walk you through the process and what to expect as you transition from a sugar-burner to a fat-burner in chapter 6.

YES, A HIGH-FAT DIET CAN BE HEALTHY

It's easy to get on board with the idea of using body fat for fuel, but many people hesitate at the idea of eating more fat. But that's a critical part of getting your body to become an efficient fat-burner. So let's look at some of the biggest concerns people have about eating a high-fat diet.

Fat Doesn't Make You Fat

There's no one nutrient that has the ability to make you gain weight—*as long as you're not overeating*. But it's easy to consume more calories than your body can use on a high-carb diet (especially a high-*refined*-carb diet), and that leads to weight gain. A high-fat diet tends to be more satiating, so it's easier to avoid overconsumption.

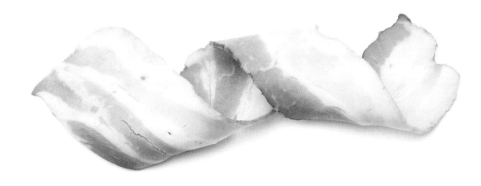

Saturated Fat Doesn't Clog Arteries

It's a common fear that saturated fat will clog your arteries and contribute to high cholesterol and heart disease. This idea often stems from the fact that saturated fat is solid at room temperature. But that notion presumes that the body's digestive and metabolic processes won't disassemble saturated fat into its components. It's almost like saying that since broccoli is solid, it will clog our arteries. I think we all can agree that sounds ridiculous!

The truth is, when we eat fats of any kind, our body breaks them down through a process called lipolysis and sends their components, fatty acids and glycerol, into the body to provide energy for our cells.

Why were we led to believe that saturated fats are unhealthy? This myth began over three decades ago when researchers mistakenly lumped together naturally occurring saturated fats and man-made trans fats, the least healthy fats you can eat.

Saturated Fat Doesn't Cause Heart Disease

The fear that saturated fat will cause heart disease stems from the idea that saturated fat raises cholesterol and that high cholesterol in turn leads to heart disease. So let's look at both of these ideas in turn.

How Saturated Fat Affects Cholesterol

One of the longest-running dietary studies in existence is the Framingham Heart Study. According to its former director, Dr. William Castelli, the study found that "the more saturated fat one ate, the more cholesterol one ate, the more calories one ate, the lower the person's serum [blood] cholesterol. . . . We found that the people who ate the most cholesterol, ate the most saturated fat, ate the most calories, weighed the least and were the most physically active."*

As long as you're not eating a diet high in refined carbs, eating more saturated fat won't increase cholesterol in an unhealthy way. In fact, eating more healthy saturated fats, like egg yolks and coconut oil, can raise both HDL ("good") cholesterol and large, fluffy LDL cholesterol particles, which are protective against heart disease. Small, dense LDL particles, which can cause inflammation in arterial walls, are not increased by eating healthy saturated fat. So eating healthy saturated fats doesn't increase the risk of heart disease.

When to Worry

Although high cholesterol isn't necessarily something to be concerned about if you're healthy, there are times when high cholesterol signals that there's another problem. If you have high cholesterol, consider if any of the following risk factors apply to you:

- excess intake of refined carbohydrates
- consumption of inflammatory oils (see page 61)
- alcohol consumption
- inflammation in the body
- poor or sluggish liver function
- stress
- physical inactivity

None of these problems have anything to do with eating fat or cholesterol, so if you have high cholesterol in combination with any of these, don't make eating low-fat or low-cholesterol your priority. Instead, address the root cause—reduce your intake of carbs, inflammatory oils, and alcohol, manage stress, increase physical activity, and so on—and see how your cholesterol changes. Eating keto can be a big help.

---

* K. Anderson, W. Castelli, and D. Levy, "Cholesterol and Mortality: 30 Years of Follow-Up from the Framingham Study," JAMA 257, no. 16 (1987): 2176–2180.

The Real Role Cholesterol Plays

High blood cholesterol levels have never proven to cause heart disease. In fact, many who experience cardiovascular disease have low cholesterol! Dr. Castelli of the Framingham Heart Study reports that "people with low cholesterol (lower than 200) suffer nearly 40 percent of all heart attacks." So why all the concern about cholesterol in the first place?

Most of us have an image of cardiovascular disease as what Dr. Michael Rothberg of the Cleveland Clinic calls the "plumbing model": dietary fat and cholesterol are slowly deposited in arterial walls, where they build up and eventually lead to blockages that cause heart attacks.* This model perpetuates misconceptions about the relationship between what we eat and what happens in our arteries.

Testing Your Cholesterol

While it may be tempting to test your fasted cholesterol and triglyceride numbers after thirty days on your Keto Quick Start, unless your weight is stable, you won't get accurate results. As you lose body fat, your cholesterol levels may increase, but not because there's a problem! Your body is simply working to release and metabolize stored fatty acids, which affects cholesterol and triglyceride readings. Wait until your weight has been stable for about three months, then get the tests run to see a more accurate number.

That said, your cholesterol readings are a snapshot in time. So if they measure higher than you were expecting, retest within a few weeks. If the results are still higher than you'd like, test once more within a few more weeks, then take the average of the three sets of results. This is a more accurate reflection of your true cholesterol state.

If you're interested in a deeper dive into cholesterol and which markers to test, I highly recommend looking into the work of Chris Masterjohn (chrismasterjohnphd.com). His explanations of the biochemistry of cholesterol and what it all means are some of the best you'll find.

First, as explained above, dietary fat is broken down and used by the body; it doesn't accumulate in our arteries. Second, dietary cholesterol has little impact on the amount of cholesterol in our blood. The liver makes 80 percent of the cholesterol in the blood; only 20 percent comes from our food. So avoiding healthy dietary fat and cholesterol is not going to have much of an effect on your arteries.

In addition, the image most of us have of a buildup of material in our arteries is inaccurate. What actually happens is that LDL particles may penetrate the walls of our arteries and become damaged by free radicals. This initiates an inflammatory response, especially at sites of damage. All this happens within the arterial walls—LDL isn't building up inside the artery itself. Inflammation ultimately causes the arterial wall to swell, which can lead to a blockage or a rupture of the arterial wall. (This is one reason why an anti-inflammatory diet is so important: eating lots of antioxidant-rich foods helps to combat this process!)

What we're taught happens

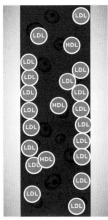

What really happens

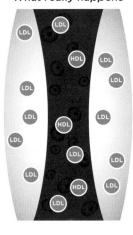

* Michael B. Rothberg, "Coronary Artery Disease as Clogged Pipes: A Misconceptual Model," Circulation: Cardiovascular Quality and Outcomes 6, no. 1 (2013): 129–132.

But know this: if cholesterol markers in your blood measure high, it's because it's combatting inflammation! It is not *causing* the inflammation.

Cholesterol is like firefighters—they are not the reason for the fire, but they show up to help put it out. So when you see a big fire (or a lot of inflammation in the body), you'll also see a lot of firefighters (high cholesterol). On the other hand, the existence of firefighters alone—even if there are a lot of them—doesn't necessarily mean a problem exists. They may be just sitting around the firehouse waiting until they are called upon to hop into a truck with a siren blaring and go fight a fire. In other words, in a body that's not experiencing inflammation, cholesterol levels that may appear high by conventional standards are likely not a cause for concern because cholesterol is responsible for hormone synthesis, maintaining cell wall integrity, and other various building and healing functions in the body. A certain level of cholesterol is not arbitrarily a cause of heart disease. Problems arise when you combine an extremely inflamed, unhealthy person with that high level of cholesterol.

The long-standing myth that eating saturated fat makes you fat and contributes to a state of poor health and nearly certain heart disease has been perpetuated by the powerful lobbying of the corn oil and soybean oil industries. And it has quite literally sent a frightened American public running away from healthy and natural saturated fats and into the welcoming arms of damaging refined vegetable oils, which I'll talk about in more detail in chapter 5.

WHY A LOW-CARB, HIGH-FAT DIET WORKS FOR FAT LOSS

Reducing your intake of carbs and replacing them with healthy fats gets your body to ramp up its fat-burning machinery and become efficient at burning not just *dietary* fat but also stored *body* fat. That means that in moments when, as a sugar-burner, you'd be feeling hangry or light-headed or dizzy and desperate to eat something, you can actually burn body fat and feel good at the same time.

Remember from chapter 1, insulin moves glucose out of the bloodstream and into storage as fat when blood sugar is high. Glucagon, on the other hand, acts when blood sugar is low: it releases fat from storage into the bloodstream so that it can be used as fuel.

So when does blood sugar drop so that glucagon can pull energy out of fat cells and into circulation?

• **When we feel hungry**   • **When we are in a fasted state**   • **When we exercise**

It's important to remember these glucagon triggers—these are the magic moments when our bodies tap into stored body fat for fuel!

Let me expand on each of the situations where glucagon kicks in and outweighs insulin in the bloodstream to help your body burn stored fat.

 FASTING: You're in a fasted state when you haven't eaten food for around eight hours or more. When you wake up each morning, provided that you slept for around eight hours or it's been at least that long since your last meal, you wake up fasted. The term *breakfast* refers to that: you're "breaking" the "fast."

Intermittent fasting is simply intentional fasting on a regular basis. There are several kinds of intermittent fasting—for example, fasting for twenty-four hours once or twice a week or limiting yourself to 500 calories for two consecutive days each week. But the most popular method of intermittent fasting is eating within an eight-hour window each day, meaning there are roughly sixteen consecutive hours when you simply don't eat. This is easiest to achieve if you fast overnight— for instance, from around 6 to 8 p.m., when you finish dinner, to 10 a.m. to noon the following day. So this is as simple as having your last meal or snack at 6 p.m. then eating again at 10 a.m. the next day, or having your last meal or snack at 8 p.m., then eating again at noon the next day.

 HUNGER: Short of fasting, we also get a boost of glucagon into our bloodstream when we feel hungry, which clearly happens well before we're in a fully fasted state. When you're fat-adapted, that boost of glucagon lets your body tap into stored body fat, and that timespan between when hunger initially kicks in and when you eventually eat is pure fat-burning! And while you'll feel hungry during that time, the fat-burning means your body is getting fuel, so hunger doesn't become "hanger" and you can easily power through.

 EXERCISE: When we exercise, we release endorphins that trigger an increase in glucagon. Exercise, especially weight training, is one of the most effective ways you can increase your body's ability to burn stored body fat. Not only will you burn fat during the activity itself, but you'll increase your muscle mass and resting metabolic rate (how many calories your body burns at rest) by increasing your insulin sensitivity. So get into the gym and lift those weights!

Low-Fat vs. Low-Carb: Which Wins for Fat Loss?

You actually *can* lose body fat through either a low-fat or a low-carb diet (among many other ways that are debatable in terms of their healthfulness).

The reason it's possible to lose weight on a low-fat, high-carb diet lies in overall energy input versus output. No, I'm not saying that fat loss is as simple as calories in versus calories out, but calories *do* matter! And so does physical activity, genetics, muscle mass, and overall health.

Even when we eat a high amount of carbs, we do occasionally burn fat, usually to fuel low- or moderate-intensity aerobic activity. In fact, our bodies rely on fat for most activities that we do day in and day out, with the exception of high-intensity exercise, which is fueled by glycogen (stored glucose). But daily activities will almost never burn more energy than we take in through food—so any body fat we burn is replenished by what we eat.

The beauty of being fat-adapted is that your overall appetite drops, so you're not consuming more calories to replace those you burn. It's also easier to lose body fat when you're eating fewer carbs because your body is trained to consistently pull energy from stored fat rather than constantly battling high blood sugar with more insulin to bring it back to baseline.

When comparing a low-fat diet to a low-carb one, the question to answer is: *Does eating low-fat work for you?* Meaning, can you maintain it long enough to lose an appreciable amount of body fat? Is eating that way enjoyable? How do you *feel* eating that way? And which way of eating feels more sustainable 80 to 95 percent of the time while allowing for an occasional off day when you eat more of the nutrient you're generally avoiding (whether carbs or fat)?

For most people, a low-carb ketogenic diet beats a low-fat diet on all counts. Eating to a ketogenic level of around 30 grams net carbs per day provides high satiety, a high level of enjoyment, and relative ease of compliance. In other words, you don't feel like you're starving all the time, as you'd often feel on a low-fat diet where you need to eat every two to three hours. You can enjoy tasty foods like bacon, steak, butter, and avocados on keto, and it's not that difficult to eat at home or eat out at a restaurant and order "around the bread," so to speak.

Calories Do Count, Even on Keto

Whether you choose to eat keto or not, the reality is that overeating causes an energy (calorie) surplus, and that will lead to weight gain. Put simply, you can't just eat keto foods or zero carbs while overeating fat and protein and expect to lose body fat. While keto is an extremely effective way to lose weight and body fat, calories still count!

I'm not going to suggest you micromanage your calorie intake, although the customization plans in chapter 7 and the SAVVY Keto Daily Trackers (pages 120 to 123) do break down calorie and macronutrient targets. These are *targets*, and aiming for the recommended grams of each macronutrient will get you there (or close enough). You don't need to count every calorie, but be aware of how much you're eating and whether you're eating because you're truly hungry or because you're trying to satisfy an emotional craving. Recognizing your own patterns will be a pivotal part of your success. Tune in to your appetite, notice how it drops over time as your body adapts to burning fat for fuel, and then, if losing body fat is your goal, keep your portions in check.

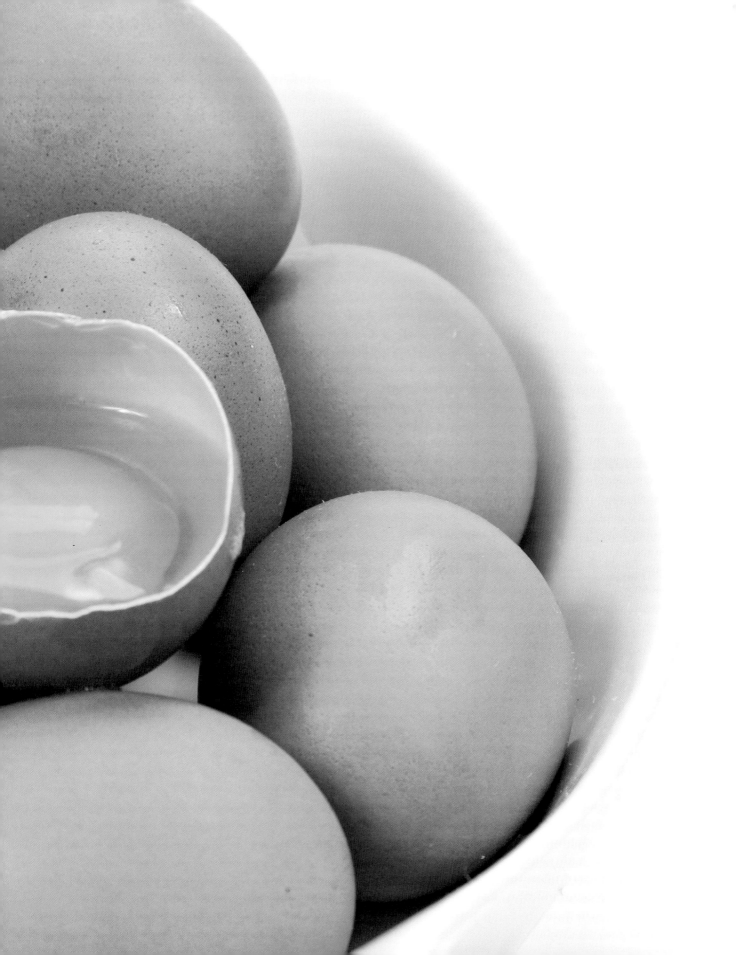

CHAPTER 3

The Lowdown on Ketosis

The low-carb, high-fat diet that helps your body become more efficient at burning fat also generates particles called ketones—hence the term "ketogenic [ketone-creating] diet."

Ketones, or ketone bodies, are created by the liver during the breakdown of fat (both dietary fat and body fat). There are three kinds of ketones that our body makes: acetoacetate, beta-hydroxybutyrate (BHB), and acetate. The presence of ketones in your blood while eating a very-low-carb diet is a normal and expected result. In the absence of glucose, ketones are used by your heart, muscles, and brain as a source of energy. In fact, while glucose is the first fuel source your brain will use when present, ketones are actually its *preferred* fuel source and are used whenever available.

Two kinds of body cells cannot use ketones: liver cells and red blood cells. So some amount of glucose is required, and in the absence of dietary glucose, to meet that need, the liver has the ability to create glucose from proteins and fatty acids in a process called gluconeogenesis (*gluco*, "glucose" + neo, "new" + *genesis,* "creation"). Some of the glucose produced this way also goes directly to the brain, while the muscles and most organs use ketones and fatty acids for fuel. After two to three days of eating a very low level of carbohydrates, the amount of glucose created through gluconeogenesis drops significantly as the tissues that can use ketones begin to do so and the body's need for glucose becomes minimal. So as ketones rise, the brain's demand for glucose decreases.[*]

---

[*] *J. C. LaManna et al., "Ketones Suppress Brain Glucose Consumption," in* Advances in Experimental Medicine and Biology *(New York: Springer, 2009), 645:301–306.*

KETOSIS VS. KETO-ADAPTATION VS. FAT-ADAPTATION

THE SCIENCE OF KETO:
Ketone Production

The breakdown of fats results in an increased presence of a molecule called acetyl coenzyme A (acetyl CoA). It's the increase in the concentration of acetyl CoA that initiates the production of ketone bodies, since in a nonketogenic state, the body would break down lower levels of acetyl CoA via the Krebs cycle in order to create cellular energy in the form of adenosine triphosphate (ATP).

Gluconeogenesis actually produces ketones—it generates acetoacetate and beta-hydroxybutyrate—as well as a small amount of glucose. So it feeds the brain two ways, with both that very small amount of glucose *and* with ketone bodies.

The creation of ketones can be triggered by any situation in which the body breaks down higher amounts of fat: fasting, starvation, long periods of exercise, alcoholism, or untreated diabetes. A very-low-carb diet, like the keto diet, is one safe, intentional way of producing ketones.

Ketosis is a metabolic state in which you have a certain amount of ketones in your blood, whether those ketones are produced by your body or come from an external source (more on that later).

Keto-adaptation is when you have ketones present in your blood and your body is also primed to use them (which is why you may no longer see them registering at as high a concentration on a urine test strip—they're being used rather than excreted). It's when you're keto-adapted that you begin to feel the neurological and metabolic benefits of being in ketosis. In other words, just because there are measurable ketones in your urine, blood, or breath doesn't mean that you're experiencing all of the metabolic and other benefits of keto-adaptation just yet!

It's also important to note that being in ketosis is not the same as being fat-adapted or being able to burn fat. All ketosis means is that there is a certain level of ketones in your bloodstream, which isn't a requirement for burning fat for fuel. You can go in and out of ketosis without changing the fact that you're fat-adapted. In fact, even as sugar-burners, our bodies are typically in ketosis in the morning after fasting overnight, and it only takes a few days of eating a very-low-carbohydrate diet to be in a consistent state of ketosis. Becoming fat-adapted, on the other hand, can take weeks or even months and does not rely on also being in ketosis.

These states—ketosis, keto-adaptation, and fat-adaptation—are often confused and referred to interchangeably, but they are distinctly different.

TO RECAP:

KETOSIS
is clinically and quantifiably measurable; it's defined by the level of ketones in your body.

KETO-ADAPTATION
is when your body is both making and using ketones as a primary fuel source.

FAT-ADAPTATION
means that your body is able to access dietary and body fat for fuel and doesn't require that ketones are present in your body.

Many people find that eating very low-carb, *without* necessarily being in ketosis, brings them the benefits they're looking for, and that lowering carbs to a level that does promote ketosis isn't necessary for goals such as fat loss or blood sugar regulation.

In fact, there are some ways to encourage ketosis that actually don't promote keto-adaptation or fat-adaptation, like adding MCT oil to your meals (more on that later in this chapter). So the goal of a ketogenic diet isn't simply to achieve a certain level of ketones in your body but rather to shift your entire metabolism away from burning glucose as a primary fuel source, for both metabolic and neurological benefits.

In the medical field, a state of ketosis is widely known as an effective nutritional treatment for neurological conditions, including epilepsy and traumatic brain injury, and for certain types of cancer. That said, it also has many other benefits that have been less widely studied or accepted (though there is emerging research on these topics), such as improvements in blood glucose sensitivity, protection against neurological conditions even before one is diagnosed, and performance improvements in endurance athletes.

The Difference Between Nutritional Ketosis and Diabetic Ketoacidosis

For people with type 1 diabetes who are not eating keto, the presence of ketones in the blood is often a sign that they don't have enough insulin to break down carbohydrates and the body has started breaking down fat for fuel. Since they're still consuming carbs, though, this means ketones are being produced *while blood sugar is also high.* This is not the case in nutritional ketosis, when the body does make enough insulin to break down any consumed carbs and only in the absence of glucose produces ketones. It's the combination of high blood sugar and ketones that's the hallmark of diabetic ketoacidosis. In nutritional ketosis, there are ketones but not high blood sugar.

Signs of diabetic ketoacidosis include nausea and vomiting, abdominal pain, excessive thirst, shortness of breath, frequent urination, foggy-headedness, and sweet, fruity-smelling breath.

If you have type 1 diabetes, the chance of getting ketoacidosis makes eating a ketogenic diet riskier, though not impossible. For tips on the safest way to eat keto with type 1 diabetes, see page 109.

Diabetic ketoacidosis is possible in type 2 diabetics as well, but it's far less likely.

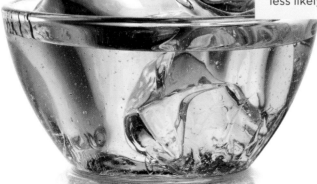

MEASURING KETONES

Since you're in ketosis when you have a certain amount of ketones in your body, the only way to know for sure if you're in ketosis is to test your ketone level. However—and this is one of the most important things I want you to know for your Keto Quick Start—*ketone levels should not be the gold standard by which you measure your progress or results on a ketogenic diet.*

The fact is, some people's bodies naturally produce more ketones than others', and there are ways to get your body to produce ketones that actually have little to do with becoming fat-adapted. I strongly urge you not to use your ketone level as proof of health or success in your Keto Quick Start. The fact of the matter is that these numbers may vary highly from person to person for various reasons, and "chasing ketones," or simply going after a certain reading, is not the ultimate goal of this dietary shift. The goal is to feel better, reduce inflammation and disease, lose the body fat you want to lose, and accomplish all of that while eating in a way that feels good and manageable as a lifestyle.

All of that said, measuring ketones can be helpful as you transition to a keto diet to help you know if you're on the right track. You're in ketosis when your blood ketone level is 0.5 to 3 mmol/L at rest or up to 5 mmol/L after a workout.

Ketone levels should not be the gold standard by which you measure your progress or results on a ketogenic diet.

One misconception is that the higher your ketone level, the better. But this isn't necessarily the case if fat loss is your primary goal. You may experience a higher level of ketones because you're eating more fat, not because your body is burning more of your stored body fat as fuel. Conversely, if you are seeking improvements in a wide variety of diagnosed health conditions, it's possible that the benefits of being keto-adapted are amplified only when a higher amount of ketones are present.

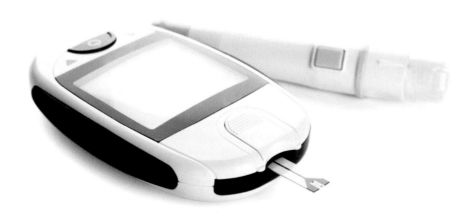

There are three ways to test your ketones:

1. **BLOOD TESTING:** This can be done at home with a relatively inexpensive device quite similar to a glucometer (which tests for blood glucose). The testing process is simple and can be done with a small finger prick. It's the most accurate method of testing ketone levels. Supplies for blood ketone testing will cost about $155 over the course of your first month. Thereafter, the cost will be around $3 per day, assuming you test three times per day.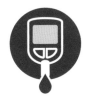

2. **URINE TESTING:** Ketone-testing strips change color depending on the level of ketones in your urine. While this method accurately gauges the amount of ketones in your urine, after several weeks to months of eating keto, they may not accurately indicate ketosis—by then, your body is using more of the ketones produced and therefore is not excreting as many in your urine. Supplies for urine ketone testing will cost $7 to $10 a month, assuming you test three times per day.

3. **BREATH TESTING:** Breath ketone meters are another way to measure ketone levels. There are only a few companies currently making these devices, and they are currently difficult to purchase. While some people love this method for testing because it's noninvasive, I found it to be cumbersome to get the software to work properly with the device for an accurate reading. For these reasons, I don't recommend breath testing at this time. Breath ketone meters may become easier to use and more widespread over time, and if so, breath testing may prove to be the easiest way to measure for ketosis.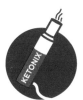

There is also another way to assess yourself and your progress that may be even more beneficial than the quantitative measures: journaling.

Keeping track of what you eat will help you to identify more than what numbers can tell you, including triggering situations (such as stressful situations at work or home, like a tight deadline or an argument with your partner), moments of weakness (grocery shopping while hungry, dining out at specific restaurants or with particular friends), and the emotional aspects of making a lifestyle change.

Over the course of days, weeks, and months, journaling will give you the best data possible on your N=1 (a subject of one) experiment. You can use the outline on page 79 as a template, or download a guide at **balancedbites.com/ketoquickstart**. If you want to take it to the next level, you can print thirty, sixty, or ninety (or more) sheets of the journal outline at an office supply or copy store and have them spiral bound.

> **There is also another way to assess yourself and your progress that may be even more beneficial than the quantitative measures: journaling.**

Now, if you were to test your blood or urine and include the results alongside other notes in your journal, you'd have superior data. But it really depends on your goals and your budget. But if you choose just one method of tracking data, make it journaling—you'll learn much more about yourself and what works for you than numbers can ever tell you.

HEALTH BENEFITS OF KETOSIS

While the ability to more easily burn fat for fuel is clearly one of the benefits of ketosis, it's not the only one!

Some other important benefits of being in ketosis are mental clarity, appetite suppression and the ability to go longer between meals, increased energy levels, improved mood, better sleep, and improved digestion for those struggling with gut imbalances due to a diet high in refined carbs.

Let me repeat part of that: mental clarity and appetite suppression are two of the main benefits of being in ketosis.

Mental clarity and appetite suppression are two of the main benefits of being in ketosis.

These benefits alone are two of the most compelling reasons why eating keto often feels easier or more manageable than eating low-fat. For those of us who struggle to maintain a low-fat diet, it's typically because we're so hungry—*all—the—time*. It's almost like it's all you can think about—when's the next time you're going to eat, what are you going to eat then. It can become all-consuming, and it makes adhering to the diet far more difficult. Furthermore, when you can think more clearly, you have more energy to do other things in your day besides focus on food. And when your mood is less erratic, you can more easily make sound, logical choices about food (and your *life*, for that matter!).

Additionally, being in ketosis can help to alleviate the potential for seizures for those with epilepsy and speed healing from traumatic brain injury. Ketosis may provide relief from symptoms of Alzheimer's and Parkinson's diseases and "could have beneficial disease-modifying activity applicable to a broad range of brain disorders that are characterized by the death of neurons."* Those diagnosed with these conditions stand to see improvements from both adhering to a ketogenic diet and including exogenous ketones or MCT oil in their diets.

---

*Maciej Gasior, Michael A. Rogawski, and Adam L. Hartman, "Neuroprotective and Disease-Modifying Effects of the Ketogenic Diet," Behavioural Pharmacology 17, nos. 5–6 (Sept. 2006): 431–439.

EXOGENOUS KETONES AND MCTS

Ketone supplements, which can be purchased in a powdered form, are known as exogenous (that is, made *outside* the body) ketones. These can be a helpful addition to your ketogenic diet, especially in the first few weeks, as you transition away from eating higher-carb. The benefit of supplementing with exogenous ketones is primarily that it makes the transition more comfortable. But for most people, the discomfort of transitioning to keto doesn't last very long—perhaps three to ten days—and many find that they can ride it out just fine without supplementing. The use of supplements is absolutely not necessary for ketosis, nor to burn body fat more effectively.

MCT is short for "medium-chain triglycerides," and these are fatty acids that are moved quickly and directly from the gut to the liver. Since these fatty acids don't need to be broken down the way other kinds of fats do before they can be used for energy, MCTs are often touted as a "functional fat," one that is used immediately as fuel for the body and brain. MCT oil is available in both a powder and a liquid supplement.

If you choose to try MCT supplementation, go *slowly*, starting with perhaps 1/2 teaspoon per day, then 1 teaspoon per day, then 1 teaspoon per meal, and so on, up to perhaps 3 tablespoons per day—or whatever amount feels good for you, included in your overall fat intake for the day. You can also blend either the powder or liquid into drinks like a Dreamy Matcha Latte (page 192) or Creamy Keto Coffee (page 193). I find that most people tolerate powdered MCT oil better than the liquid form. Note that overdoing it on MCT oil can lead to an urgent and uncomfortable trip to the bathroom! Your body may adjust to higher doses over time, however, so start slowly and you can add more as time goes on, perhaps increasing incrementally each week.

If you want to increase your ketone level for the potential neurological benefits (mental clarity and sharpness in the short term, as well as improved brain health in the long term), you may consider adding supplemental MCT or exogenous ketones to your diet. But if you're looking to burn body fat, taking supplemental ketones simply to see a higher ketone reading is defeating the purpose of changing your diet—you won't lose body fat any faster with a higher ketone reading. If these supplements make you feel better and you enjoy consuming them, then go for it. But don't think that they're essential to your success with your Keto Quick Start or to burn body fat.

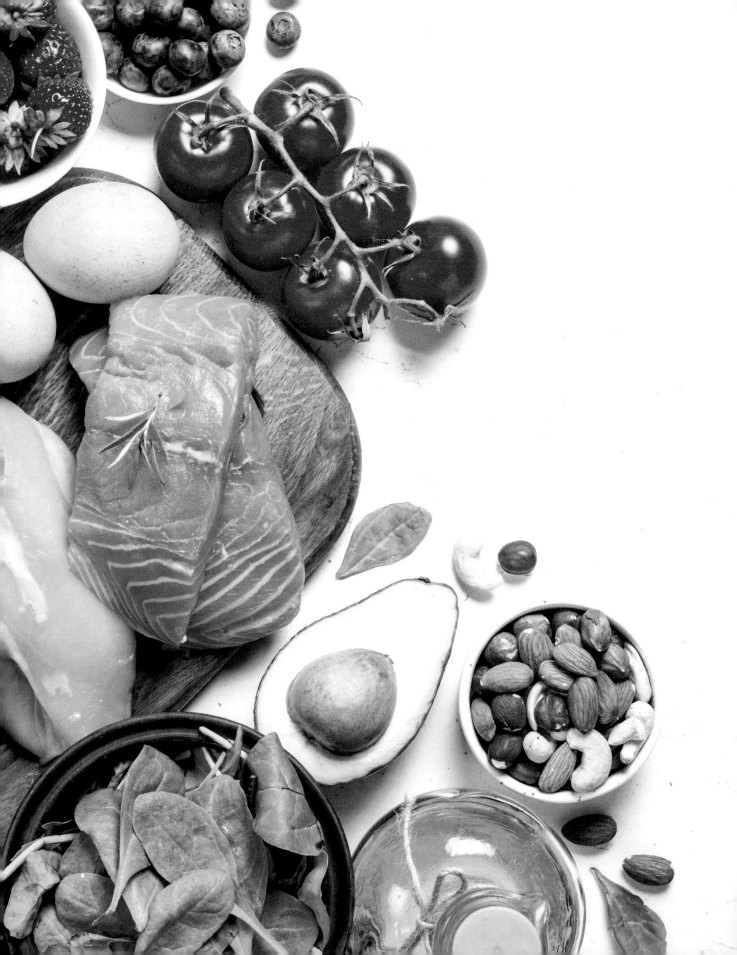

CHAPTER 4

What to Eat: SAVVY Keto

When you eat keto, you'll be eating foods that you may have feared in the past. Eating keto means including foods that are rich in naturally occurring saturated fat and avoiding foods rich in "complex carbs," which long held the base of the famous food pyramid.

While getting into a state of ketosis is not reliant on the quality of your food but rather on the absence of carbohydrates, if your goal with keto is to become a healthier person, the foods you eat do matter. Your overall health and long-term success on keto will be far better if you focus on nutritious, keto-friendly whole foods than if you focus *only* on macronutrients. You'll also find it easier to lose body fat, and your levels of inflammation will also be lower.

The chart below gives a few examples comparing the standard American diet, what we've been taught is healthy according to conventional wisdom, the Paleo diet (which focuses on real, whole foods and eliminates most grains), and keto. Of course, what you eat on keto may not be *exactly* what's here, but it will give you an idea of what a keto diet looks like.

	Standard American Diet	"Healthy" according to conventional wisdom	Paleo	Keto
BREAKFAST	A bowl of cereal, or a breakfast bar or granola bar, or a bagel, muffin, or pastry; coffee with milk and sugar	Oatmeal with raisins and brown sugar or maple syrup, or fat-free strawberry yogurt with low-fat granola; coffee or tea with skim milk	Eggs and bacon or sausage with arugula and sauerkraut; coffee with coconut milk; banana or apple	Eggs and bacon or sausage with arugula and sauerkraut; coffee with coconut milk or heavy cream
LUNCH	Salad of iceberg lettuce with breaded chicken, tomato, cucumber, and premade ranch dressing; chips; cookie; soda	Salad of mixed greens with grilled chicken and fat-free dressing; low-fat chips; diet soda	Salad of mixed greens with chicken breast, avocado, apple, nuts, extra-virgin olive oil & lemon dressing; flavored sparkling water	Salad of mixed greens with grilled chicken thighs, goat cheese, nuts, extra-virgin olive oil & lemon dressing; flavored sparkling water
SNACK	Bag of chips or a cookie or candy bar; sweetened iced tea, soda, or coffee with milk and sugar	Low-fat pretzels or cookie; no-calorie sweetened iced tea or iced coffee with skim milk	Fruit & nut bar (e.g., LÄRABAR) and jerky; unsweetened iced tea or coffee with coconut milk	Pork rinds; unsweetened iced tea or coffee with cream or coconut milk
DINNER	Out to dinner for Mexican food, or order pizza in	Grilled chicken tacos with corn shells, fat-free sour cream, salsa, and guacamole	Steak tacos in grain-free shells with guacamole, and salsa; fresh cabbage slaw	Steak tacos in lettuce wraps, full-fat sour cream, salsa, guacamole; fresh cabbage slaw
DESSERT	Ice cream or cookies	Low-fat ice cream or low-fat cookies	Sweet potato with ghee and cinnamon or banana "nice cream" (ice cream made from blended frozen bananas)	Berries with cream; Salted PB Bites (page 354) or other keto treat

SAVVY Keto is an approach I developed to help you be mindful about what you're eating and guide you in building your plate. That said, if every meal doesn't look perfect according to the SAVVY framework, don't sweat it! This approach is meant to guide and support your decisions and keep you focused on real, whole foods. There will always be times when you need to throw together a snack or meal on the go or when your available options aren't ideal. In all of your food choices, your goal for achieving ketosis is to not exceed your maximum carb count for the day.

The basic tenets for building your plate during your Keto Quick Start are easy to remember if you keep the word SAVVY in mind.

 START WITH PROTEIN. Protein is your primary focus for building each meal. That doesn't mean that it makes up the bulk of your meal, just that it's what you need to think about first—everything else will follow.

 ADEQUATE FAT. Be sure there's some healthy fat on your plate. If you're eating lean protein or plain veggies, add some olive oil, butter, nuts or seeds, or cheese (if you can eat it).

 VEGGIES! Eat lots of non-starchy vegetables. Remember, you'll be able to subtract fiber from your total carbs for the day, so pile on the high-fiber veggies.

 VARIETY. Change up what you're eating regularly. It helps you get a good balance of vitamins and minerals, and it keeps you from getting bored!

 YES TO HERBS AND SPICES. To get lots of vitamins, minerals, and phytonutrients in your meal—as well as tons of flavor!—always season your food with fresh herbs and a variety of spices.

Let's look at each of these points one by one.

To Track or Not to Track

This chapter is about building your plate, not tracking your macros. It's about learning to make good food choices and knowing what a keto diet looks like. Depending on your goals, tracking may be important. For example, if you want to lose more than 30 pounds, you can likely see some great progress without tracking. If you're aiming to lose less than 30 pounds or are more interested in fine-tuning your body composition, then tracking is likely to help you achieve that.

But if you want to avoid tracking your food intake and are mostly interested in improving your overall health, just following the guidelines in this chapter will help you get many of the benefits of the keto diet.

START WITH PROTEIN

Keto is known as a high-fat, low-carb diet, but the best place to start is actually with *protein*. While some keto protocols recommend eating less protein, eating enough protein is the key to (1) feeling full after a meal and (2) increasing your ability to burn fat, which is what keeps you from feeling hungry between meals. Those are the two biggest factors to making a keto diet work, so focus first on getting adequate protein onto your plate.

Guidelines for calculating your personal protein goal are in chapter 7, but if you don't want to spend much time tracking your macros, a good rule of thumb is to get 20 grams of protein per meal for women, 30 grams for men. This is probably much more than you're used to eating, so you'll need to make a concerted effort to hit that number. Getting more protein into your diet will likely be the biggest adjustment you make for your Keto Quick Start.

⚠ IMPORTANT! If you're following a therapeutic ketogenic diet for the treatment of neurological conditions or traumatic brain injury, a higher protein intake is not the way to go. I'll address the best macronutrient breakdown for these cases on page 89.

It's unlikely you'll regularly eat more protein than your goal because protein is highly satiating, so it's tough to overeat. But if you go over your protein target for the day, not to worry—it's highly unlikely to interfere with your goal of being in ketosis.

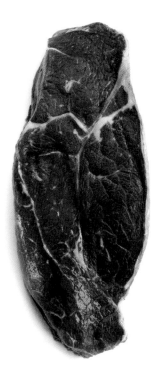
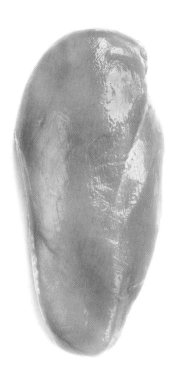
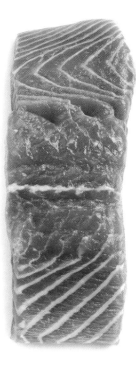

The Importance of Protein

The reason you often see nutritionists like myself focusing on carbs and fat, whether advocating for a low-carb or a low-fat approach, is that the need for adequate protein remains constant while carbs and fat can be tweaked to help you feel fuller, enjoy your meals more, lose or gain weight, and so on. Whether you're burning carbs or fat as your primary fuel source hinges on the amount of carbs you eat, not on the amount of protein!

But you need to get enough protein in order to feel full after a meal and increase your ability to burn fat, so protein is a crucial part of a keto diet. In fact, Keto Quick Start calls for more protein than some other keto advocates advise, to make sure you get the full benefits and avoid overeating.

Protein and Parkinson's

A note about following a ketogenic diet with Parkinson's disease: If you take levodopa with carbidopa or benserazide (brand names Sinemet and Madopar), it's important to moderate your protein intake according to your doctor's recommendations. Protein can prevent the absorption of these medications.

While it's true that insulin is released in response to the consumption of protein (though far less than is released in response to carbs), the context of protein consumption may be essential: research shows that in a fasted state (which ketosis mimics in terms of insulin and glucagon levels), the introduction of protein does *not* spike insulin levels but *does* increase glucagon. This is important to understand for your keto diet! Since glucagon triggers the release of fat from storage so that it can be burned for fuel, eating protein on keto can keep you satiated *and* burning more fat; without a spike in insulin and with a minimal increase in glucose from gluconeogenesis, it won't kick you out of ketosis.

Eating primarily fat and protein, with limited carbohydrates, will still allow insulin to do its job and get nutrients to your cells, without the inflammation and systemic stress–promoting spikes in blood sugar and insulin that come from refined carbs—and without the weight gain that can accompany them. You'll be hard-pressed to find a diet that better supports fat-burning than one that's a combination of very low carb, high fat, and substantial protein.

Why Animal Protein Matters

Protein is found in both plant and animal foods, but it turns out that for keto, animal protein has an advantage over plant protein.

The reason is that in plants, the protein is packaged with—you guessed it!—carbohydrates. A 1-cup serving of lentils, arguably one of the plant-based crowd's favorite sources of protein, packs about 18 grams of protein and 40 grams of carbohydrate. Compare this to a 3-ounce portion of wild salmon, which packs around 22 grams of protein with zero carbohydrates! The carbohydrates in plants cause a spike in blood sugar and insulin, which protein alone does not—and which makes it much harder for your body to become (or stay) fat-adapted.

The popular myth that too much red meat isn't healthy is just that, a myth. There is nothing inherently unhealthy about red meat.

Why the persistent myth, then? Often, observational studies that deem red meat bad for you look at conventional grain-fed beef or processed meats, without considering grass-fed beef. They're also frequently based on dietary recalls (can you remember what you ate all day three or four days ago?) or look at red meat in the context of an overall *unhealthy* diet, not one that includes a plethora of plant foods alongside the meat. When red meat is eaten as part of a diet rich in refined carbs, it's nearly (if not entirely) impossible to identify what health effects are rooted in the meat and which come from the refined carbs.

Can Too Much Protein Trigger Hypoglycemia?

According to Dr. Ben Bickman, a professor of pathophysiology and a biomedical scientist at Brigham Young University in Utah, in the context of a very-low-carb diet, the response your body has to protein will be very little insulin and more glucagon. This means that your body will pull nutrients from stores to keep blood sugar even, so eating protein should not result in a hypoglycemic state. If you feel at all hypoglycemic after consuming protein, I'd suspect another underlying metabolic issue is at the root of it, because that wouldn't be an expected physiological response in someone who is eating a very-low-carb diet. If this happens to you, I recommend working one-on-one with a functional medicine practitioner or naturopathic doctor to get to the root of it.

No scientific study has ever found a cause-and-effect relationship between red meat and poor health. And, in fact, many who run away from red meat out of fear end up replacing it with more refined carbohydrates, which—unlike red meat—have been proven to increase inflammatory markers and risk of cardiovascular disease.

If you are prone to excess iron in your body, then eating foods rich in iron (like red meat) frequently or in large quantities is clearly not a good idea. If you have an intolerance to the proteins found in red meat (rare, though possible), then of course you should avoid it.

However, red meat, especially when humanely raised on pasture and grass-fed, is one of the most nutrient-dense foods we can eat. Red meat is rich in iron, B vitamins, zinc, and carnitine, and the fat from 100 percent grass-fed meat contains anti-inflammatory omega-3 fatty acids and is rich in conjugated linoleic acid, which has anticarcinogenic, antiobese, antidiabetic, and antihypertensive properties. Rather than focusing on fear-based reporting or marketing against a whole, unprocessed, ancestral food like red meat, shift your attention to eating the best-quality meat you can for its amazing health benefits.

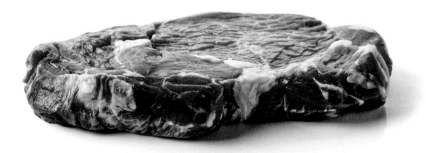

Vegetarianism Isn't the Health Panacea You've Heard It Is

While eating a plate that's built of a large proportion of plant foods, like vegetables, nuts, and some fruits, is absolutely healthy and recommended, avoiding animal foods completely can lead to long-term, deeply rooted nutritional deficiencies if your plants-only diet is not very carefully balanced and supplemented.

Plant foods are a fantastic source of vitamins and minerals, phytonutrients, and fiber, and they carry relatively few calories. This means that, ounce for ounce, plant foods tend to be very nutrient-dense—which is a great thing!

The problem is that the human body more readily absorbs certain essential nutrients from animal sources than from plants. Nutrients that humans should be getting from animal sources include iron, omega-3 fatty acids, vitamin D, and B vitamins. The difficulty in getting these nutrients from plants is due to a variety of factors: the way our digestive system works, the absence of necessary nutrient cofactors in plants, and enzymatic and detoxification activities in the body.

Over time, a poorly constructed animal-foods-free diet can lead to diseases caused by nutrient deficiency. But the symptoms can take many years to become manifest, by which point the disease state is extremely difficult to reverse, not to mention painful and potentially debilitating.

While many people may feel great *initially* when they remove animal foods from their diets, it's likely that this is because they're also avoiding inflammatory foods like sugar and poor-quality oils. An improvement in health may also come about because they're avoiding unhealthy foods that are normally paired with animal foods—like the refined-grain bun that comes with a burger.

If you want to eat a healthy plant-based diet, then build your plate *largely* of plant foods while also including well-raised, high-quality animal foods. You'll feel fuller, longer, from the dense protein, and you'll get better nutrition from the vitamins and minerals in animal foods.

Your Keto Quick Start was designed to include animal foods, and I don't recommend avoiding animal foods if optimal health is your goal.

Can I Still Eat Keto If I Can't Afford Grass-Fed and Organic Everything?

Yes! It's important not to let perfect be the enemy of the good when it comes to making healthy choices. Making shifts away from refined foods and slowly starting to swap in better-quality ingredients not only is perfectly fine but will also get you feeling better right away.

Start by prioritizing healthy fats (see chapter 5 for the details, or the guide on page 69), then proteins, then produce. Using the guide to food quality on page 66, begin at the baseline and move up from there as your budget allows.

Over time, you may find you spend less on things like over-the-counter and even prescription medications, dining out, or even alcohol, allowing more wiggle room in your budget for better-quality food.

And if that's never the case for you, it's still completely okay! The main goal is to get real, whole foods onto your plate and to remove the processed and refined foods—there's no need to stress yourself out worrying about perfection.

Practical Tips for Increasing Your Protein Intake

To make hitting your protein goals easier, I recommend having more protein on hand and ready to eat than you may have had before. Here are some easy and practical ways to stock up on healthy proteins.

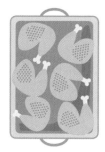

Precook/batch cook your proteins.

Whenever you cook, make a double or triple batch. Putting two pans of chicken thighs, for example, into the oven takes no more effort than putting in one pan, and it's just as easy to brown two pounds of ground meat as it is to brown one. With the extra food on hand, you'll save time down the line, and it's much easier to grab proteins for future meals or snacks.

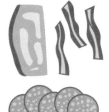

Stock up on deli meats like turkey, ham, roast beef, prosciutto, and salami.

These are easy to grab in a pinch for snacking or adding to a meal. I especially love adding ham to breakfast as an extra protein source. Remember that bacon isn't so much a protein source as a fat source! Also, don't worry about the sodium content of deli meats. While eating keto, you need to get more electrolytes—sodium, potassium, and magnesium—so this is one easy way to do that. (I'll talk more about electrolytes on page 76.)

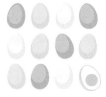

Hard-boil a dozen eggs each week.

Hard-boiled eggs are a fantastic portable snack. If eating them cold doesn't sound appealing, try this: peel the egg, then place it in a cup or bowl of hot tap water for several minutes to take the chill off before eating. You can also prep poached eggs ahead of time: after placing them in the ice bath after poaching, transfer them, still in the cold water, to an airtight container and store them in the refrigerator for up to two days. To reheat, place them in a cup or bowl of hot water for several minutes.

ADEQUATE FAT

Your target should be between 30 and 75 grams of healthy fat at each meal (for the average person, the target will be around 150 grams each day—see page 90 for how to calculate your individual number). This may come as a bit of a surprise if you're already familiar with keto, but you don't need to add a ton of fat to your meals in order to eat a high-fat diet. It's mostly about choosing fattier cuts of meats and adding some healthy fat sources to salads and vegetables.

For example, a big salad with about 1 cup of chopped chicken thighs (with the skin on), lots of leafy greens, a quarter of an avocado (or a tablespoon of sunflower or pumpkin seeds, or an ounce of cheese), and a vinaigrette dressing that includes a tablespoon of olive oil will yield 30 to 40 grams of fat! If your total for the day is anywhere in the range of 90 to 150 grams, you can see how you're already well on your way to your daily fat intake in that one meal, without adding much of what we typically think of as "fatty foods." It's a common misconception that you need to consistently add a lot of extra fat to your meals to hit your fat-intake goals for the day.

To stay on top of your fat intake, buy bone-in, skin-on chicken thighs or breasts instead of boneless, skinless breasts (yes, you'll eat the skin!). Look for fattier cuts of steak, like rib-eye, instead of flank or sirloin steak. Choose 80 or 85 percent fat grass-fed ground beef and skip the "extra-lean" 93 percent fat ground beef. Pick ground pork or lamb or at least ground dark-meat turkey over ground turkey breast.

If you are eating lean meats (for instance, grilled chicken or turkey breast, lean pork chops, or flank steak) or seafood, I recommend adding 1 tablespoon of fat per 4 ounces of protein. But you can skip this if there is adequate fat provided by other parts of the meal, such as cooking fats or bacon used in a dish, cheese melted on some vegetables, or cheese, avocado, nuts or seeds, and salad dressing.

In salads, add at least one source of healthy fat (in addition to dressing), such as avocado slices, nuts, seeds, or crumbled chicharrones (yes, fried pork skins—they're a great crouton replacement!).

Plant Fats or Animal Fats?

The healthiest fats are those which are naturally occurring. This includes *both* animal fats from well-raised animals (in their most natural environment, like 100 percent grass-fed, pastured beef and pastured pork), as well as the dairy from those animals, *and* plants like avocados and avocado oil, olives and olive oil, nuts, and seeds. Certain types of plant fats that are isolated from their original form or source are extremely unhealthy.

Not all plant fats are the same, and they're certainly not healthy just because they come from plants! Unhealthy plant fats include any that are highly processed, like vegetable oils (soybean, canola, and cottonseed, for example), hydrogenated or partially hydrogenated vegetable shortening (like Crisco), margarine and other fake butter spreads, fryer oils that have been repeatedly used (all restaurant fryers), and mayonnaise and salad dressings made from vegetable oils.

I'll talk about healthy and unhealthy fats in much more depth in chapter 5.

Just by including a few healthy fats in your meals, you'll easily reach your fat-intake goals for the day. But notice that I said "healthy fats": "healthy" is crucial. In the next chapter, I'll talk a lot more about what makes a fat healthy and how to choose the right fats for your keto diet.

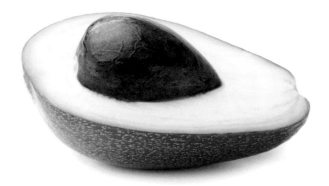

VEGGIES!

On keto, veggies are likely to be your primary source of carbs. A good goal is 10 grams of net carbs—that's total carbs minus fiber—per meal, for 30 grams of net carbs per day.

Don't fear vegetables because of their carb counts! If you've searched online for keto recipes, you may have noticed that they are often very meat- and cheese-heavy (when they're not recipes for treats and baked goods). Don't forget that fresh whole foods are keto, too!

Starchy vegetables should be limited, true. That includes potatoes, sweet potatoes, plantains, some winter squash like butternut and kabocha, yucca/cassava, and taro. (I'll talk about how to incorporate some of these into your meals in a healthy way on pages 88 to 89.)

Non-starchy vegetables, on the other hand, don't need to be limited the way starchy vegetables do, and there is an extremely wide array to choose from. Non-starchy vegetables include but are not limited to:

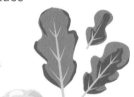
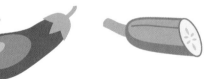

- all leafy greens, such as kale, arugula, spinach, and lettuce
- bell peppers
- broccoli
- Brussels sprouts
- cabbage
- cauliflower
- celery
- eggplant
- green beans
- hearts of palm
- jicama
- mushrooms
- spaghetti squash
- sprouts, such as broccoli sprouts, sunflower sprouts, radish sprouts
- zucchini and other summer squash

If you're still hungry at the end of the day after eating everything you planned for, or if you're looking at what's for dinner and feeling stressed that you've already eaten most of your allotted carbs, you are always welcome to add more non-starchy vegetables to your plate. While the carb grams do add up eventually, so does the fiber—and since you can subtract fiber from your total carb count, the veggies won't contribute much in the way of carbs. And eating an extra cup of bell peppers, for example, is not going to destroy your metabolism or make fat-burning impossible, I promise! In fact, the vitamins and minerals you'll get from those vegetables will likely push you even further along your path to health. Just keep in mind that if you're eating roasted veggies that have been cooked in fat or adding more salad dressing to leafy greens, those extra fats do need to be counted in your daily totals.

Here's the caveat, though: while real foods rich in carbs are nutrient-dense and we needn't fear or demonize them, in large quantities, they are antagonistic to the goals of a ketogenic diet. Therefore, when eating a keto diet, it's best to avoid large quantities of even healthy carbs (unless you've planned a higher-carb meal or day, as I'll talk more about in chapter 7). That said, a healthy body can be metabolically flexible, and a high-carbohydrate portion of food now and then will not be a disaster. If you are healing insulin resistance, it's best to avoid too many carbs until your body is able to process them in a balanced way. However, once your metabolism is working as expected, it's natural to be mostly in ketosis and then come out of that for a short period of time before slipping back into it. The human body is adaptable, and you don't need to turn keto eating into a religion.

If you become fearful of carbs to the point that it makes you want to throw in the towel even though you're feeling amazing and experiencing great results, then reconsider how strict you want to be about keto. If you feel best simply drawing a hard line and never eating carbs again, then so be it. If the idea of having too much restriction makes you want to rebel against any rules, then consider a more flexible approach where you plan a day or a meal here or there that allows for more carbs (more on that in chapter 7).

You'll likely find that, over time, you crave high-carb foods less and less, and certainly unhealthy refined carbs become less appealing once you've been avoiding them for a while. Enjoying those foods as a treat now and then becomes easier when your everyday meals are balanced and healthful.

Net Carbs vs. Total Carbs

Net carbs are equal to total carbs minus fiber. Since fiber is indigestible and therefore isn't absorbed, it won't spike blood sugar or insulin. So if you're eating high-fiber vegetables and you want to just count total carbs, you can shoot for 40 to 50 grams total carbs per day. However, if you want to subtract the fiber, you'd shoot for around 30 grams net carbs. When I first ate keto, I only counted total carbs and often ate in the 30 to 35 gram range, but I allowed myself to go up to 40 to 50 grams just for the sake of my sanity, since we can't ever really know *exactly* how many carbs a single natural food holds. Even nutrition facts are always going to be a best approximate!

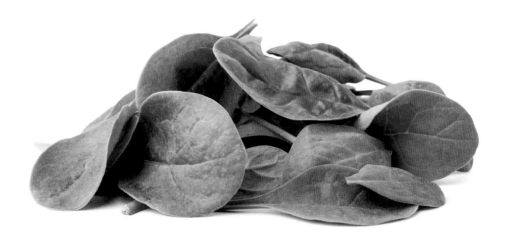

VARIETY

Do your best each week to buy a variety of vegetables when grocery shopping. Aim for at least three colors, including green—so perhaps something purple and something red as well! When selecting vegetables, vary between those that are deeply colored all the way through (like purple cabbage, for example) and those that have deeply colored skins but a white flesh (like zucchini). While all are great choices, there are different vitamins and phytonutrients in each type and color of vegetable.

Varying proteins can be a bit tricky at first since we're mostly creatures of habit, and, let's face it, grocery stores tend to sell the same handful of cuts all the time! But look for what's on sale each week, and maybe try a new cut or protein type you haven't before. If you've never had lamb, give it a shot! It's especially easy to try new types of ground meat: they tend to be inexpensive, and they're easy to season and brown in a skillet or make into meatballs.

Visit your local farmers market or ask the butcher at your grocery store what's good that week. See if they have some great ideas for how to prepare new cuts of meat. Most butchers are quick to tell you their favorites and the best way to prepare them.

Also, seek out new recipes! The vast majority of recipes in all of my books—*Practical Paleo*, *The 21-Day Sugar Detox* series, and *Mediterranean Paleo Cooking*—are either keto-friendly as written or can be made keto with an ingredient swap or two. If you find keto recipes elsewhere, just make sure that they use healthy whole foods.

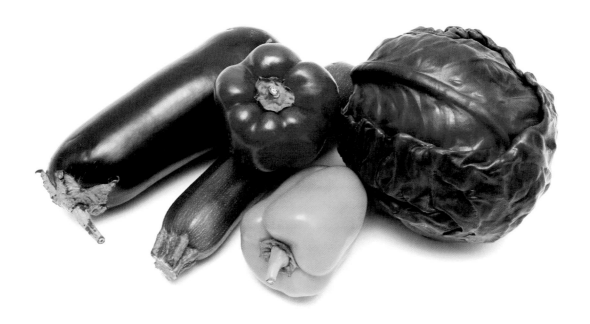

YES TO HERBS AND SPICES

It can be easy to get stuck on the same flavors, just as it's easy to always buy the same foods at the store. But a few shakes of a new spice blend or the addition of new herbs can add not just excitement but also nutrients that are often tough to find in foods when we're eliminating lots of carbs.

For example, 1/4 cup of cilantro (about how much I sprinkle into a salad) contains 16 percent of the recommended daily amount of vitamin K and 5 percent of the recommended daily amount of vitamin A, as well as some vitamin C and E, both antioxidants that help fight inflammation. Or take chives, which are rich in vitamin C, potassium, iron, and calcium, and also contain beta-carotene, folate, niacin, thiamin, and riboflavin.

Those are just two examples, but all fresh herbs carry amazing nutrition, so play around with them in the kitchen and add them to your meals. Try using herbs as a garnish, or to eat larger amounts, blend them into a pesto (see the recipe on page 343). Herbs carry almost no calories and virtually no carbs unless you're eating a cup at a time, and at that point it's about 1 gram, which is negligible—and almost no one eats a whole cup at a time!

In the spices category, just a teaspoon of paprika, for example, packs a hit of vitamins A, C, E, K, and B_6, among others, with just 1 gram of carbs. In most recipes, you probably won't use a full teaspoon, but still, gram for gram, it's a powerhouse! Ground ginger is another great example: it's packed with manganese, a nutrient that's essential for several body processes, including metabolism and joint health, and that helps prevent anemia.

Ounce for ounce, herbs and spices are one of the absolute best ways to add flavor and nutrition to your meals!

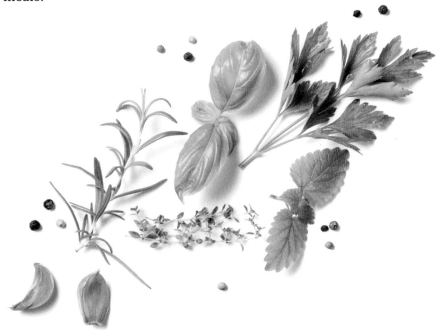

KETO FOODS LIST

FOOD	SERVING	SERVING WEIGHT	TOTAL CARBS (g)	FIBER (g)	NET CARBS (g)	PROTEIN (g)	FAT (g)
ZERO-CARB VEGGIES (<1 g per serving)							
Bamboo shoots (cooked)	1/2 cup	60 g	1.15	0.6	0	0.0	0.0
Celery (raw)	1/2 cup	50 g	1.49	0.8	0	0.0	0.0
Daikon / white icicle radish (raw)	1/2 cup	50 g	1.32	0.7	0	0.0	0.0
Garlic (raw)	1 tsp	3 g	0.99	0.06	0	0.0	0.0
Fresh herbs (cilantro, mint, parsley, etc.)	1/4 cup	variable	0.66	0.36	0	0.0	0.0
Leafy greens (arugula, bok choy, endive, lettuce, spinach, turnip greens, watercress, etc.)	1 cup raw or 1/2 cup cooked	variable	1.44	1.04	0	0.0	0.0
Mushrooms, white (raw)	1/2 cup raw or 1/4 cup cooked	35 g	1.14	0.35	0	1.1	0.0
Rapini / broccoli raab / broccoli rabe (cooked)	1/2 cup	42 g	1.31	1.18	0	1.6	0.0
Spices	n/a	-	-	-	0	-	-
Sprouts (alfalfa, broccoli, radish, etc.; raw)	1/2 cup	17 g	0.36	0.32	0	0.0	0.0
VERY-LOW-CARB VEGGIES							
(1–2 g net carbs per serving)							
Asparagus (cooked)	1/2 cup	90 g	3.7	1.8	1.9	2.2	0.0
Cauliflower (cooked)	1/2 cup	62 g	2.55	1.43	1.1	1.1	0.0
Chard (cooked)	1/2 cup	88 g	3.63	1.85	1.8	1.7	0.0
Collard greens (cooked)	1/2 cup	95 g	5.37	3.8	1.6	2.6	0.0
Cucumbers (raw)	1/2 cup	52 g	3.7	1.8	1.6	0.0	0.0
Fennel bulb (raw)	1/2 cup	44 g	3.21	1.36	1.9	0.0	0.0
Green onions	1/4 cup	24 g	1.76	0.64	1.1	0.0	0.0
Hearts of palm (canned)	1/2 cup	73 g	3.37	1.75	1.6	1.8	0.0
Kohlrabi (raw)	1/2 cup	68 g	4.22	2.45	1.8	1.2	0.0
Leafy greens (purslane, radicchio, etc.)	1 cup raw or 1/2 cup cooked	42 g	1.63	0.18	1.5	0.0	0.0
Mushrooms, portobello (raw or cooked)	1/2 cup	43 g	1.66	0.56	1.1	0.0	0.0
Mustard greens	1 cup raw or 1/2 cup cooked	70 g	3.16	1.4	1.8	1.8	0.0
Okra (cooked)	1/2 cup	80 g	3.61	2	1.6	1.5	0.0
Radishes (raw)	1/2 cup	58 g	1.97	0.93	1.0	0.0	0.0
Shallots (raw)	1 tbsp chopped	10 g	1.68	0.32	1.4	0.0	0.0
(2–3 g net carbs per serving)							
Artichokes (cooked)	1/2 cup	84 g	10.04	7.22	2.8	2.4	0.0
Broccoli (cooked)	1/2 cup	78 g	5.6	2.57	3.0	1.9	0.0
Cabbage	1 cup raw or 1/2 cup cooked	70 g	4.06	1.75	2.3	0.0	0.0
Dandelion greens (raw)	1 cup	55 g	5.06	1.93	3.1	1.5	0.0
Eggplant (cooked)	1/2 cup	50 g	4.37	1.25	3.1	0.0	0.0
Green beans / snap beans (cooked)	1/2 cup	63 g	4.96	2.02	3.0	1.2	0.0
Jicama / yambean (raw)	1/2 cup	60 g	5.29	2.94	2.4	0.0	0.0
Peppers (raw or cooked)	1/2 cup	75 g	4.52	1.58	2.9	0.0	0.0
Sprouts, mung bean (raw)	1/2 cup	52 g	3.09	0.94	2.2	1.6	0.0
Summer squash (zucchini, yellow squash, etc.; cooked)	1/2 cup	90 g	3.88	1.26	2.6	0.0	0.0
Tomatoes and tomatillos (raw)	1/2 cup	90 g	3.5	1.08	2.4	0.0	0.0

FOOD	SERVING	SERVING WEIGHT	TOTAL CARBS (g)	FIBER (g)	NET CARBS (g)	PROTEIN (g)	FAT (g)
(3–5 g net carbs per serving)							
Brussels sprouts (cooked)	1/2 cup	78 g	5.54	2.03	3.5	2.0	0.0
Carrots (raw or cooked)	1/2 cup	61 g	5.84	1.71	4.1	0.0	0.0
Kale (raw or cooked)	1 cup	67 g	5.57	1.14	4.4	1.9	0.0
Kohlrabi (cooked)	1/2 cup	83 g	5.55	0.91	4.6	1.5	0.0
Leeks (cooked)	1/2 cup	52 g	3.96	0.52	3.4	0.0	0.0
Rutabagas (cooked)	1/2 cup	85 g	5.81	1.53	4.3	0.0	0.0
Snow peas / snap peas	1 cup raw or 1/2 cup cooked	80 g	3.45	1.37	4.0	1.6	0.0
Spaghetti squash (cooked)	1/2 cup	78 g	5.04	1.09	4.0	0.0	0.0
Tomatoes (cooked)	1/2 cup	120 g	4.81	0.84	4.0	1.1	0.0
Turnips (mashed and cooked)	1/2 cup	115 g	5.82	2.3	3.5	0.0	0.0
LOW-CARB VEGGIES (7–10 g net carbs per serving)							
Arrowroot (raw)	1/2 cup	60 g	8.03	0.78	7.3	2.5	0.0
Beets (cooked)	1/2 cup	85 g	8.47	1.7	6.8	1.4	0.0
Green peas (cooked)	1/2 cup	80 g	12.5	4.4	8.1	4.3	0.0
Lotus roots (cooked)	1/2 cup	60 g	9.61	1.86	7.8	0.0	0.0
Onions (raw)	1/2 cup	80 g	7.47	1.36	6.1	0.0	0.0
Onions (cooked)	1/2 cup	105 g	10.66	1.47	9.2	1.4	0.0
Parsnips (raw)	1/2 cup	67 g	12.05	3.28	8.8	0.0	0.0
Winter squash (butternut, kabocha, pumpkin, etc.)	1/2 cup	103 g	8.85	1.55	7.3	0.0	0.0
MODERATE-CARB VEGGIES (10–15 g net carbs per serving)							
Parsnips (cooked)	1/2 cup	78 g	13.27	2.81	10.5	1.0	0.0
Sunchokes / Jerusalem artichokes	1/2 cup	75 g	13.08	1.2	11.9	1.5	0.0
White potato (cooked)	1/2 cup	78 g	16.5	1.72	14.8	2.0	0.0
HIGH-CARB VEGGIES & TUBERS (>15 g net carbs per serving)							
Cassava / yucca (raw)	1/2 cup	103 g	39.2	1.85	37.4	1.4	0.0
Plantains (cooked)	1/2 cup	77 g	23.99	1.77	22.2	0.6	0.0
Sweet potatoes (cooked)	1/2 cup	100 g	20.71	3.3	17.4	2.0	0.0
Taro (cooked)	1/2 cup	66 g	22.84	3.37	19.5	0.3	0.0
VERY-LOW-CARB FRUITS							
(<3 g net carbs per serving)							
Avocados (raw)	1/2 avocado	73 g	6.31	4.96	1.4	1.43	11.25
Coconut meat, dried, unsweetened	1 ounce	28 g	6.62	4.56	2.1	1.93	18.07
Coconut meat, raw	1/2 cup	40 g	6.09	3.6	2.5	1.33	13.4
Coconut milk (full-fat)	1 tbsp	15 g	0.42	0.0	0.0	0.0	3.2
Kumquats (raw)	1 kumquat	19 g	3.02	1.24	1.8	0.0	0.0
Lemon juice (raw)	1 fluid ounce	30 g	2.07	0.09	2.0	0.0	0.0
Lime juice (raw)	1 fluid ounce	31 g	2.61	0.12	2.5	0.0	0.0
Olives	1 ounce	28 g	1.75	0.9	0.0	0.0	3.0
Rhubarb (raw)	1/2 cup	61 g	2.77	1.1	1.7	0.0	0.0
Starfruit / carambola (raw)	1/2 cup	54 g	3.63	1.51	2.1	0.0	0.0
Yams (cooked)	1/2 cup	68 g	18.69	2.65	16.0	1.0	0.0
(3–5 g net carbs per serving)							
Blackberries (raw)	1/2 cup	72 g	6.92	3.82	3.1	1.0	0.0
Cranberries (raw)	1/2 cup	55 g	6.71	2.53	4.2	0.0	0.0
Raspberries (raw)	1/2 cup	62 g	7.4	4.03	3.4	0.0	0.0
Strawberries (raw)	1/2 cup	76 g	5.84	1.52	4.3	0.0	0.0

Note that some items have been assigned an approximate value within about 1–2 grams.

When more than one kind of a food is listed in a single row (e.g., more than one kind of steak), the nutritional information is an average of all the kinds specified. Averages were only calculated when the difference between the varieties was negligible. Foods that come in packages (e.g., sardines and tuna) are not listed; read package labels for nutritional data. Protein and fat are not listed if the amounts are negligible.

FOOD	SERVING	SERVING WEIGHT	TOTAL CARBS (g)	FIBER (g)	NET CARBS (g)	PROTEIN (g)	FAT (g)
LOW-CARB FRUITS (5–10 g net carbs)							
Apples (raw)	1/2 cup	55 g	7.6	1.32	**6.3**	0.0	0.0
Apricots (raw)	1/2 cup	78 g	8.67	1.56	**7.1**	1.1	0.0
Blueberries (raw)	1/2 cup	74 g	10.72	1.78	**9.0**	0.0	0.0
Canteloupe (raw)	1/2 cup	89 g	7.26	0.8	**6.5**	0.0	0.0
Guavas (raw)	1/2 cup	83 g	11.89	4.48	**7.4**	2.1	0.0
Honeydew melon (raw)	1/2 cup	89 g	8.09	0.71	**7.4**	0.0	0.0
Nectarines (raw)	1/2 cup	72 g	7.6	1.22	**6.4**	0.0	0.0
Oranges (various kinds; raw)	1/2 cup	90 g	10.58	2.16	**8.4**	0.0	0.0
Papayas (raw)	1/2 cup	70 g	7.57	1.19	**6.4**	0.0	0.0
Peaches (raw)	1/2 cup	77 g	7.35	1.16	**6.2**	0.0	0.0
Pears (raw)	1/2 cup	81 g	12.34	2.51	**9.8**	0.0	0.0
Persimmons (raw) 1 small persimmon		25 g	8.38	0	**8.4**	0.0	0.0
Pineapples (raw)	1/2 cup	83 g	10.89	1.16	**9.7**	0.0	0.0
Plums (raw)	1/2 cup	83 g	9.48	1.16	**8.3**	0.0	0.0
Pomegranate seeds (raw)	1/2 cup	44 g	8.23	1.76	**6.5**	0.0	0.0
Watermelon (raw)	1/2 cup	77 g	5.81	0.31	**5.5**	0.0	0.0
MODERATE-CARB FRUITS (10–15 g net carbs)							
Cherries (raw)	1/2 cup	77 g	12.33	1.62	**10.7**	0.0	0.0
Grapefruit (pink/red; raw)	1/2 cup	115 g	12.26	1.84	**10.4**	0.0	0.0
Grapes (raw)	1/2 cup	76 g	13.76	0.68	**13.1**	0.0	0.0
Kiwis (raw)	1/2 cup	89 g	13.05	2.67	**10.4**	1.0	0.0
Lychees / litchis (raw)	1/2 cup	95 g	15.7	1.24	**14.5**	0.0	0.0
Mangoes (raw)	1/2 cup	83 g	12.43	1.33	**11.1**	0.0	0.0
Tangerines (raw)	1/2 cup	98 g	13.07	1.76	**11.3**	0.0	0.0
HIGH-CARB FRUITS (15–25 g net carbs)							
Bananas (raw)	1/2 cup	75 g	17.13	1.95	**15.2**	0.0	0.0
Figs (raw)	1/2 cup	153 g	29.35	4.44	**24.9**	1.2	0.0
Passionfruit / granadilla (raw)	1/2 cup	118 g	27.59	12.27	**15.3**	2.6	0.0
Plantains (cooked)	1/2 cup	77 g	23.99	1.77	**22.2**	0.0	0.0
VERY LOW-CARB NUTS & SEEDS (<2g net carbs per serving)							
Brazil nuts (unblanched)	1 ounce	28 g	3.44	2.1	**1.3**	4.0	18.6
Macadamia nuts (dry roasted, with salt)	1 ounce	28 g	3.59	2.24	**1.4**	2.1	21.3
Pecans (dry roasted, without salt)	1 ounce	28 g	3.79	2.63	**1.2**	2.7	20.8
Pumpkin seeds / pepitas	1 tbsp	9 g	1.54	0.34	**1.2**	2.12	3.96
Sesame seeds (dried)	1 tbsp	9 g	2.11	1.06	**1.1**	1.6	4.5
Sunflower seeds (dried)	1 tbsp	9 g	1.8	0.77	**1.0**	1.9	4.6
MODERATE CARB NUTS & SEEDS (>2 g net carbs per serving)							
Almond butter (with salt)	2 tbsp	32 g	6.02	3.3	**2.7**	6.7	17.8
Almonds (dry roasted, with salt)	1 ounce	28 g	5.94	3.05	**2.9**	5.9	14.6
Chestnuts (roasted)	1 ounce	28 g	14.83	1.43	**13.4**	0.0	0.0
Hazelnuts (dry roasted, without salt)	1 ounce	28 g	4.93	2.63	**2.3**	4.2	17.5
Pine nuts	1 ounce	28 g	3.66	1.04	**2.6**	3.8	19.1
Walnuts	1 ounce	28 g	3.84	1.88	**2.0**	4.3	18.3
Peanuts (dry roasted, with salt)	1 ounce	28 g	6.02	2.24	**3.8**	6.6	13.9
Peanut butter (smooth, with salt)	2 tbsp	32 g	6.26	1.92	**4.3**	8.0	16.1
Pistachios (dry roasted, with salt)	1 ounce	28 g	8.02	2.77	**5.3**	5.9	12.6
Sesame seed butter / tahini	2 tbsp	30 g	7.86	2.8	**5.1**	5.3	14.4
Sunflower seed butter (with salt)	2 tbsp	32 g	7.46	1.82	**5.6**	5.5	17.7

FOOD	SERVING	SERVING WEIGHT	TOTAL CARBS (g)	FIBER (g)	NET CARBS (g)	PROTEIN (g)	FAT (g)
ZERO-CARB DAIRY							
Butter (salted)	1 tbsp	14 g	0	0	**0.0**	0.0	7.7
Cheese, hard (cow or goat)	1 ounce	28 g	0.9	0	**0.0**	10.0	7.2
Cheese, soft (cow or goat)	1 ounce	28 g	0.13	0	**0.0**	5.8	7.8
Ghee / clarified butter	1 tbsp	13 g	0	0	**0.0**	0.0	12.9
Mozzarella cheese, whole milk (cow)	1 ounce	28 g	28 g	0	**0.0**	6.2	6.3
VERY-LOW-CARB DAIRY (<5 g per serving)							
Cottage cheese (cow)	1/2 cup	113 g	3.82	0	**3.8**	12.6	4.9
Ricotta cheese, whole milk (cow)	1/2 cup	124 g	3.77	0	**3.8**	14.0	16.1
MODERATE-CARB DAIRY (10–15 g per serving)							
Yogurt (full-fat)	1 cup	246 g	11.46	0	**11.46**	4.3	4.0
Milk, whole (cow or goat)	1 cup	244 g	11.66	0	**11.7**	7.7	8.0
Milk, whole (sheep)	1 cup	245 g	13.13	0	**13.1**	14.7	17.2
Yogurt (full-fat)	1 cup	246 g	11.46	0	**11.46**	4.3	4.0
PROTEINS							
Beef, brisket, 1/8" fat (cooked)	4 ounces	112 g	-	-	0	30.0	20.6
Beef, ground (80% lean) (cooked)	4 ounces	112 g	-	-	0	30.0	20.0
Beef, ground (85% lean) (cooked)	4 ounces	112 g	-	-	0	30.0	17.3
Beef, ground (90% lean) (cooked)	4 ounces	112 g	-	-	0	30.0	13.1
Beef, lean steak (flank, chuck roast / pot roast, NY strip; cooked)	4 ounces	112 g	-	-	0	30.0	10.0
Beef, fattier steak (beef ribs, rib eye / Delminico, short loin / T-bone, skirt steak; cooked)	5 ounces	112 g	-	-	1	30.0	20.0
Bison, ground (cooked)	4 ounces	112 g	-	-	0	28.5	9.7
Bison, steak or roast (cooked)	4 ounces	112 g	-	-	0	32.0	6.0
Chicken, light/white meat (breast, boneless, skinless; cooked)	4 ounces	112 g	-	-	0	34.7	4.0
Chicken, dark meat (thighs or drumstick, bone-in, skin-on; cooked)	4 ounces	112 g	-	-	0	25.4	16.6
Chicken, wings (bone-in, skin-on; cooked)	4 ounces	112 g	-	-	0	30.1	21.8
Egg (white and yolk)	1 large egg		0.6-	0-	0	6	5
Pork, bacon (cooked)	1 slice	8 g	-	-	0	3.0	3.3
Pork, ground or ribs (meat only, cooked)	4 ounces	112 g	-	-	0	28.8	23.3
Pork, ham roast (bone-in; cooked)	4 ounces	112 g	-	-	0	29.1	3.4
Pork, loin chops, lean (cooked)	4 ounces	112 g	-	-	1	29.3	7.6
Pork, spare ribs (cooked)	4 ounces	112 g	-	-	0	32.6	33.9
Turkey, white meat	4 ounces	112 g	-	-	0	28.0	1.0
Turkey, dark meat	4 ounces	112 g	-	-	0	28.0	2.5
Cod (cooked)	4 ounces	112 g	-	-	0	22.9	0.3
Crab (cooked)	4 ounces	112 g	-	-	0	20.0	0.8
Lobster (cooked)	4 ounces	112 g	-	-	0	21.3	1.0
Salmon (cooked)	4 ounces	112 g	-	-	0	25.0	4.7
Scallops (cooked)	4 ounces	112 g	-	-	1	26.0	1.5
Shrimp (cooked)	4 ounces	112 g	-	-	1.7	25.5	1.9
Snapper (cooked)	4 ounces	112 g	-	-	0	29.5	1.9
Tuna, fresh (cooked)	4 ounces	112 g	-	-	0	33.5	7.0
VERY-LOW-CARB PROTEINS (<5g net carbs per serving)							
Oysters (raw)	4 ounces	112 g	-	-	4.3	8.5	2.3

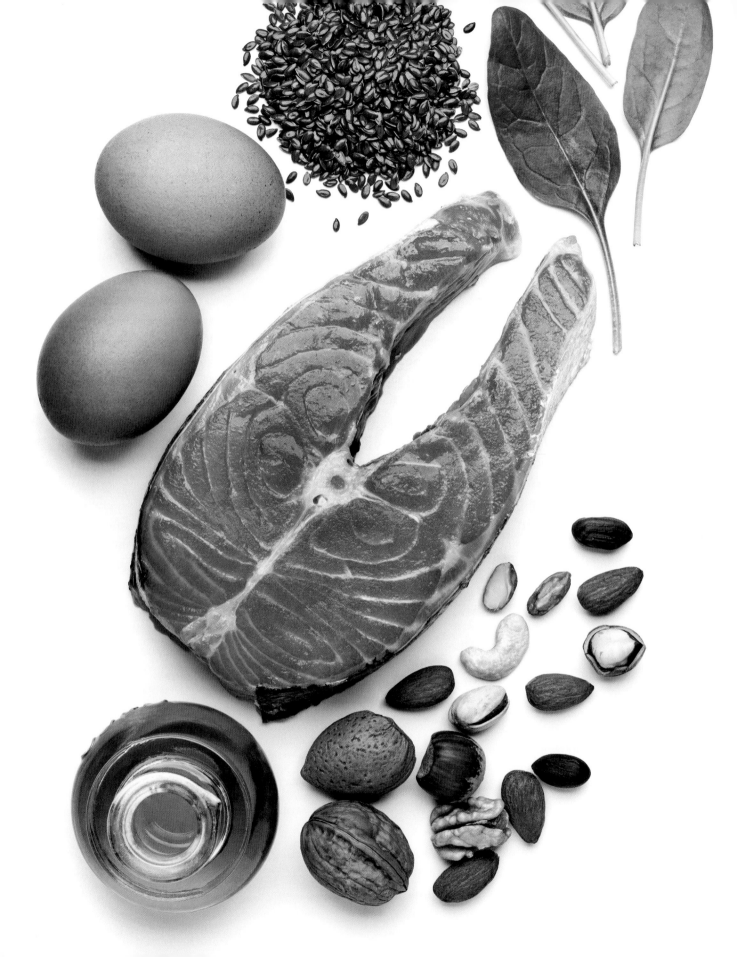

CHAPTER 5

Choosing Healthy Fats

Cleaning up your diet and focusing on including more fats doesn't mean adding just *any* fats! You want to eat the highest-quality fats and oils that you can.

These are the questions I ask when deciding which fats to eat and which to avoid, in order of importance:

1. **Is it in a whole food?**

2. **How is it made?**

3. **What is its fatty acid composition and stability?**

4. **What is its source?**

5. **What is its micronutrient content?**

Now, you don't need to know why these questions matter to pick healthy fats—if you simply want to know which fats to eat and which to avoid, use the guide on page 69, or visit balancedbites.com/ketoquickstart for a list of well-sourced and well-respected brands of fats and oils.

But I believe there's value in knowing *why* certain fats are healthy and others can actually harm you. If you're interested in diving deeper, read on!

1. IS IT IN A WHOLE FOOD?

If a fat or oil is found as is in nature, in real, whole foods—like fatty fish, avocado, or dairy—it's among the healthiest fats to eat. I consider both butter and ghee to be naturally occurring, real-food fats. Yes, both require some processing, but that processing is purely mechanical (churning) and doesn't introduce anything that isn't present in fresh whole milk, straight from the cow. That's about as naturally occurring as you can get when talking about a food that isn't in its original, from-the-cow form.

Real, whole foods rich in healthy fats include the following:

- avocado
- bacon (yes, really! *Especially* from pastured pork!)
- beef
- cacao
- chicken with the skin on (especially dark meat)
- coconut chips
- dark-meat turkey

- eggs
- fatty fish, like salmon and herring
- lamb
- nuts
- olives
- plain, full-fat yogurt (without flavors, sweeteners, stabilizers, or additives)
- pork
- seeds

No need to buy lean cuts of meat (which tend to be more expensive anyway)—you can rely on the less-expensive fattier cuts for your keto diet. Of course, quality does matter when choosing these foods, which I'll get into shortly.

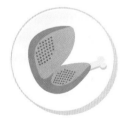 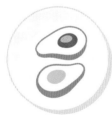 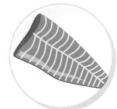 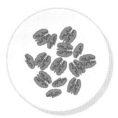 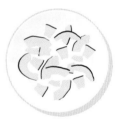

BOTTOM LINE

Choosing whole-food sources of naturally occurring fats will always be the absolute best option for getting more healthy fats in your diet.

Budget Tip

The most cost-effective cuts of meat are stew and braising cuts, as well as those that have been less processed—like a whole chicken instead of only the thighs. The more specific and popular the cut, the more expensive it will be. For example, boneless, skinless chicken breasts and breast tenders are the most expensive cuts of chicken; buying a whole chicken is the least expensive, *and* it'll include the best, fattiest cuts for your keto diet.

2. HOW IS IT MADE?

If you're not getting fat from a whole food, the next best option is a healthy oil. Some oils are made with minimal processing, while others go through *extreme* processing in order to be bottled and put on a grocery store shelf.

Traditional oils like extra-virgin olive oil and coconut oil go through a pressing process to extract the oil from the fatty fruit of the plant. This process, while mechanical, doesn't damage the resulting oil, and the oils retain their antioxidant levels. Examples of other healthy cold-pressed oils are avocado, peanut, and sesame oil. (Not all cold-pressed oils are the best choices, though; I'll explain why on page 62.)

More-modern oils like canola, soybean, sunflower, safflower, grapeseed, rice bran, and cottonseed oil—collectively referred to as "vegetable oils"— are extracted via a process that requires many steps, several of which may be problematic both for the resulting oil and for human health.

Vegetable oils are processed using solvent extraction. The complete process of making vegetable oils includes these steps:

Refined Coconut Oil

While some refined coconut oil is best avoided because it's gone through an RBD process that's similar to the one used for vegetable oils, there are refined coconut oils that have been steam-processed instead. Steam processing is not harmful to the stable fats in coconut oil, so steam-processed refined coconut oil is a good option if you want the high-heat-stable properties of coconut oil without the coconut scent and flavor. No chemicals, additives, or hexane are used in steam processing. Nutiva, Tropical Traditions, and Wilderness Family Naturals / Wildly Organic all make steam-processed refined coconut oils that are good choices.

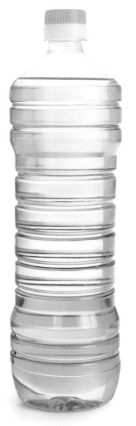

1. cleaning the seeds
2. preconditioning and flaking the seeds
3. cooking the flaked seeds
4. pressing the flake to mechanically remove a portion of the oil
5. using a chemical solvent to extract the remaining oil from the press cake
6. desolventizing and toasting the meal
7. degumming, bleaching, and deodorizing the oil

Collectively, these steps are often referred to as "refining, bleaching, and deodorizing," or RBD. The oil can be damaged in steps 2, 3, 5, 6, and 7. Even worse, the solvent used in step 5 is hexane, a chemical known to have toxic effects on human health (including but not limited to neurotoxicity, peripheral polyneuropathy, color vision defects, and testicular atrophy). Furthermore, this processing strips away disease-fighting antioxidants, thus rendering the oils more heavily loaded with disease-promoting free radicals.

Buyer Beware

Some low-quality olive oils may go through additional processing, and that processing may include enzymes, steam, hexane, or other solvents. Better-quality olive oils don't use any of these processes or chemicals, so it's important to purchase the highest-quality oils possible. Some signs of a high-quality oil are a "pressed-on" date (different from a "use by" or "bottled on" date) and a dark-colored or opaque glass bottle or tin (not clear and not plastic). Ideally you want to consume an extra-virgin olive oil that was pressed within the last 24 months. My favorite brand is Kasandrinos, but other brands you may want to try include Coppetti, Nuñez De Prado, and Papa Vince.

While cold-pressing avoids the refining, bleaching, and deodorizing that happens in solvent extraction, some heat is generated during the process. In the EU, that heat cannot exceed 80.6°F, but olive oil bottled outside the EU is not guaranteed to have had low-temperature extraction. This is important because high heat can damage the fats in olive oil, and the polyphenol, antioxidant, and vitamin content of oils processed at higher heat will be lower.

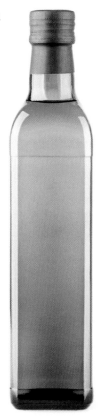

Compare this to the cold-pressing process by which extra-virgin olive oil is made:

1. cleaning the olives and removing the pits
2. grinding the olives into a paste
3. malaxing (mixing) the paste
4. pressing the paste to separate out the oil

Virgin (unrefined) coconut oil is made in a similar method. None of these steps damage the oil or are harmful to health.

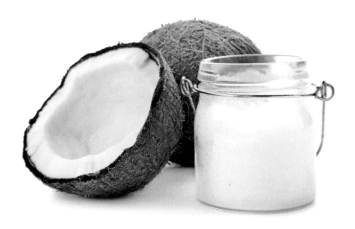

BOTTOM LINE

Choose oils that have gone through the least damaging process from plant to bottle. Avoid all vegetable oils and opt for organic, extra-virgin, cold-pressed plant-based oils.

3. WHAT IS ITS FATTY ACID COMPOSITION AND STABILITY?

You don't need to worry about the fatty acid composition of real, whole foods. But when choosing an oil, especially a cooking oil, it's important to understand what it's made of.

There are three main types of fatty acids, which make up all fats and oils:

- saturated fatty acids (SFAs)
- monounsaturated fatty acids (MUFAs)
- polyunsaturated fatty acids (PUFAs)

Of the three, MUFAs are the least controversial, and their beneficial impact on human health is well known—which is why olive oil has been touted as a healthy oil for decades. Saturated and polyunsaturated fatty acids are more controversial.

As you read in chapter 2, it's a common misconception that avoiding saturated fat is ideal for optimal health. In fact, saturated fats are more stable than unsaturated fats. That means they're less likely to be damaged or oxidized—and oxidized oils are some of the most inflammatory foods. In fact, whether or not a fat is healthy often comes down to how likely it is to be oxidized.

What Does It Mean When a Fatty Acid Is Oxidized?

Oxidation occurs when something—light, heat, air, or a combination of these—disrupts the molecular structure of a fatty acid. Because our bodies use the fatty acids we eat to create and repair our own cells, an oxidized fatty acid can end up compromising cell structures and affecting overall health.

For example, according to nutrition expert Chris Masterjohn, "the oxidation of polyunsaturated fatty acids in the lipoprotein membrane is what drives the oxidation of the particle that makes it contribute to atherosclerosis."[*] In other words, oxidized PUFAs in our cell membranes is one factor that leads to atherosclerosis, the buildup of plaque in our arteries.

The More Stable the Fat, the Better It Is for Cooking

Ever wonder why high-quality olive oils are sold in dark-green glass bottles? It's to keep light from oxidizing the oil. Ever wonder why coconut oil doesn't smell rancid after sitting on the counter without a lid but vegetable oil does? Air damages vegetable oil and makes it rancid.

---

[*] Chris Masterjohn, "Is Coconut Oil Killing Us?," Mastering Nutrition (podcast), June 24, 2017, https://chrismasterjohnphd.com/2017/06/24/coconut-oil-killing-us.

Eat. Your. Fish!

There is one PUFA that is known to be good for you: omega-3. It has an anti-inflammatory effect in the body that's very beneficial. However, it's still important to get omega-3 from high-quality whole foods, like wild-caught salmon, walnuts, and chia seeds. When isolated from whole foods, omega-3, like any PUFA, becomes highly susceptible to oxidation.

While not everyone has a taste for seafood, I highly recommend attempting various recipes using omega-3-rich fish until you find a way to enjoy it. The health benefits of the whole-food form of this anti-inflammatory fat really can't be overstated, and supplementing is not the route that I recommend. Since we know how susceptible to damage omega-3 fatty acids are, it's extremely difficult to guarantee that what you are getting in a supplement is of high quality and also in a stable, unoxidized form. There may be some situations where acute supplementation with omega-3s can be helpful, as in the case of a traumatic brain injury, but for everyday use in promoting overall health, we must look for this nutrient in our whole foods.

I highly recommend Vital Choice as a source of quality wild seafood that's accessible nationwide via their website, or use the Monterey Bay Aquarium's Seafood Watch guide to find a good choice in your local market. Salmon, mackerel, and sardines are all great sources of omega-3 fatty acids.

The difference in how these oils respond to oxidizing and rancidifying elements like light and air primarily results from how stable they are. (Micronutrient content also matters to some extent—some polyphenols, for example, help protect the fat from oxidation.) Saturated fats, like coconut oil, are the most stable. Monounsaturated fats, like olive oil, are less stable, and polyunsaturated fats, like vegetable oil, are highly unstable and are likely to become oxidized and go rancid.

This means that for cooking, which exposes fats to heat as well as light and air, naturally occurring saturated fats are safest. Monounsaturated fats like olive oil are fairly safe for cooking, depending on other factors in this list, but PUFAs are particularly unsafe to cook with, especially at high heat, and are best for cold uses (if appropriate for consumption at all).

Man-made trans fats are never healthy to eat. Foods that contain these trans fats include margarine, Crisco, Earth Balance (including the new version that claims to be a coconut product but actually contains soybean oil), Smart Balance, Benecol, Country Crock, and I Can't Believe It's Not Butter. Trans fats are associated with an increased risk of heart attack, stroke, and type 2 diabetes, and they have absolutely no health benefits or nutritional value.

Vegetable oils are extremely high in PUFAs, making them unsuitable for cooking. Flax and fish oils are typically purchased in the refrigerated section of a store, and knowing they're kept cold to avoid damage, you wouldn't cook with them, would you? Why would you want to cook with other oils that are very high in PUFAs?

And yet many refined vegetable oils are marketed as ideal for cooking because they have a high smoke point—the temperature beyond which an oil becomes burned. A high smoke point only tells you that the oil won't be unpalatable when cooked at certain temperatures. It's a culinary and flavor measure, and it's higher or lower based on the free fatty acid content of the oil, but it doesn't tell you about the healthfulness of the oil. Many natural oils tend to have a higher free fatty acid content, which causes their smoke points to be lower, but that doesn't make them less healthy, just more easily burned!

High temperatures and repeated use (particularly in frying) also decrease the stability of an oil, so when they're combined with heat, oils that are highly unsaturated immediately become even less stable. Thermal or heat degradation of oils (particularly those used in fryers) produces inflammatory free radicals as well as other compounds that are potentially toxic, atherosclerosis-promoting, and even carcinogenic (particularly in oils that have been through a deodorization process).*

Here's a quick reference of commonly eaten fats and oils and their fatty acid composition.

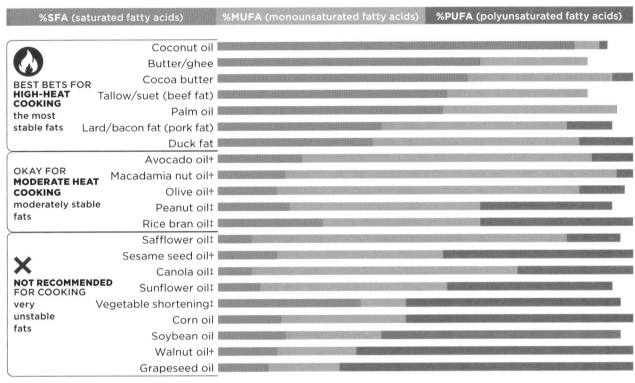

%SFA (saturated fatty acids)	**%MUFA** (monounsaturated fatty acids)	**%PUFA** (polyunsaturated fatty acids)

BEST BETS FOR HIGH-HEAT COOKING
the most stable fats

- Coconut oil
- Butter/ghee
- Cocoa butter
- Tallow/suet (beef fat)
- Palm oil
- Lard/bacon fat (pork fat)
- Duck fat

OKAY FOR MODERATE HEAT COOKING
moderately stable fats

- Avocado oil†
- Macadamia nut oil†
- Olive oil†
- Peanut oil‡
- Rice bran oil‡

NOT RECOMMENDED FOR COOKING
very unstable fats

- Safflower oil‡
- Sesame seed oil†
- Canola oil‡
- Sunflower oil‡
- Vegetable shortening‡
- Corn oil
- Soybean oil
- Walnut oil†
- Grapeseed oil

 † While not recommended for cooking, cold-pressed nut and seed oils that are stored in the refrigerator may be used after cooking for flavor.

 ‡ While the fatty acid profile of these oils may seem appropriate at first glance, the processing method they go through makes them unhealthy—they are not recommended for consumption, whether hot or cold.

BOTTOM LINE

Choose fats and oils that are rich in SFAs (like coconut oil, ghee, or tallow) first, and use these for cooking in most cases. MUFAs (like olive oil or lard) are the next best choice. Stay away from isolated PUFAs (like vegetable oils) as much as possible. Whole-food forms of PUFAs, like omega-3s in wild-caught salmon or organic walnuts and chia seeds, are protected from oxidation within the food and are a great choice as well.

---

*Samantha A. Vieira, David Julian McClements, and Eric A. Decker, "Challenges of Utilizing Healthy Fats in Foods," Advances in Nutrition 6, no. 3 (May 2015): 309S–317S; Wei-wei Cheng et al., "Glycidyl Fatty Acid Esters in Refined Edible Oils: A Review on Formation, Occurrence, Analysis, and Elimination Methods," Comprehensive Reviews in Food Science and Food Safety 16 (2017): 263–281.

4. WHAT IS ITS SOURCE?

You know now that whole foods are your absolute best sources for healthy fats, whether animal-based, like the fat in ground pork, or plant-based, like the fat in an avocado.

When choosing animal-based foods with higher fat content, it's important for general health (though not *critical* to your keto success) to select those from animals that were raised in environments and on feed best matched to what nature dictates. Cows, for instance, are meant to eat grass, not grain, and chickens are not natural vegetarians (though many egg cartons tout that they're from vegetarian-fed hens)—they're meant to eat bugs, grubs, and grass as well as grain. The foods (meat, eggs, dairy, etc.) that result from animals raised on their natural diets are more nutritious and have more beneficial, anti-inflammatory omega-3 fatty acids than those raised in other conditions or given feed.

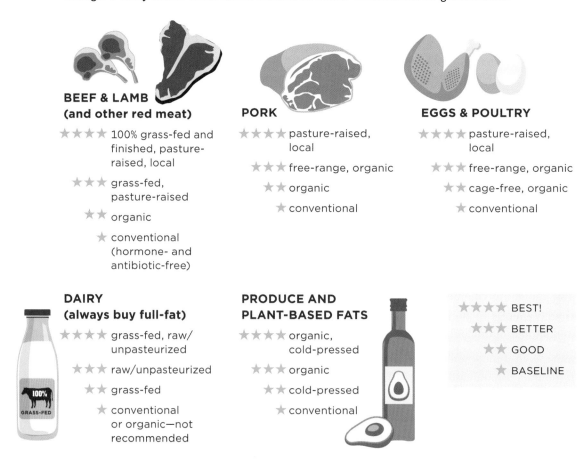

BEEF & LAMB (and other red meat)

★★★★ 100% grass-fed and finished, pasture-raised, local

★★★ grass-fed, pasture-raised

★★ organic

★ conventional (hormone- and antibiotic-free)

PORK

★★★★ pasture-raised, local

★★★ free-range, organic

★★ organic

★ conventional

EGGS & POULTRY

★★★★ pasture-raised, local

★★★ free-range, organic

★★ cage-free, organic

★ conventional

DAIRY (always buy full-fat)

★★★★ grass-fed, raw/unpasteurized

★★★ raw/unpasteurized

★★ grass-fed

★ conventional or organic—not recommended

PRODUCE AND PLANT-BASED FATS

★★★★ organic, cold-pressed

★★★ organic

★★ cold-pressed

★ conventional

★★★★ BEST!

★★★ BETTER

★★ GOOD

★ BASELINE

"Best" is the ideal to aim for. So, for example, you'll *ideally* want to buy local, pasture-raised pork and bacon. If you can't find pasture-raised pork at a local farmers market, from a local farmer, or at your grocery store, then free-range organic pork is your next best bet. If you can't find organic pork at all, then any pork will do.

But don't let the perfect be the enemy of the good!

If you can't find the "perfect pork" or organic oils, or if they're out of your price range, don't sweat it. Get the best quality you can and continue looking for higher-quality foods. Since you'll be eating more animal foods than you likely did in the past, you'll naturally want to find ones that are higher-quality. But again, while the quality of your food matters, it is not critical to your keto success.

BOTTOM LINE

The quality of the source is important for your overall health and the health of the planet, but it's not critical for getting into a fat-burning, ketogenic state.

Choosing Healthy Fats at a Restaurant

When dining out, you'll be faced with the chance to choose items on a menu that naturally contain more fat (like chicken with skin or a fattier cut of steak) or to add fats to your meal through sauces and other elements.

Here is a quick list of ways to add **high-quality** fats to a meal, rather than low-quality fats.

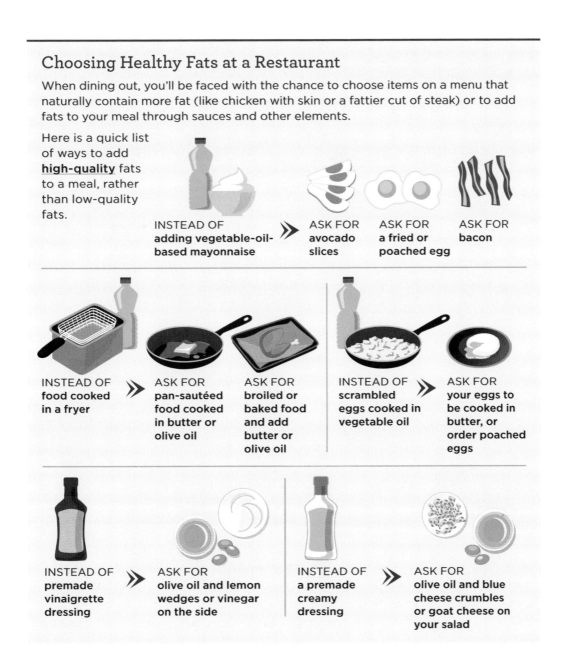

INSTEAD OF **adding vegetable-oil-based mayonnaise** » ASK FOR **avocado slices** ASK FOR **a fried or poached egg** ASK FOR **bacon**

INSTEAD OF **food cooked in a fryer** » ASK FOR **pan-sautéed food cooked in butter or olive oil** ASK FOR **broiled or baked food and add butter or olive oil**

INSTEAD OF **scrambled eggs cooked in vegetable oil** » ASK FOR **your eggs to be cooked in butter, or order poached eggs**

INSTEAD OF **premade vinaigrette dressing** » ASK FOR **olive oil and lemon wedges or vinegar on the side**

INSTEAD OF **a premade creamy dressing** » ASK FOR **olive oil and blue cheese crumbles or goat cheese on your salad**

5. **WHAT IS ITS MICRONUTRIENT CONTENT?**

The final factor in determining which fats and oils are ideal choices is its micronutrient content—which (and how many) vitamins, minerals, and phytonutrients are present in it. As you know, fat itself is a macronutrient; it's responsible for the calories (energy) the food delivers. But the part of fat that delivers deeper nutrition to fuel our cellular processes are the *micro*nutrients. I'd even argue that the micronutrient content in all food, not just fats, can help you feel fuller after a meal, so getting as many micronutrients in our diet as possible is always ideal.

Now, this is the last factor to consider, so it's the least important and may seem like minutia or perfectionism. But here's the thing: when you are deciding between two fats that are nearly identical in every other factor, nutrient density is a smart thing to consider—especially because fats make up a large percentage of your keto diet!

Which fats contain more vitamins and minerals? Some of this depends on the quality of the fat. When it comes to animal foods, the way an animal was raised, its diet, its environment, and whether or not it was administered any medications all play into the healthfulness of its fat. For example, if you're eating a fatty cut of beef, it will have more beneficial nutrients if it's from a grass-fed cow than if it's from a grain-fed cow—it will have a better ratio of omega-6 to omega-3, and it will have more conjugated linoleic acid, a fat that's well-documented to support fat loss. This is also true for the fat in grass-fed dairy versus grain-fed.

In terms of cooking fats, again, consider the source. Coconut oil and ghee, for example, are both traditionally made, minimally processed fats that are great for cooking at high temperatures. But ghee from grass-fed cows contains small amounts of fat-soluble nutrients like vitamins A, E, and K, whereas coconut oil doesn't have those vitamins. Now, coconut oil *does* contain medium-chain triglycerides, which are known to have some great benefits on a keto diet (see page 41), but these aren't vitamins or minerals, and I wouldn't make coconut oil the only cooking oil you use if you can tolerate ghee. It's a good idea to change up which fats you use to get the benefits from them all.

Another example would be if you're choosing between a high-quality extra-virgin olive oil and a high-oleic sunflower oil. While this specially bred sunflower oil may have more monounsaturated fatty acid than traditional sunflower oil, it doesn't contain the high level of antioxidants that extra-virgin olive oil does. Extra-virgin olive oil also contains vitamin E and polyphenolic compounds like oleuropein, which has potent antioxidant, antitumor, and anti-inflammatory properties. So if given the choice between high-oleic sunflower oil and extra-virgin olive oil, the clear choice is extra-virgin olive oil.

GUIDE TO **HEALTHY FATS & OILS**

Consult this guide when you're wondering what fats and oils to use in recipes. For information on whole foods rich in healthy fats, such as well-raised animals, avocados, nuts and seeds, and coconut, see page 60.

Plant-based fats and oils should, ideally, be organic, extra-virgin (when applicable), cold-pressed (when applicable), and unrefined. Animal-based fats and oils should, ideally, be pasture-raised, grass-fed, and organic.

Visit balancedbites. com/ ketoquickstart for recommended brands of fats and oils.

✔ HEALTHY FATS

BEST FOR COOKING
like sautéing, roasting, or frying
(primarily saturated and monounsaturated)

ANIMAL-BASED

Bacon fat/grease

Butter

Duck fat

Ghee/clarified butter

Lamb fat

Lard

Schmaltz (chicken fat)

Tallow

PLANT-BASED

Avocado oil

Cacao butter

Coconut oil

MCT oil

Olive oil

Palm oil (from sustainable sources)

Peanut oil

Sesame oil

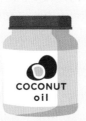

COCONUT oil

BEST FOR COLD USES
like salads, smoothies, or drizzling
(primarily mono- and polyunsaturated)

PLANT-BASED

Flaxseed oil*

Macadamia nut oil†

Pecan oil†

Walnut oil†

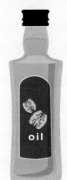

oil

Flaxseed oil is higher in polyunsaturated fatty acids, so I recommend consuming it in limited amounts. For the benefits of the oil without the potential downsides of isolated PUFAs, eat whole or ground flax seeds instead.

† While not recommended for cooking, cold-pressed nut and seed oils that are stored in the refrigerator may be used to finish recipes or after cooking is completed, for flavor.

✗ FATS TO AVOID

MAN-MADE SATURATED FATS

Man-made fats are never healthy. Trans fats are particularly harmful.

"Buttery spreads," including Earth Balance, Benecol, and I Can't Believe It's Not Butter

Hydrogenated and partially hydrogenated oils

Margarine

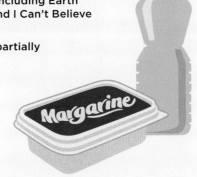

Margarine

REFINED UNSATURATED FATS & OILS

Collectively known as "vegetable oils," these are highly processed and easily oxidized.

Canola oil (aka rapeseed oil)‡	Safflower oil
Corn oil‡	Soybean oil‡
Grapeseed oil	Sunflower oil
Rice bran oil	"Vegetable" oil‡

‡ I don't recommended these oils for consumption, whether hot or cold, but they are listed here for your reference, as they are commonly used in processed foods and at restaurants.

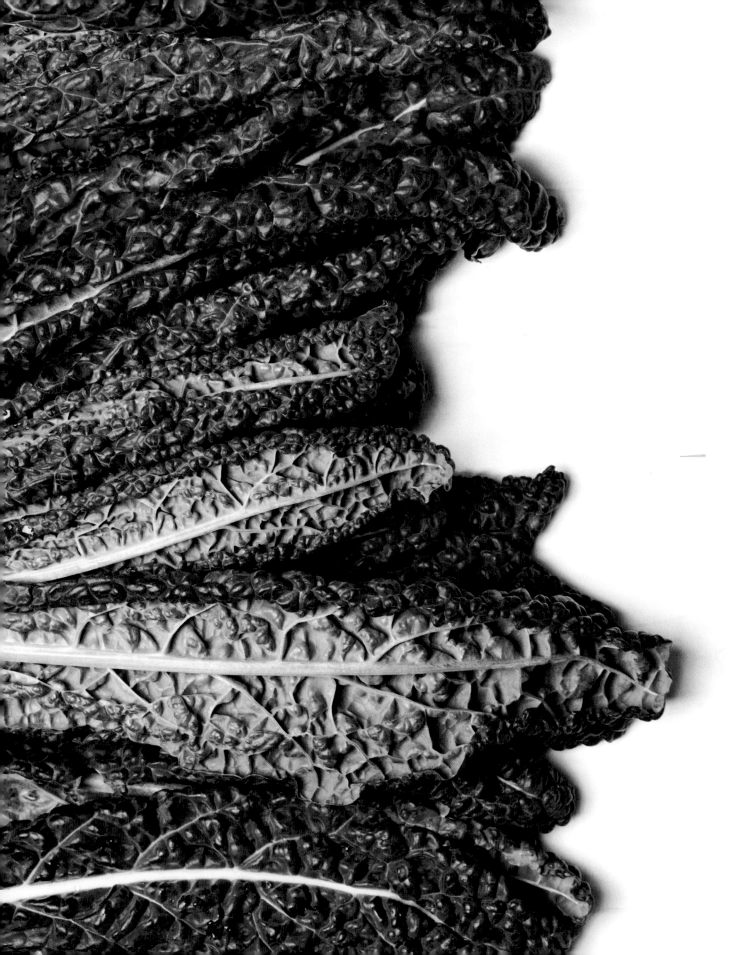

CHAPTER 6

Getting Started on Your Keto Quick Start: What to Do and What to Expect

The first four weeks of eating keto can be tough—there's no denying that it's a major change from the way most of us are currently eating. But it doesn't have to be stressful or take over your life. The Keto Quick Start is about easing into keto and learning to build your plate to get the benefits of keto without measuring, weighing, or tracking everything you eat.

This chapter will walk you through your first month of eating keto. It's all about keeping things simple, planning ahead, and knowing what to expect.

BEFORE YOU BEGIN

Jumping Ahead

While I recommend easing into keto over four weeks, you don't have to! If you feel comfortable with your new diet after a week or two and are eager to start tracking macros and customizing your diet for your individual needs, go ahead and jump to chapter 7, which talks in detail about calculating your intake of carbs, protein, and fat and adjusting your diet depending on your goals and activity level. If you're eating keto as a way of addressing a particular health concern, this may be especially helpful for you.

Before you dive into your first week on keto, you'll find that doing some prep work will make your transition much easier. Take a look at what you have in your pantry and swap keto-friendly items for non-keto items, using the guides on pages 73 and 74. You may choose to either throw away or donate unopened items, or save them for times when you'll make a meal that's not strictly keto. If you find that you have trouble resisting items that are kept in the house, then I recommend that you get them out! Don't allow yourself to be derailed because these items are sitting around and leading to temptation.

Some of the pantry recommendations may be easily found in local grocery stores, while others may not. This is a great time to take advantage of online resources like Amazon to do some pantry-stocking so that you're ready to go for day 1 and not left scrambling for ingredients.

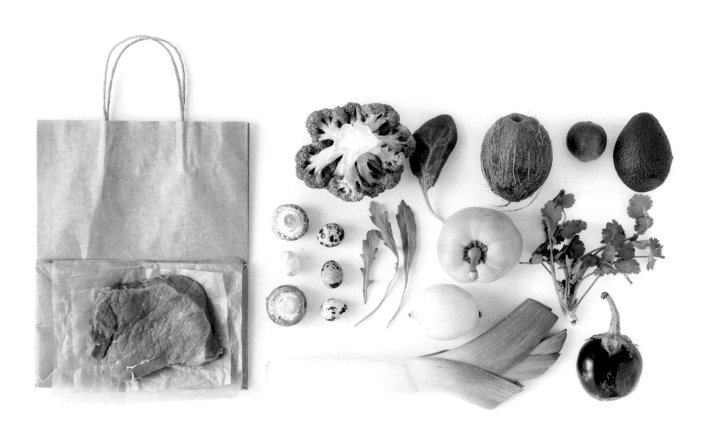

PANTRY CLEANOUT

1. Using the Keto Foods List (pages 56 to 57) and checking labels for carbs and sugar, audit your pantry for non-keto ingredients and foods. Set them aside and plan to remove the day before you start your Keto Quick Start. If you don't want to throw them away, you can donate them, or if your family will still be using them, label them "not keto" and set them somewhere safely out of sight.

Many of the items you'll need to toss or set aside will be sauces, dressings, and some spices and spice blends. These are the biggest culprits when it comes to hidden sugars and carbs. Oh, and of course you'll be getting rid of anything carb-heavy, like crackers, chips, cookies, and bread!

2. Next, make a list of the pantry items that you're tossing or won't be using, so that you can replace them with keto-friendly versions or alternatives (see Keto Swaps for Everyday Favorites, pages 74 to 75). Restock and refill your pantry with keto items such as tuna, capers, healthy mayonnaise, and spices so that you have lots to choose from on busy nights when you're low on fresh groceries and need to mix pantry items with fresh, or when you've just returned from traveling, you don't have time for a big grocery shopping trip, and cooking from fresh ingredients feels impossible!

If you aren't able to find pantry items locally, order online.

KETO PANTRY SHOPPING LIST

Below is a list of items that are great to have on hand, though they're not required for all of your keto cooking! If you're following a meal plan in this book, shopping lists on pages 150 to 153 note which pantry items you'll need. Of course, you may already have them on hand if you've got a well-stocked pantry.

When stocking your keto pantry, you may need to replace non-keto versions of some of the items listed, such as some types of canned pumpkin (if you have a sweetened version), nut butter, pasta sauce (if it has added sugars), or mayonnaise (if you have one made with unhealthy oils).

almond butter

apple cider vinegar

avocado oil *(for making homemade mayonnaise, page 335)*

avocado oil mayonnaise *(look for only avocado oil in the ingredients)*

balsamic vinegar

broth, chicken *(look for organic versions without additives; avoid low-sodium versions)*

cacao powder

canned diced tomatoes

canned pumpkin

capers

chicharrones / pork rinds *(great as a breadcrumb replacement when ground up)*

coconut flour

coconut aminos *(a healthy soy sauce replacement—soy is often inflammatory for many people, and I recommend avoiding it when possible)*

coconut cream

coconut milk, full-fat

coffee

dark chocolate *(100% cacao is ideal; some great brands are Francois Pralus, Domori, Creo, Eating Evolved, and the Montezuma variety from Trader Joe's)*

extra-virgin olive oil *(I recommend Kasandrinos brand, found online at kasandrinos.com)*

fish sauce *(I recommend Red Boat brand)*

hot sauce, sugar-free/sweetener-free *(I recommend Frank's or Tabasco)*

mayonnaise

mustard

nutritional yeast *(if you can't eat dairy; store in the refrigerator once opened)*

nut butter *(store in the refrigerator after opening)*

nuts, roasted or raw *(store raw nuts in the refrigerator)*

olives, various kinds

pasta sauce *(look for clean ingredients: sugar-free, no unhealthy oils like canola oil or soybean oil)*

peanut butter

red wine vinegar

salmon, canned *(preferably wild, stored in water, no salt added)*

salsa

sardines, canned, with skins on *(preferably wild, stored in water, no salt added)*

sesame oil

shredded coconut

spices! Some basics: ground black pepper, ground cinnamon, granulated garlic, granulated onion, ginger powder, dried ground oregano, paprika

tahini

tea

tomato paste

tuna, canned *(preferably wild, stored in water, no salt added)*

vinegars, various kinds *(check for added sugar or high sugar content)*

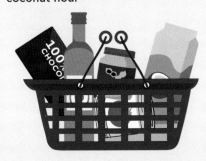

KETO SWAPS FOR EVERYDAY FAVORITES

HIGH-CARB / NON-KETO FOOD	KETO SWAP

Collard or lettuce wraps (per ounce)
TOTAL CARBS	DIETARY FIBER	NET CARBS*
1.6 g	1.0 g	0.6 g

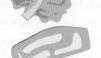

Bread (per slice)
TOTAL CARBS	DIETARY FIBER	NET CARBS*
11.9 g	0.9 g	11.0 g

Deli meat (to wrap cheese or veggies)
TOTAL CARBS	DIETARY FIBER	NET CARBS*
0.0 g	0.0 g	0.0 g

Buns and rolls (each)
TOTAL CARBS	DIETARY FIBER	NET CARBS*
21.3 g	0.9 g	20.4 g

Portobello mushrooms (per 2 portobello caps)
TOTAL CARBS	DIETARY FIBER	NET CARBS*
7.35 g	3.3 g	4.05 g

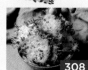

Nut- or seed-based crackers (per 15 crackers)
TOTAL CARBS	DIETARY FIBER	NET CARBS*
18.0 g	15.0 g	3.0 g

Crackers made from grain flours (per 15 saltines)
TOTAL CARBS	DIETARY FIBER	NET CARBS*
33.6 g	1.2 g	32.4 g

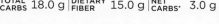
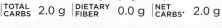

Baked Cheese Crisps (page 308)
TOTAL CARBS	DIETARY FIBER	NET CARBS*
2.0 g	0.0 g	2.0 g

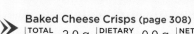 308

Thinly sliced cucumbers (per 1/2 cup)
TOTAL CARBS	DIETARY FIBER	NET CARBS*
1.9 g	0.3 g	1.6 g

Breakfast cereal (per cup)
TOTAL CARBS	DIETARY FIBER	NET CARBS*
24.4 g	0.7 g	23.7 g

Matcha Chia N'Oatmeal (page 182)
TOTAL CARBS	DIETARY FIBER	NET CARBS*
19.0 g	13.0 g	6.0 g

 182

Cookies (per 1-ounce cookie)
TOTAL CARBS	DIETARY FIBER	NET CARBS*
16.3 g	0.0 g	16.3 g

No-Bake Carrot Cake Bites (page 366)
TOTAL CARBS	DIETARY FIBER	NET CARBS*
5.0 g	1.0 g	4.0 g

 366

Donuts (per 4 1/4" donut; 75 grams)
TOTAL CARBS	DIETARY FIBER	NET CARBS*
38.0 g	1.6 g	36.4 g

Salted PB Bites (page 354)
TOTAL CARBS	DIETARY FIBER	NET CARBS*
3.0 g	2.0 g	1.0 g

 354

Bars made from meats and/or nuts and seeds (per Chicken Sriracha EPIC Bar)
TOTAL CARBS	DIETARY FIBER	NET CARBS*
2.0 g	2.0 g	0.0 g

Granola bars (per 1.5-oz soft granola bar with chocolate chips)
TOTAL CARBS	DIETARY FIBER	NET CARBS*
30.2 g	1.6 g	28.6 g

Macadamia nuts (per handful)
TOTAL CARBS	DIETARY FIBER	NET CARBS*
3.6 g	2.2 g	1.4 g

Pancakes made from grain flours (per three 4-inch pancakes)
TOTAL CARBS	DIETARY FIBER	NET CARBS*
41.7 g	1.5 g	40.2 g

Pumpkin Spice Keto Pancakes (page 186)
TOTAL CARBS	DIETARY FIBER	NET CARBS*
24.0 g	13.0 g	11.0 g

 186

Nutritional info source: NutritionData.com

Net carbs = total carbs – fiber

HIGH-CARB / NON-KETO FOOD	KETO SWAP

Zucchini noodles
| TOTAL CARBS | 6.6 g | DIETARY FIBER | 2.2 g | NET CARBS* | 4.4 g |

Spaghetti squash
| TOTAL CARBS | 10.0 g | DIETARY FIBER | 2.2 g | NET CARBS* | 7.8 g |

Carrot noodles (per 1 cup cooked)
| TOTAL CARBS | 12.8 g | DIETARY FIBER | 4.6 g | NET CARBS* | 8.2 g |

Cucumber noodles (per 1 cup raw)
| TOTAL CARBS | 3.8 g | DIETARY FIBER | 0.6 g | NET CARBS* | 3.2 g |

Shirataki noodles (per 1 cup)
| TOTAL CARBS | 1.0 g | DIETARY FIBER | 2.0 g | NET CARBS* | 0.0 g |

Roasted vegetables (per 1 cup broccoli; as a base for sauces with protein)
| TOTAL CARBS | 11.2 g | DIETARY FIBER | 5.2 g | NET CARBS* | 6.0 g |

Pasta made from grain flours
(per 1 cup spaghetti)
| TOTAL CARBS | 43.2 g | DIETARY FIBER | 2.5 g | NET CARBS* | 40.7 g |

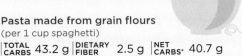

Sweeteners (such as sugar, honey, maple syrup) (per teaspoon)
| TOTAL CARBS | 4–6 g | DIETARY FIBER | 0.0 g | NET CARBS* | 4–6 g |

Stevia (see page 162)
| TOTAL CARBS | 0.0 g | DIETARY FIBER | 0.0 g | NET CARBS* | 0.0 g |

Rice
(per 3/4 cup white long-grain rice)
| TOTAL CARBS | 33.5 g | DIETARY FIBER | 0.6 g | NET CARBS* | 32.9 g |

Riced cauliflower (per 3/4 cup)
| TOTAL CARBS | 4.0 g | DIETARY FIBER | 2.0 g | NET CARBS* | 2.0 g |

Shredded cabbage (per 3/4 cup cooked)
| TOTAL CARBS | 6.2 g | DIETARY FIBER | 2.1 g | NET CARBS* | 4.1 g |

Meal replacement shakes
(per 1 cup of Ensure Plus)
| TOTAL CARBS | 50.1 g | DIETARY FIBER | 0.0 g | NET CARBS* | 50.1 g |

Chocolate Raspberry Smoothie
(page 188)
| TOTAL CARBS | 27.0 g | DIETARY FIBER | 19.0 g | NET CARBS* | 8.0 g |

188

Meal replacement shakes
(per 8 oz Glucerna Rich Chocolate Shake)
| TOTAL CARBS | 16.0 g | DIETARY FIBER | 4.0 g | NET CARBS* | 12.0 g |

Pumpkin Spice Smoothie
(page 190)
| TOTAL CARBS | 10.0 g | DIETARY FIBER | 2.0 g | NET CARBS* | 8.0 g |

190

Full-fat plain yogurt with 1/4 cup chopped walnuts, ground cinnamon, and pinch of stevia
(per 6 oz Stonyfield plain yogurt)
| TOTAL CARBS | 12.0 g | DIETARY FIBER | 2.0 g | NET CARBS* | 10.0 g |

Yogurts with fruit or sweeteners
(per 6 oz Yoplait Strawberry Yogurt)
| TOTAL CARBS | 25.0 g | DIETARY FIBER | 0.0 g | NET CARBS* | 25.0 g |

Full-fat plain yogurt with 1/4 cup sliced fresh strawberries (per 6 oz Stonyfield plain yogurt)
| TOTAL CARBS | 11.2 g | DIETARY FIBER | 0.8 g | NET CARBS* | 10.4 g |

Nutritional info source: NutritionData.com

REPLACE
Low-fat and nonfat dairy
Nondairy milks, like soy- and oat-based

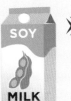

WITH
Full-fat dairy
Unsweetened nut milks**
Unsweetened coconut milk yogurts**
Unsweetened hemp milk**
Products made from unsweetened nut milk, coconut milk, or hemp milk

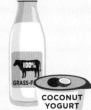

** There are many recipes available online; most store-bought brands have too many additives.

KETO FLU?
ELECTROLYTES TO THE RESCUE!

It's completely normal to experience flu-like symptoms upon lowering your carb intake, and it usually doesn't last more than a few weeks, tops! Most people experience these symptoms about four days to one week into keto eating, and they last for a week or two.

But not all symptoms are just part of adjusting to the switch. If you consistently experience headaches, muscle cramping or twitches, increased heart rate (outside of exercising), fatigue (and you're not undereating), or dizziness, you are likely experiencing an electrolyte imbalance. When your body shifts from processing primarily carbs to primarily fat, it needs more sodium and chloride to help regulate the balance of water and hydration within the body, potassium to support the heart, nerves, and muscles, and magnesium to help regulate over three hundred enzymatic processes in the body. These minerals are collectively referred to as electrolytes.

You can get these nutrients in real foods (see the box below), which I of course recommend first and foremost. Mineral water is also a great source as well (Gerolsteiner and San Pellegrino are rich in many electrolytes), but you may find you also need to supplement. Several brands combine electrolytes specifically for those on a keto diet. If you need to supplement, your best bet is to try one of these and see how you feel, then increase or decrease your dosage as needed.

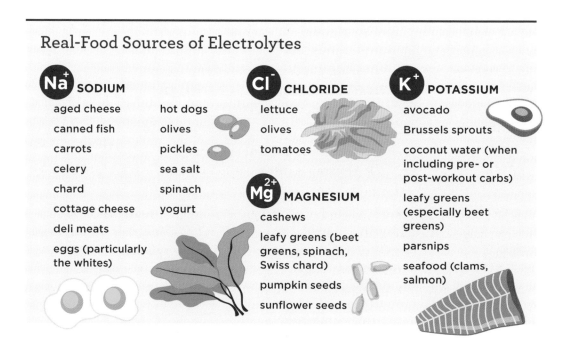

Real-Food Sources of Electrolytes

Na⁺ SODIUM

aged cheese	hot dogs
canned fish	olives
carrots	pickles
celery	sea salt
chard	spinach
cottage cheese	yogurt
deli meats	
eggs (particularly the whites)	

Cl⁻ CHLORIDE

lettuce
olives
tomatoes

Mg²⁺ MAGNESIUM

cashews

leafy greens (beet greens, spinach, Swiss chard)

pumpkin seeds

sunflower seeds

K⁺ POTASSIUM

avocado

Brussels sprouts

coconut water (when including pre- or post-workout carbs)

leafy greens (especially beet greens)

parsnips

seafood (clams, salmon)

WEEKS 1 AND 2

What You'll Do

For your first two weeks of keto, keep things simple! Avoid high-carb foods, build your plate with the SAVVY approach you learned about in chapter 4, and do not even think about counting anything!

Yes, you read that right! Do not count anything on weeks 1 and 2!

In your first two weeks transitioning to keto, the goal is to familiarize yourself with your options and take a positive, "Oh, I can eat this!" approach without constantly feeling like you have to agonize over every decision. If you stress about counting calories or macronutrients while you're building your pantry, getting used to preparing more protein than before, and buying new-to-you vegetables, it'll all feel like too much. There's no reason to add more to your to-do list at this point. You'll do fine just avoiding carbs as best you can.

This does not mean these weeks are open for you to "accidentally" eat carbs. "Accidentally" is in quotes because, while there can be accidental consumption— for instance, a restaurant may have put some sugar in a sauce you didn't anticipate, which is a legitimate accident and something you can learn from— many people will simply want to eat carby foods because carbs aren't being counted this week. *If I'm not counting them, they don't count, right?* Wrong.

Weeks 1 and 2 are no-counting weeks to keep your stress levels in check, but this is definitely still a time to lower your carb intake so that you are preparing your body for what's to come once you do start counting carbs. And to prepare your mind, review the recommended macronutrient goals in chapter 4.

For these two weeks, eat anything in the green sections on the Keto Foods List (pages 56 to 57). If it's protein or fat, eat it. If it's a non-starchy vegetable, eat it. If it's nuts, seeds, or avocado, eat it.

For these two weeks, eat anything in the green sections on the Keto Foods List (pages 56 to 57).

Avoid starchy foods, sugary foods, all fruit except lemons and limes, and all alcoholic beverages (the trace amounts of alcohol in something like vanilla extract are okay).

Read the labels on everything in your pantry and at the grocery store to find hidden sugars and carbs—sugars you don't expect to be included in certain items but that are added as preservatives or to enhance flavor (especially in sauces, dressings, jerky, and other packaged items). Don't use or buy anything without knowing if it contains sugar or carbs, and avoid the foods that won't fit into your keto eating.

Get prepped with snacks! Buy keto-friendly snacks to have on hand if you get stuck without something to eat. Nuts, seeds, cheese, chicharrones (pork rinds/ cracklings), precut veggies, 100% dark chocolate, and jerky are all good options.

Drink plenty of water—always important, but especially during your first couple of weeks on keto. The drastic decrease in carbohydrates means that less water is coming into your body through your food, since the carbohydrate molecule actually contains H_2O as part of it. It may seem counterintuitive, since most carb-rich foods don't seem to be watery, but this is one reason why you may initially lose some water weight when going keto.

If you exercise regularly at high intensity, it's a good idea to scale back your workouts a bit for weeks 1 and 2. You can definitely exercise, but don't expect to go all-out. These should be 50 percent effort weeks as your body begins to acclimate to a lower carb intake.

This is also the time to begin keeping notes and journaling about your experience.

This is also the time to begin keeping notes and journaling about your experience, using the template at right if you like. It may seem like there are some days when not much is happening in terms of feeling differently, whether positive or negative, but that's all information to track! I talked about the benefits of journaling for noting how your body adapts to a keto diet in chapter 3, but there are less quantitative benefits, too.

As you move forward, this record will be a powerful tool in self-assessment because it can help you remember how you felt early on and how that has changed. For example, your first two weeks may be very challenging, but you may find that by weeks 3 and 4 you're hitting your stride. Knowing that the beginning was difficult will make maintaining your healthy habits easier, since you'll be able to recall that the transition was a difficult time that you want to avoid going through again! Alternatively, you may find that you felt much better out of the gate and your energy has faltered a bit over time. What you may discover through your notes is that you were eating more the first few weeks and have reduced your intake a bit too much as your appetite has decreased. This information will help you to personally fine-tune your approach to strike the right balance for you.

Another benefit to keeping a written record of your experience: sharing it with others! When a friend or family member asks for your recommendation about going keto, you may initially tell them to just "go for it," forgetting how that early time felt now that you've been doing it for a while. Your records will help you to gain that perspective back and allow you to more clearly communicate realistic expectations to others. Chances are, as you improve your own health, others will ask about it, so it's great to be able to give them a fair and balanced perspective without sugarcoating or forgetting some of the bumps you may have hit along the way.

And finally, as you move ahead on your journey, the record of your experience will be evidence of your ability to accomplish a major change in your life, and that can naturally propel you to make other positive changes. When we recognize our successes—and acknowledge where we hit some roadblocks—we can more easily set ourselves up for success in the future.

DAY

SLEEP TIME & QUALITY

in bed: _____

_____

woke up: _____

_____

☐ excellent   ☐ fair

☐ good   ☐ poor

EXERCISE

time: _____

duration: _____

type: _____

how it felt: _____

MOOD & ENERGY

☐ excellent   ☐ fair

☐ good   ☐ poor

WHAT I ATE FOR...

breakfast _____

_____

_____

_____

lunch _____

_____

_____

_____

snack (if any) _____

_____

_____

dinner _____

_____

_____

TODAY'S CRAVINGS (IF ANY)

I think I may have been craving this food because: _____

_____

_____

I managed this craving by: _____

_____

_____

TODAY'S WIN: _____

_____

_____

TODAY'S CHALLENGE: _____

_____

_____

OTHER NOTES ABOUT TODAY: _____

_____

_____

_____

_____

_____

_____

_____

How You'll Feel

You can expect to feel excited, a bit nervous, but mostly hopeful and empowered. It's natural to be feeling mostly positive but also unsure about the decisions you're making. This is why the first two weeks on your Keto Quick Start are ease-in, get-to-know-keto weeks. You are going to do just fine!

Physically, you can expect a low-grade headache, general lethargy, and either an increase or decrease in overall appetite. It's normal to feel generally tired around three to four days in and then to bounce back a bit. Your digestive process may speed up or slow down a bit while you lower your carb intake. Your workouts may feel a bit sluggish as you adapt to this new way of eating. But none of these ill effects will last long! By about seven to ten days in, most of these issues will have subsided and your body will start to feel more balanced again. If by the end of week 2 you're not feeling like the fatigue is lifting, it may be a good time to consider adding some electrolyte supplements (see page 76).

WEEKS 1–2 RECAP

Keep It Simple

- Eat protein, healthy fats, vegetables, nuts, seeds, and avocados to satiety without measuring.

- Avoid starchy and sugary foods.

- Read labels for hidden sugars and carbs.

- Stock up on keto-friendly snacks.

- Drink plenty of water.

- Don't worry if you're experiencing some mild symptoms of discomfort—this is normal.

- Scale back your exercise routine temporarily.

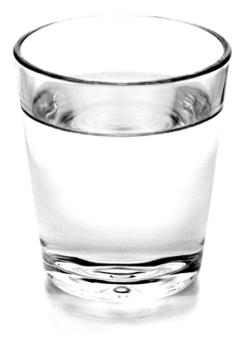

WEEKS 3 AND 4

What You'll Do

In week 3, you're going to start counting carbs. Not *everything* you're eating—only carbs!

Continue to build your plate according to the SAVVY Keto method (page 45), but when you serve yourself anything that has carbs in it, it's time to measure!

Use the Keto Foods List (pages 56 to 57) to determine how many carbs are in the portion of food you're having. If a food you're eating isn't on the list, look it up online (use nutritiondata.com or, for packaged foods, the back of the package or the manufacturer website). You can measure your serving of food in cups, pieces, or servings per the package description (e.g., if the bag contains two servings and you eat half, it's one serving), but using a food scale is the absolute most accurate way to measure. You won't always need to measure your food, however. Once you're used to what portions look like, you'll be able to more easily estimate the amount of food just by eyeballing it, instead of constantly using a food scale or measuring cups or spoons.

Your target starting point is 30 grams of net carbs per day (with, ideally, at least 10 grams of fiber, for 40 grams of total carbs).

If you end up a bit under or over 30 grams, don't worry. You are not aiming for perfection; you just want to get close to that goal and become accustomed to what 30 grams of carbs looks like—how portions of different foods tally up over the day—and what it feels like for your hunger and energy levels. Remember, net carbs = total carbs – fiber, so you can eat "more carbs" if you are eating higher-fiber foods.

Your target starting point is 30 grams of net carbs per day (with, ideally, at least 10 grams of fiber).

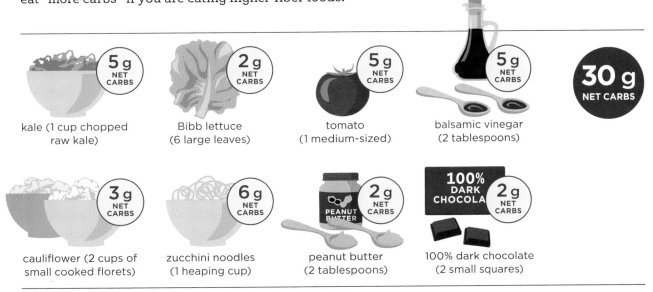

kale (1 cup chopped raw kale) — 5 g NET CARBS

Bibb lettuce (6 large leaves) — 2 g NET CARBS

tomato (1 medium-sized) — 5 g NET CARBS

balsamic vinegar (2 tablespoons) — 5 g NET CARBS

30 g NET CARBS

cauliflower (2 cups of small cooked florets) — 3 g NET CARBS

zucchini noodles (1 heaping cup) — 6 g NET CARBS

peanut butter (2 tablespoons) — 2 g NET CARBS

100% dark chocolate (2 small squares) — 2 g NET CARBS

Tracking Options

If you'd like to track your food online, you can use any number of calculators. I recommend FitDay.com: you can quickly enter custom foods at any time that will save into your own personal database, and you can access it via your computer or an app on a mobile device. Both features make it easy to use over a long period of time because you don't need to enter custom foods that aren't part of the standard database over and over again.

Additionally, over time, you may find that your own personal carb threshold to maintain ketosis is a bit higher than 30 grams. (It's not likely to be lower than 30 grams, but that is possible.) Review ways to test for ketosis or track signs of fat-burning on page 39.

If you want to use the SAVVY Keto Daily Tracker (pages 120 to 123), feel free to track just your carbs that way—but don't worry about tracking fats and proteins yet.

During these weeks you can try to hit fat and protein targets, based on the calculations on page 90, but do not stress over this! If you're keeping track of your fat and protein intake this week, make sure it's only for informational purposes, not to encourage yourself to eat more or less protein and fat. Just get a sense for what you eat naturally. You may be pleasantly surprised to see that you're eating fairly close to the targets—or you may even need to eat more than you were before.

Continue drinking plenty of water, and consider adding electrolytes into the mix if you're feeling off in your workouts or have persistent headaches, muscle cramps, or trouble sleeping (see page 76 for more on electrolytes).

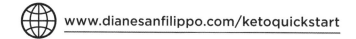

www.dianesanfilippo.com/ketoquickstart

Carb Up? (A Word of Exception)

If you are feeling very run-down, lethargic, or physically stressed, consider eating between 50 and 100 grams of carbs for just one day on or around days 12, 13, or 14 (near the end of week 2). You may find that a brief reprieve feels good for you. This won't ruin your efforts! Remember, each morning when we wake up, we are in a fasted, fat-burning state.

While every day matters, in the big nutritional picture for both your Quick Start and your lifestyle beyond, you want to find a place of metabolic flexibility, where you can enjoy a higher-carb meal or day now and then without worry. Just make sure you're eating real-food carbs like fruit, winter squash, potatoes, or sweet potatoes—ideally, grain-free foods.

Why grain-free? To avoid the inflammation that often accompanies eating grains. Grains contain some particularly gut-irritating types of carbohydrates. While, yes, they do have some vitamins and minerals, they also contain antinutrients, which are known to interfere with mineral absorption.

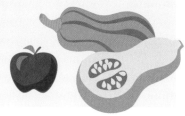

How You'll Feel

You can expect to feel a bit more self-assured, confident, and comfortable with your food choices. Sorting through which foods are higher and lower in carbs becomes much easier by the end of week 3.

Physically, you can expect your appetite to decrease slightly. This may be due to the lower carb intake as well as a generally lower "food reward"—the endorphin rush you were previously getting from a carb-based meal or snack. The pleasure from eating those foods is diminished, and the feeling of eating for fuel instead of pleasure kicks in a bit. This doesn't mean that keto foods aren't pleasurable to eat! But you'll begin to approach your next meal thinking, "Am I hungry now? Hmm, I guess I am!" as opposed to "I AM SO HUNGRY WHERE IS THE FOOD"—often referred to as feeling *hangry* ("hungry" + "angry").

That said, you may not experience a decreased appetite. And if you don't, do not fret! While decreased appetite is a hallmark of keto, it takes some people longer to experience it than others.

You may also continue to experience a low-grade headache, general lethargy, and either an increase or decrease in overall appetite. Your digestive process may speed up or slow down a bit while you lower your carb intake.

Some positives you may experience physically in weeks 3 and 4 include clearer thoughts, less afternoon fatigue, and more regulated blood sugar throughout the day.

If you exercise regularly, you were working at around 50 percent effort for the first two weeks, so for weeks 3 and 4 you can try to take yourself back toward your normal level of effort. You may find that you still need to scale back a bit, perhaps to 75 to 80 percent of your normal effort, but you should be finding exercise more comfortable than perhaps it was for weeks 1 and 2.

WEEKS 3–4 RECAP

Start Counting, but Don't Aim for Perfection

- Eat protein and fat to satiety without measuring.

- Measure portions / serving sizes of carb foods, including vegetables, nuts, seeds, and avocados.

- Avoid starchy and sugary foods, but consider having one "carb up" day if necessary.

- Drink plenty of water. Consider adding electrolyte supplements.

- Don't worry if you're still experiencing some mild symptoms of discomfort— this is normal.

- Increase your exercise effort for these two weeks, either back to normal or to about 75 to 80 percent of your norm.

WHAT'S NEXT?

Where you go from here is entirely up to you. After four weeks on a low-carb keto diet, your body has become more efficient at burning fat, your blood sugar has stabilized, your mental clarity has improved, and you're probably feeling less hungry, less often, than before. You may also have seen some weight loss, but what's certain is that you've been feeding your body a healthier diet, and it's benefiting from it!

If you're feeling good and you're happy with your new way of eating, keep it up!

If you're feeling good and you're happy with your new way of eating, keep it up! Just keeping an eye on your carb intake, along with avoiding unhealthy fats and focusing on whole foods, can be very effective. Once you understand the basics of which foods fit easily into a very-low-carb ketogenic diet, you don't always have to track your macros to enjoy the benefits of eating keto.

But you may find that you need to dial in your macros more precisely to see the benefits you're looking for. Maybe you're concerned about a specific health condition, such as type 2 diabetes or Parkinson's, and want to make sure your diet is optimizing the benefits of keto for that condition. Maybe you haven't seen the scale move as much as you were hoping it would. Or maybe you're an athlete and you need to tweak your diet to optimize your performance. The next chapter is a deep dive into customizing keto for your personal needs.

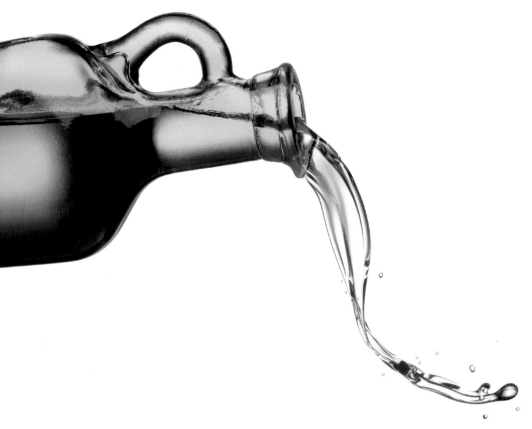

STEPS TO GOING KETO

Right now, you may be sitting at home, looking at your fridge, pantry, and even your current grocery list, feeling a bit overwhelmed, and thinking, *Where do I start?!*

The steps here offer an overview of the Quick Start: how you can ease into keto by changing what's on your plate and focusing on keeping carbs low. After that, you can fine-tune your diet for your personal needs.

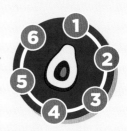

1 Focus on real, whole foods that are rich in healthy fats and protein and low in carbs.

The SAVVY Keto guidelines in chapter 4 explain how to build a plate that's full of healthy nutrients and promotes ketosis. Look at the Keto Foods List on pages 56 to 57 for a wide variety of options, and choose healthy fats according to the guide on page 69.

For the first two weeks, just keep your focus on building a healthy low-carb plate—don't worry about counting anything yet!

2 Start counting carbs.

After two weeks, begin tracking your carb intake. Keeping carbs low is the most critical element of a keto diet. This means sidelining the sweet stuff, especially grains, refined and packaged foods, and treats. The Keto Foods List on pages 56 to 57 will show you how different foods stack up in terms of carb counts. Aim for 30 grams net carbs per day.

Remember two things: fiber is subtracted from total carbs to get net carbs, and 30 grams is a target, not a hard-and-fast rule! Give yourself a little flexibility, but be sure to keep carbs minimal.

3 Think about counting fat and protein, too.

After four weeks on a very-low-carb diet, you may find that you're feeling great and want to keep it up. Go for it! But dialing in your fat and protein may also be necessary to meet certain goals. If you want to zero in on your macros because you aren't seeing the progress you were hoping for, each SAVVY Keto Daily Tracker (pages 120 to 123) gives the amounts of carb, fat, and protein to shoot for based on your daily calories goal. Alternatively, you can calculate your target macros according to the instructions on page 90.

4 Consider your goals and activity level.

If you really want to narrow down your target macros, take into account your goals and activity level—they'll affect how high or low you can go on carbs while staying in the keto-friendly range. The plans on pages 88 and 89 will help you tailor your macros, and they'll give you options for increasing carbs as needed. Because these plans are based on your goals and activity level, not just your calorie intake, they'll help you think about your real day-to-day needs—which is especially important for sticking with keto in the longer term.

You certainly don't have to follow any of these plans, but you may find them helpful in tweaking the keto diet to best fit your lifestyle and what you want to get out of the diet.

5 Factor in any special concerns.

If you have a specific health concern or diagnosed condition—such as type 2 diabetes, Hashimoto's thyroiditis, adrenal health, hormonal imbalances, neurological health, etc.—or you have unique dietary needs because you're an endurance athlete or are aiming to lose body fat, read through the recommendations on pages 98 to 111. There are considerations to take into account for each issue, and you may want to emphasize certain nutrients in your diet.

6 Tweak as needed!

It's all about making keto work for you—and discovering if eating keto for the longer term is your best path to feeling great. The troubleshooting tips on pages 132 to 134 can help you address any concerns, and chapter 6 walks you through what to expect as you get started and how to adjust to your new way of eating. Plus, all the customization options in this book are there to help you figure out what fits your needs best. Figure out what you need to feel your best, and then stick with it!

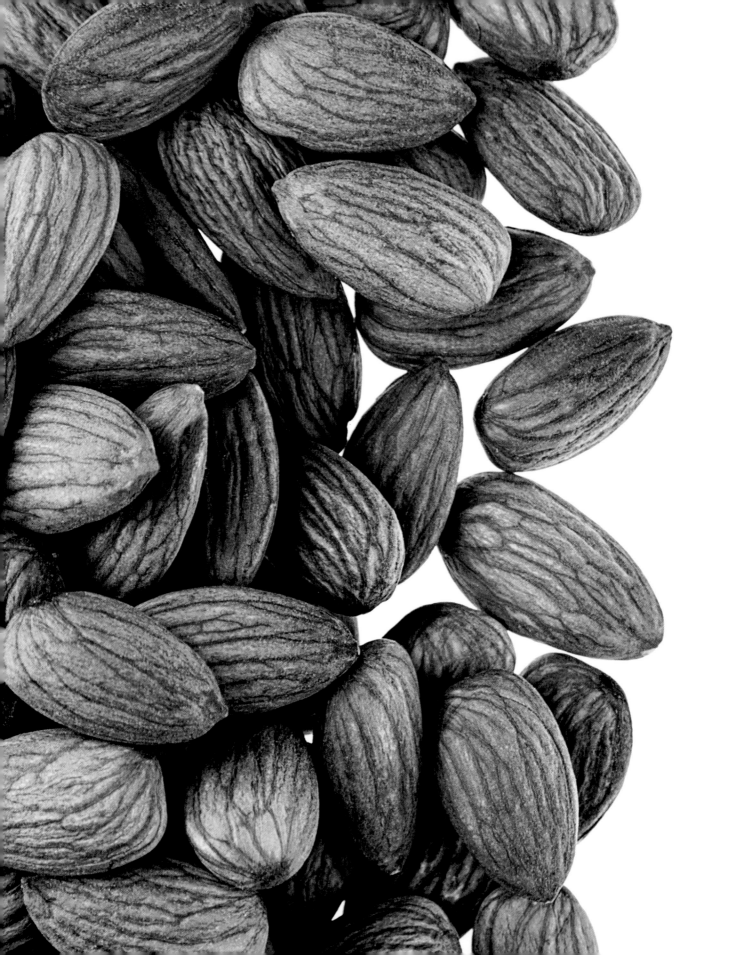

CHAPTER 7

Customizing Keto: Beyond the Quick Start

After following a keto diet for four weeks, as outlined in the previous chapter, you may feel great and decide you don't want to dive into the nitty-gritty details of tweaking and measuring your macros. That's great! In that case, feel free to skip this chapter and the next. You can freely eat keto foods, keeping your carb count low, and see some amazing health benefits.

But attaining some goals requires more precise measuring and tracking of macros. I've created three plans, based on goals and activity levels, that will help you dial in your intake of carbohydrate—and therefore fat, and protein—to meet your particular needs:

- **Everyday Fat Burner:** Your primary focus is fat loss, and you have a low to moderate amount of activity.

- **Fat-Fueled Athlete:** Your primary focus is athletic performance, and you have a moderate to high amount of activity.

- **Therapeutic Keto Eater:** Your primary focus is managing a metabolic condition (such as insulin resistance or type 2 diabetes), neurological condition (such as Parkinson's or Alzheimer's), or traumatic brain injury.

Each plan has a different target for protein, fat, and carbohydrate intake, but they all fall into the following ranges:

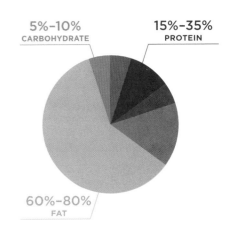

5%–10%
CARBOHYDRATE

15%–35%
PROTEIN

60%–80%
FAT

PROTEIN: 15%–35% of daily calories

FAT: 60%–80% of daily calories

CARBOHYDRATE: 5%–10% of daily calories

Remember, these numbers are ballparks! The exact number isn't critical, though I do recommend hitting within 10 to 20 grams of your target for each macronutrient whenever possible.

All three plans and their macronutrient goals are explained in more detail below. In two of the three plans, there are options for adding higher-carb days into the mix. This is what I recommend for most people who want to gain the benefits of keto while living in a way that feels doable for the longer term. (If you're a Therapeutic Keto Eater, having higher-carb days is not a good idea—see the facing page.)

But! Higher-carb days DO NOT equal sugar-and-carb free-for-alls! On these days, you'll simply be including more carbs from healthy sources or enjoying a food item or two that you normally wouldn't. I'll explain much more about adding carbs on page 91.

KETO QUICK START PLANS

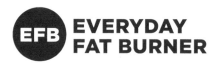 **EVERYDAY FAT BURNER**

PRIMARY FOCUS:
Fat loss, increased metabolism, improved health

ACTIVITY:
Low to moderate level of training or exercise intensity anywhere from 2 to 5 days per week.

KETO GOAL
If your primary goal is increased metabolism / fat loss and improved health, aim for a moderate amount of protein and keep carbs very low.

MACRO BREAKDOWN

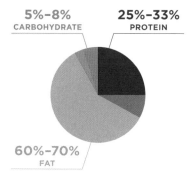

5%–8% CARBOHYDRATE
25%–33% PROTEIN
60%–70% FAT

OPTION 1:
Cyclical higher-carb days after at least two weeks of strict keto

Add more carbs, beyond 8% of total calories, roughly 1 to 1.5 consecutive days per week. The exact amount isn't critical, but don't approach this as an all-out carb fest, either. If you want a number to shoot for, try staying below about 150 grams for the day. For example: Eat a normal keto diet Sunday afternoon through Friday evening; eat higher-carb all day Saturday through Sunday morning. On days when you eat higher-carb, eat a bit less fat. Again, the exact amount isn't critical; choose leaner meats and add a bit less fat to meals. (Consider not counting your macros at all on your higher-carb days to give yourself a mental break as well.) This approach is known as a Cyclical Ketogenic Diet (CKD).

OPTION 2:
Targeted higher-carb meals around workouts after at least two weeks of strict keto

Add 5–15 grams of carbs to your day pre-workout and another 20–50 grams post-workout. Exactly how many carbs you'll eat depends on your total daily calories. Women should target the lower end of the range, 25–35 grams total (~1/2 cup of white rice), and men should target the higher end, 40–50 grams total (~1 cup of white rice). This approach is known as a Targeted Ketogenic Diet (TKD).

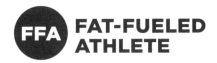

FAT-FUELED ATHLETE

PRIMARY FOCUS:
Athletic performance

ACTIVITY:
Moderate to high level of training or exercise intensity anywhere from 3 to 6 days per week

KETO GOAL

If your primary goal is improved athletic performance, aim for a higher amount of protein and increase carbs to as much as 10% of daily calories.

MACRO BREAKDOWN

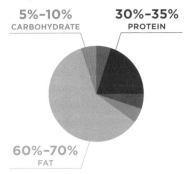

5%–10% CARBOHYDRATE

30%–35% PROTEIN

60%–70% FAT

OPTION 1:
Targeted higher-carb meals around workouts after at least two weeks of strict keto

Add 5–15 grams of carbs to your day pre-workout and another 20–50 grams post-workout. Exactly how many carbs you'll eat depends on your total daily calories. Women should target the lower end of the range, 25–35 grams total (~1/2 cup of white rice), and men should target the higher end, 40–50 grams total (~1 cup of white rice). This approach is known as a Targeted Ketogenic Diet (TKD).

OPTION 2:
Cyclical higher-carb days after at least two weeks of strict keto

Add more carbs, beyond 10% of total calories, roughly 1 to 1.5 consecutive days per week. The exact amount isn't critical, but don't approach this as an all-out carb fest, either. If you want a number to shoot for, try staying below about 150 grams for the day. For example: Eat a normal keto diet Sunday afternoon through Friday evening; eat higher-carb all day Saturday through Sunday morning. On days when you eat higher-carb, eat a bit less fat. Again, the exact amount isn't critical; choose leaner meats and add a bit less fat to meals. (Consider not counting your macros at all on your higher-carb days to give yourself a mental break as well.) This approach is known as a Cyclical Ketogenic Diet (CKD).

THERAPEUTIC KETO EATER

PRIMARY FOCUS:
Managing a metabolic condition, neurological condition, or traumatic brain injury

ACTIVITY:
N/A

KETO GOAL

If your primary goal is to treat a metabolic condition, neurological condition, or traumatic brain injury, aim for less protein and a high amount of fat, and keep carbs minimal.

MACRO BREAKDOWN

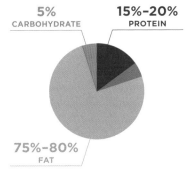

5% CARBOHYDRATE

15%–20% PROTEIN

75%–80% FAT

To optimally manage your health condition, it's essential to keep carbs low. Do not add more carbohydrates to a TKE plan.

After at least three months on this plan: If you started this plan with a metabolic condition but your condition has reversed and you're now able to manage your blood glucose without medications and your fat loss has stabilized (i.e., you've lost a significant amount of weight and are finding your progress is continuing but at a slower pace than before), then you can consider switching to the Everyday Fat Burner or Fat-Fueled Athlete plan.

Calculating Your Macros

PROTEIN: As the SAVVY Keto guidelines say, start with protein—so first, calculate how much protein you want to get each day. Here's a simple way to begin nailing down a target based on your *ideal* body weight/composition. (If you aren't aiming to lose or gain weight, simply use your current body weight.)

0.8 X **DESIRED BODY WEIGHT** = **daily grams of PROTEIN**

FOR EXAMPLE: *If your goal weight is 150 pounds, you'd aim for 120 grams of protein each day (0.8 x 150 = 120).*

OR

1.2 X **DESIRED LEAN MUSCLE MASS** in pounds = **daily grams of PROTEIN**

FOR EXAMPLE: *If your goal for lean muscle mass is 105 pounds, you'd aim for 126 grams of protein each day (1.2 x 105 = 126).*

Lean muscle mass is weight minus body fat, so to calculate it, you'll need to know your body fat percentage.* If you weigh 150 pounds and you have 30 percent body fat (average for a nonathletic woman), your lean body mass would be 105 pounds (30% of 150 = 45; 150-45 = 105 pounds).

Notice that calculating either way will yield a similar result, though using lean muscle mass will provide a more *precise* result. But it's not always a number that's easy or practical to determine, so don't get too hung up on it.

Make hitting your protein goal your priority when you plan what you'll be eating each day. Carbs and fat are much easier to fit in and find quickly, whereas preparing protein or having it on hand requires that extra bit of forethought. (For tips on getting more protein in your diet, see page 50.)

Protein and carbs both have 4 calories per gram, so once you know how many grams of protein you're aiming for, you can calculate the calories. For example, if your goal is 126 grams of protein per day, you should be eating 504 calories of protein per day (126 grams x 4 calories per gram).

CARBS: For carbs, aim for no more than 30 grams of net carbs (total carbs minus fiber) per day. (However, depending on your goal and activity level, you may end up adding some carbs to your day, as explained on pages 88 to 89.) Remember to use total carbs when you're calculating calories!

FAT: Once you have targets for protein and carbs, the rest of your daily calories will come from fat. When you're calculating how many grams of fat you'll be eating, remember that fat has 9 calories per gram—but macros are tallied up by percentage of daily *calories*, not grams. The Daily Trackers on pages 120 to 123 show how target macros add up to percentages of your total daily calories.

You'll select which Daily Tracker to use based on your approximate total calories for the day.

You can find many visual examples of different body fat percentages online. I find they're pretty accurate, so you can find the one that most closely matches your body and use it as an estimate for your body fat percentage.

WHY ADD CARBS TO YOUR KETO QUICK START?

There are several reasons to add more carbs to certain days of your overall keto plan:

1) To tune in to your body's signals and respond to them

2) To fuel high-intensity exercise

3) To create a lifestyle plan for long-term success, not just a short-term diet

4) To avoid excessive amounts of noncaloric sweeteners

You will not forgo the benefits of eating keto by conscientiously including healthy carbs in your diet. The key is to add them thoughtfully and in a specific way—cycling them on particular days or around workouts, as described on pages 88 to 89—so that you give your body what it needs but also support your overall healthy-lifestyle goals. Being healthy and including carbs in your diet are not mutually exclusive concepts, and finding a balance that allows you to eat primarily keto with some higher-carb days will allow you the metabolic flexibility to avoid any ill effects. If you are healing insulin resistance, it's best to avoid too many carbs until your body is able to process them in a balanced way. However, once your metabolism is working as expected, it's natural to be mostly in a fat-burning state and then come out of that for a short period of time before slipping back into it. The human body is adaptable, and you don't need to turn keto eating into a religion.

> **You will not forgo the benefits of eating keto by conscientiously including healthy carbs in your diet.**

If you become fearful of carbs to the point that it makes you want to throw in the towel even though you're feeling amazing and experiencing great results, then reconsider how strict you want to be about keto. If you feel best simply drawing a hard line and never eating carbs again, then so be it. If the idea of having too much restriction makes you want to rebel against any rules, then consider a more flexible approach like the ones outlined here, where you plan a day or a meal here and there that allows for more carbs.

You'll likely find that, over time, you crave high-carb foods less and less, and certainly unhealthy refined carbs become less appealing once you've not eaten them for a while. Enjoying those foods as a treat now and then becomes easier when your everyday meals are balanced and healthful.

Let's look in more detail at the reasons listed above for adding more carbs on certain days.

Respond to Your Body's Signals

After the first two weeks of keto eating, the way you feel will tell you if you need extra carbs to feel more balanced or to fuel your workouts (or both!). (Since everyone tends to feel a bit off for the first two weeks, that period can be a misrepresentation of how you'll feel in the longer term while eating keto.)

Once you're past the first two weeks, some short-term signs that your body is asking for more carbs include the following:

- **Lethargy or fatigue despite eating sufficient calories and drinking plenty of water.** Low calorie intake and dehydration are the main causes of fatigue and lethargy, so if you're sure these aren't the issue for you, then adding more carbs may help.

- **A sense of internal physical stress or elevated heart rate for no reason (not during exercise) that's alleviated by a serving of about 30 grams of carbs.** If you test this when you're feeling physically stressed, you'll feel a sense of calm wash over you after you eat; you can almost feel the relief deep in your body. This is not about emotions or cravings—after two weeks on keto, the desire for sugar or sweets should have diminished a lot, but be clear and honest with yourself about the source of this feeling. If you're having a hard-to-identify, deeper level of "body hunger" that doesn't pass in thirty to sixty minutes, then adding carbs can help.

- **Trouble falling or staying asleep**

- **Poor exercise performance**

On top of these short-term signs that you need more carbs, there are also longer-term signs that your body is not doing well with a very-low-carb intake that may not present for several months. If you experience any of the following, you should either add more carbs according to the plans on pages 88 to 89 or stop eating keto in general:

- Dysregulated hormones, altered menstrual cycles that do not feel positive, amenorrhea

- Thinning hair or hair loss

- Increased acne

- Irritability, moodiness, or mood swings

- Chronic fatigue

- Shortness of breath

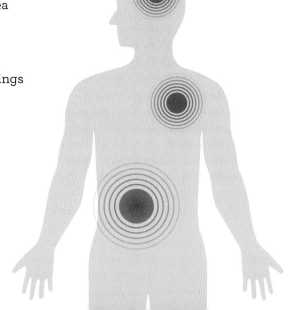

Fuel High-Intensity Exercise

High-intensity exercise is any type of movement that pushes your heart rate to 80 percent or higher of your max heart rate for an extended period of time. You can also think of it as exertion that nears your max capacity for any amount of time.

For example, many standard weight-lifting programs may not qualify as high-intensity unless you're lifting between 80 percent and 95 percent of your max for certain lifts, causing your heart rate to spike and maintain the spike for a period of time before you recover.

Many endurance activities (long-distance running or hiking, for instance) are considered moderate intensity, but if you are sprinting, for example, that is considered high intensity.

An aerobic exercise class generally will have you moving and operating in your aerobic (or fat-burning) heart-rate zone, about 70 to 80 percent of your maximum heart rate, for the majority of the time, with short dips into your anaerobic (or carbohydrate-burning) zone, which is about 80 to 90 percent of your maximum heart rate.

If you notice any of the short-term symptoms listed at left after two weeks on keto, it's a good sign that your training intensity is high, at least on some days of the week, and you can benefit from some higher-carb days with either a TKD or CKD approach (described on page 89).

Create a Lifestyle Plan for Long-Term Success

As a holistic nutritionist, I absolutely see benefits to eating a strict keto diet for both short and long periods of time. However, with any diet, the more dogmatic, rules-based, and inflexible it is, the more it sets us up for failure in the long term.

This doesn't mean that adhering to a strict keto diet isn't possible, nor does it mean that I am discouraging it. What I am discouraging is deciding right away that you need to adhere to an overly strict plan for the rest of your life. That often results in simply throwing in the towel when it becomes difficult. On the other hand, what I've seen in practice for nearly a decade is that if we're given some wiggle room, we can and will stick to a dietary principle we agree with for a very long period of time, perhaps our entire lives.

So if we give ourselves some flexibility that allows us to adhere to a keto way of eating for, let's say, 90 percent of the time, we're more likely to stick to it over the long term. And over the long term, we'll reap more benefits from that 90 percent than we would get from being 100 percent strict for a short amount of time.

I want to show you how great you can feel when you change what you eat—and show you how you can make it work in the long term. Giving yourself higher-carb days, as described on pages 88 to 89, can help.

Avoid Excessive Amounts of Noncaloric Sweeteners

If you endeavor to remain at 5 percent carbohydrates for a very long period of time, unless you are extremely disciplined and have no trouble avoiding sweets, you will find that the only way to enjoy a sweet treat, aside from some berries or other low-carb fruit now and then, will be to use noncaloric sweeteners.

If you want to use a naturally derived noncaloric sweetener now and then, that's up to you. I personally use *small* amounts of stevia (preferably in green powder or liquid extract form, as these are the least processed and have no or few additives) and monk fruit from time to time. But I have a very hard time recommending noncaloric sweeteners in large quantities. Whether they're naturally derived— like stevia, monk fruit, chicory root fiber, and erythritol—or lab-created—like aspartame, sucralose, or saccharin—I think we simply don't know enough about the potential long-term negative effects of these sweeteners to consume them with wild abandon. Furthermore, countless people report experiencing digestive distress with nearly every variety of sweetener, and some sweeteners have been shown to disrupt the balance of bacteria in the gut.

When it comes time to enjoy a sweet treat, which doesn't need to be every single day, having wiggle room for some real-food carbs truly comes into play!

When it comes time to enjoy a sweet treat, which doesn't need to be every single day, having wiggle room for some real-food carbs truly comes into play! If you are staying on your keto plan most of the time and you want to enjoy an occasional non-keto treat, it's better to find a way to do that without being thrown completely off track than to feel like you've failed if you eat a more carb-heavy whole food or even a sweetened food.

Some people may feel that this approach gives too much freedom or flexibility to a keto way of eating, but I don't see it that way at all. Not allowing any grey areas in a dietary plan sets us up for failure over and over again. As much as I love 100 percent cacao dark chocolate and recommend it for a more regular treat, not everyone enjoys it, and sometimes you do want a bite of something sweeter. A truly sustainable healthy-eating plan gives us enough flexibility that we can maintain it for a long time, perhaps for life!

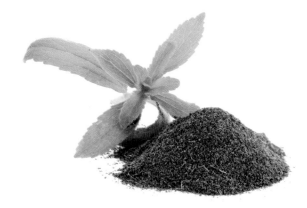

KETO FOR WOMEN

Many consider keto to be a potential hormonal stressor because it's a kind of "starvation" (clearly you aren't starving for nutrition, but you are starving your cells of carbohydrates for the most part). For this reason, some question whether this way of eating is appropriate for women, whose hormonal systems work differently from men's.

> **Many women see benefits for hormonal balance on keto, starting with the regulation of blood sugar, which has a supportive effect on hormones.**

Yes, keto is safe for women. In fact, many women see benefits for hormonal balance on keto, starting with the regulation of blood sugar, which has a supportive effect on hormones. Women who struggle with premenstrual cramps or other symptoms, polycystic ovary syndrome (PCOS), and other hormonal issues may find great relief when eating a keto diet for at least two to three months.

If eating only 30 grams of net carbs per day does not feel good for you, then increase it. You may discover that you can eat a lot more net carbs and remain in ketosis—or not. You may also find that you feel better eating very low-carb even when you're not in ketosis—and that is okay! A very-low-carb but not ketogenic diet is still extremely healthy and therapeutic in many ways.

In terms of approaching keto differently than men do, it's important to pay attention to the impact it may be having on your menstrual cycle and how nutritional cravings due to your cycle may impact how it feels to eat lower-carb all month long. For example, if your body is seeking vitamin C, it can provoke a carb craving (which is not the same as an emotional craving for carbs!). If you notice a connection between your cycle and cravings, you may want to add more real-food carbs on certain days of your cycle to feel more balanced and not crave sugar. And while you may find that your cycle is a bit off the first month or two, by about three to four months into keto, it should become regular again.

If you're experiencing problems with your cycle many months into keto, I recommend troubleshooting by asking yourself the following questions:

1. **Are you overconsuming caffeine?** If you are drinking caffeinated beverages at all, it may be too much for you.

2. **Are you undereating?** If you are eating fewer calories than you're burning, this can be a stressor. This question is especially important for busy moms and women who tend to skip meals when things get busy.

3. **Are you fasting too often?** If you've been thinking intermittent fasting is the be-all, end-all approach but your hormones are telling you otherwise, I recommend not fasting.

Seed Cycling

Our world today is filled with stress and estrogenic compounds in our environment, both of which can throw hormones off balance. Seed cycling is one way to balance hormones naturally, by eating different types of seeds at different times during your menstrual cycle. And since you're eating more fat on a keto diet and seeds are a great source of healthy fats, seed cycling is one way to easily add healthy fats to your meals.

During the first half of your cycle (the follicular phase, starting the first day of your period and continuing to day 14 or ovulation), add a total of 2 tablespoons (1 tablespoon each) of whole or freshly ground pumpkin and flax seeds to your meals. These seeds contain nutrients like magnesium, B vitamins, and omega-3 fatty acids, all of which naturally support a healthy estrogen level, which is required in this follicular phase of menstruation.

During the second half of your cycle (the luteal phase, days 15 to 28 or menses), add a total of 2 tablespoons (1 tablespoon each) of whole or freshly ground sunflower and sesame seeds to your meals. These seeds contain zinc, vitamin E, and omega-6 fatty acids, which naturally support healthy progesterone levels, which is required for this luteal phase of menstruation.

It's ideal to consume fresh raw seeds in their whole form and chew them until they're liquid. But you can also grind them or add them to salads, smoothies, and other foods, which is a much easier way to eat them.

You can grind fresh raw seeds in batches, but don't purchase them pre-ground, because their omega-3 fatty acids are sensitive to the effects of light, heat, and air. Grind the seeds in a coffee or spice grinder—if possible, one you use only for seeds—and keep them in an airtight glass container in your refrigerator. The ground seeds are most easily consumed in smoothies, as a salad topping, or sprinkled over roasted vegetables.

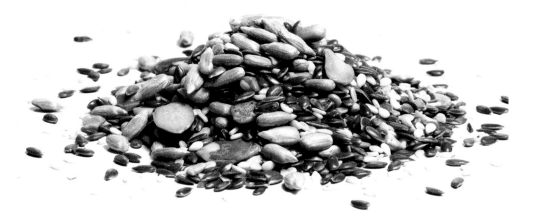

Note that if you are amenorrheic before beginning keto—you aren't having a period at all—you can seed cycle to match to the cycles of the moon (new moon to full moon first, then full moon to new moon). If you are amenorrheic upon changing your diet to keto and that persists for more than three months, please consult your physician.

For more on this topic and other hormonal regulation and period recovery topics, I recommend the works of Dr. Jolene Brighten.

Keto and Women's Hormones

Stabilizing blood sugar is well known to help to regulate cortisol, and cortisol dysregulation is a major contributing factor to imbalanced sex hormones. Therefore, low-carb and keto eating can be very therapeutic for many women who struggle with hormonal imbalances, PCOS, and infertility. That said, it's not right for everyone. Different levels of carbs affect individual women differently, so there is no specific amount of carbs that works for everyone.

Different levels of carbs affect individual women differently, so there is no specific amount of carbs that works for everyone.

If you aren't experiencing hormonal balance improvements after a few months of keto, I recommend increasing carbs in 50-gram (net) increments for one month at a time, remembering to scale back your fat so your calories remain consistent. If you don't feel better after a month at the higher carb amount, increase your intake by another 50 grams for the next month. Continue this process until you have a month where you feel good, healthy, and balanced. Eating 100 to 150 grams of net carbs per day is still a relatively low-carb diet! This may feel easier and better for you, and you'll still reap some benefits of a lower carb intake. (You may be in ketosis in this range; you'd have to test your ketones to know for sure.)

Regarding child-bearing years, there is no one right way to eat for every woman who is looking to conceive or who wants to support healthy menstruation. Some women truly thrive on keto or a very-low-carb diet, and some simply do not. The same goes for women in menopausal years.

There is no direct cause-and-effect relationship between carb intake and hormones that is true for every woman—context always matters! For example, for an overly stressed, perhaps underfed, and regularly exercising woman, a low-carb keto diet may not be the best idea. But for a woman who is managing her stress pretty well, is eating enough, and is exercising regularly, keto may feel great.

There is just not a simple prescriptive answer that works for everyone. You'll need to do some experimenting to figure out what works for you.

KETO AND SPECIFIC HEALTH CONCERNS

Since the keto way of eating seems to run counter to what conventional wisdom tells us (incorrectly) is healthy, naturally many folks have questions about how increasing fat and drastically lowering carbohydrate intake may have an impact on various health concerns.

Following are my suggestions for those who want to address a particular health condition or concern. If you're interested in detailed meal plans for these concerns, you'll find them in my book *Practical Paleo*, second edition. Just keep in mind that, while all the foods recommended in that book support good health, not all are right for a keto diet.

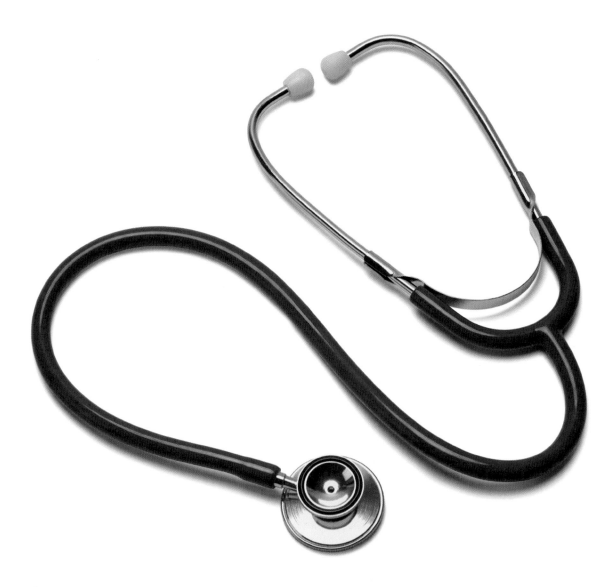

Adrenal Fatigue

It's often debated whether keto is appropriate for those with adrenal fatigue or exhaustion. That keto is a potential stressor for the body is an argument against it, while the fact that many experience systemic stress *relief* on keto is clearly an argument for it. The truth of the matter is: it depends. If your body feels better with a lower carb intake, then you will experience increased energy, improved sleep, and better moods, just like most who eat keto. However, we are all different, and there are always folks for whom keto simply doesn't feel great, and it's hard to know exactly why that happens. It can be that they're not getting balanced nutrition; it can also be that asking the body to reregulate to low levels of carbohydrates is one more stressor and simply doesn't have the beneficial impact for them that it does for others. That said, I think the best approach to keto if you're concerned with fatigue is to seek quality whole-food sources of the nutrients that best support adrenal health.

If you're concerned about or healing from adrenal fatigue, the most important thing you can do is make sure you're getting adequate nutrition. Your adrenal glands need several nutrients for support.

While eating keto, be sure to include foods rich in these nutrients:

- **B vitamins:** liver, bison, lamb; flounder, haddock, salmon, trout, tuna; nutritional yeast, mushrooms, hazelnuts, walnuts
- **Vitamin C:** bell peppers, broccoli, Brussels sprouts, cauliflower, collard greens, daikon radishes, garlic, kale, mustard greens, parsley, spinach, lemons, limes, strawberries
- **Vitamin E:** avocados, broccoli, Brussels sprouts, spinach; extra-virgin olive oil, pecans
- **Magnesium:** kale, other green leafy vegetables; pumpkin seeds (pepitas)
- **Omega-3 fats:** cold-water fish, such as salmon, herring, and mackerel; pecans, walnuts, chia seeds, flax seeds
- **Zinc:** oysters, shellfish; lamb, red meat, pumpkin seeds (pepitas)

For some people, eating keto is a stressor that does not result in improved health. Initially, as you transition to being a fat-burner, you may feel bouts of increased fatigue or stress. This is normal during the first four to six weeks, but it should even out over time. If you don't feel an improvement in your energy levels after about eight weeks, then consider adding more carbs to your diet for a month, for a total of between 50 and 150 grams net carbs per day. (This also means lowering fat intake to keep the number of calories the same.)

The only way to truly know how eating keto is affecting your adrenal glands is to have your hormones tested before, during, and after (if you decide to stop). That said, tracking qualitative data like your energy levels, mood, recovery from exercise, and sleep patterns can tell you a lot about your adrenal health! (See page 78 for more on journaling to track your health.)

If, after testing and trial-and-error experimenting with your nutrition, you decide that you want to add more carbs, I recommend using the adrenal health meal plan outlined in my book *Practical Paleo*, second edition.

Autoimmune Conditions

Keto can be extremely effective in lowering systemic inflammation, improving digestion, and improving mental clarity and energy levels. That said, your body's response to keto depends on your particular autoimmune disease and symptoms.

I would recommend adhering to a keto diet for three months and then, if you are not seeing benefits or feeling better, rebalancing your diet to add more carbs—for a total of between 50 and 100 grams net carbs per day—for a month. (This will also mean lowering fat intake to keep the number of calories the same.) After a month on the higher-carb program, assess how you feel and rebalance your macros again as needed.

If you're concerned about or have a diagnosed autoimmune condition, one of the most important things you can do is make sure you're getting adequate nutrition. Your immune system needs several targeted nutrients for support.

While eating keto, be sure to include foods rich in these nutrients:

- **Vitamin A (retinol):** liver, eel; clarified butter or ghee (page 336)

- **Butyric acid:** clarified butter or ghee (page 336; eliminating dairy proteins is advised for those with AI conditions as they can be inflammatory for some)

- **Vitamin C:** broccoli, Brussels sprouts, cauliflower, collard greens, daikon radishes, garlic, kale, mustard greens, parsley, spinach, lemons, limes, strawberries

- **Vitamin D:** cold-water fish, such as salmon, herring, and mackerel; grass-fed butter or ghee (page 336)

- **Glycine:** bone broth (page 220); gelatin (see page 160)

- **Omega-3 fats:** cold-water fish, such as salmon, herring, and mackerel

- **Prebiotic fiber:** jicama, Jerusalem artichokes, dandelion greens, asparagus, onions

- **Probiotics:** fermented vegetables, such as cabbage (sauerkraut/kimchi), carrots; low-sugar kombucha (fermented tea)

- **Selenium:** garlic, red Swiss chard, turnips

- **Zinc:** oysters, shellfish; lamb, red meat

Keto eating isn't right for everyone, and it isn't even right for everyone with a particular health condition. It's best to try it for yourself and see how you feel, knowing that if you're not feeling better, losing body fat, or reaching other goals, then it may just not be the right approach for you.

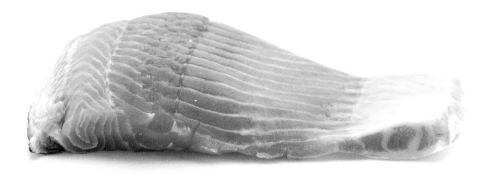

Cancer

There are some forms of cancer for which a ketogenic diet may enhance the benefits of chemotherapy and radiation. Cancerous cells have a different metabolic process than normal cells, and, as a result, a keto diet may sensitize cancer cells to traditional therapies.

Research also shows that cancer cells proliferate when provided with more glucose, so starving them of that glucose by eating a very-low-carb diet may provide benefit. According to one study, "Dietary modifications, such as high-fat, low-carbohydrate ketogenic diets that enhance mitochondrial oxidative metabolism while limiting glucose consumption could represent a safe, inexpensive, easily implementable, and effective approach to selectively enhance metabolic stress in cancer cells versus normal cells."*

If you're concerned about cancer prevention specifically or are currently diagnosed, the most important thing you can do if you decide to eat keto is make sure you're getting adequate nutrition. Your immune system needs several targeted nutrients for support.

While eating keto, be sure to include foods rich in these nutrients:

- **Vitamin A (retinol):** liver, eel; grass-fed butter, clarified butter or ghee (page 336); egg yolks

- **Vitamin C:** broccoli, Brussels sprouts, cauliflower, collard greens, daikon radishes, garlic, kale, mustard greens, parsley, spinach, lemons, limes, strawberries

- **Carotenoids:** pumpkin, citrus, tomato, watermelon, pink grapefruit; kale, spinach, collard greens, beet greens, broccoli, carrots, red peppers

- **Curcumin:** turmeric (dried or fresh)

- **Vitamin D:** cold-water fish, such as salmon, herring, and mackerel; grass-fed butter, ghee (page 336)

- **Flavonoids:** green tea

- **Limonene:** citrus

- **Diindolylmethane (DIM):** broccoli, broccoli sprouts, Brussels sprouts, cauliflower, kale, chard, collards

- **Vitamin E:** avocados, broccoli, Brussels sprouts, spinach; extra-virgin olive oil, pecans

- **Magnesium:** kale, other green leafy vegetables; pumpkin seeds (pepitas)

- **Omega-3 fats:** salmon, herring, mackerel; flax and chia seeds, pecans, walnuts

- **Polyphenols:** blueberries, strawberries

- **Proteolytic enzymes:** papayas and pineapples (which are not specifically keto-friendly, so I recommend supplementing instead if you can)

While I would never state that a keto diet can cure cancer, I would recommend it for anyone who is currently undergoing cancer treatment, based on the existing research.**

---

* Bryan G. Allen et al., "Ketogenic Diets as an Adjuvant Cancer Therapy: History and Potential Mechanism," Redox Biology 2 (2014): 963–970.

** Daniela D. Weber, Sepideh Aminazadeh-Gohari, and Barbara Kofler, "Ketogenic Diet in Cancer Therapy," Aging 10, no. 2 (February 2018): 164–165.

Digestive Issues (SIBO and IBS)

You'll likely feel relief eating keto if you've been diagnosed with small intestinal bacterial overgrowth (SIBO) or irritable bowel syndrome (IBS) because you'll be removing the most irritating-to-digestion foods: higher-carb ones!

Often SIBO and IBS are aggravated by highly fermentable carbohydrates, and most of those are eliminated on keto. That said, some very keto-friendly vegetables, like cauliflower and broccoli, may still be problematic with these conditions. There's never a one-question, one-answer solution when it comes to digestive function, since every person has a unique digestive system and gut microbiome—even individuals with the same diagnosis.

The best way to know how keto will affect you if you have SIBO or IBS is, as always, to test it. If you find you struggle to digest the higher amount of fats, see the troubleshooting recommendations on page 133. If you find you need more fiber, you can add ground flax or chia seeds to a smoothie each day to see if that helps. Beyond that, I definitely recommend working one-on-one with the health-care practitioner who diagnosed you to fine-tune your eating approach.

If digestive health is your primary concern, your system needs several targeted nutrients for support.

While eating keto, be sure to include foods rich in these nutrients:

- **Vitamin A (retinol):** liver, eel; grass-fed butter, clarified butter or ghee (page 336), egg yolks

- **Butyric acid:** grass-fed butter, clarified butter or ghee (page 336)

- **Vitamin C:** broccoli, Brussels sprouts, cauliflower, collard greens, daikon radishes, garlic, kale, mustard greens, parsley, spinach; lemons, limes, strawberries

- **Vitamin D:** cold-water fish, such as salmon, herring, and mackerel; grass-fed butter, ghee (page 336)

- **Glycine:** bone broth (page 220), collagen peptides, gelatin (see page 160)

- **Omega-3 fats:** cold-water fish, such as salmon, herring, and mackerel; pecans, walnuts, chia seeds, flax seeds

- **Probiotics:** fermented vegetables, such as cabbage (sauerkraut/kimchi), carrots, beets; low-sugar kombucha (fermented tea)

- **Selenium:** eggs; garlic, red Swiss chard; Brazil nuts

- **Soluble fiber:** artichokes, asparagus, onions; shirataki noodles; chia and flax seeds

- **Zinc:** oysters, shellfish; lamb, red meat; pumpkin seeds (pepitas)

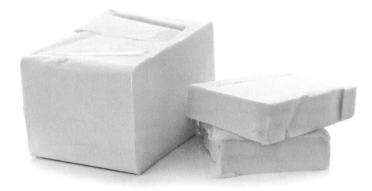

Endurance Athletes

Keto is a fantastic idea for endurance athletes because it will allow your body to adapt to burning fat instead of glycogen (stored carbohydrates). Fat is a more sustainable fuel source: aerobic rates of activity (versus anaerobic, high-intensity interval training) allow the body to naturally use fat for energy. And when you can allow your body to tap into your fat stores to sustain you during your training or events, you give yourself a longer duration during which to perform without "bonking"—what happens when you run out of glycogen when you're not fat-adapted.

Ideally you'd spend at least two to three months adapting to a ketogenic diet before attempting any longer-format races, to be sure your body has made the transition to burning fat and is fueling optimally. From there, provided that you do not push into higher-intensity exercise, like sprinting, too often, your body should be able to sustain you for several hours of endurance work by burning body fat.

The Fat-Fueled Athlete plan on page 89 will show you how to include carbohydrates in a targeted way in order to optimize your performance.

I recommend testing ketones regularly to make sure your body is burning fat optimally and then playing around with varying levels of pre-workout carbs—these will fuel some of your initial movement but will be quickly burned. For more information on keto and endurance athletics, I recommend *The Art and Science of Low Carbohydrate Performance* by Drs. Stephen Phinney and Jeff Volek.

If you're an endurance athlete, your system needs several targeted nutrients for support.

While eating keto, be sure to include foods rich in these nutrients:

- **Vitamin A (retinol):** liver, eel; grass-fed butter, clarified butter or ghee (page 336); egg yolks

- **B vitamins:** organ meats, red meat, seafood (including shellfish and mollusks), cheese, nutritional yeast

- **Vitamin C:** broccoli, Brussels sprouts, cauliflower, collard greens, daikon radishes, garlic, kale, mustard greens, parsley, spinach; lemons, limes, strawberries

- **Carnitine:** Red meat (darker meat has more)

- **Conjugated linoleic acid (CLA):** Grass-fed beef and lamb

- **Vitamin D:** cold-water fish, such as salmon, herring, and mackerel; grass-fed butter or ghee (page 336)

- **Vitamin E:** avocados, broccoli, Brussels sprouts, spinach; extra-virgin olive oil, pecans

- **Iron:** red meat, liver

- **Alpha lipoic acid (ALA):** red meat, organ meats

- **Omega-3 fats:** cold-water fish, such as salmon, herring, and mackerel; pecans, walnuts

- **Zinc:** oysters, shellfish; lamb, red meat; pumpkin seeds (pepitas)

Fat Loss

Many argue that simply avoiding carbohydrates leads to a reduction in overall caloric intake and therefore counting calories isn't necessary. And if you have more than thirty pounds you want to lose, simply making the switch to keto should support fat loss even if you don't pay much attention to portions or overall caloric intake. However, if you have fewer than thirty pounds to lose, I strongly encourage tracking your overall caloric intake. As a half-Italian woman from New Jersey whose family always cooked delicious food, I can tell you firsthand that spontaneous calorie reduction upon going keto doesn't always happen. While some who aren't used to cooking may find it hard to eat as many calories on keto as they did before, for many people, it's not hard to maintain the same calorie intake or even eat more calories now that they're not shying away from fats.

If fat loss is your goal, the ideal approach is to combine keto eating with some portion management. The Daily Tracker (pages 120 to 123) will be your best tool to use. Select the tracker template that best aligns with your target daily calories and go from there.

If you feel insanely hungry while following the plan you've selected, either bump up your intake slightly, by about 200 calories, or simply add a serving of protein and green vegetables to your day. See how you feel and go from there. You don't want to be starving, but you also don't want to eat for the sake of eating if you aren't truly hungry. And remember that while your body is primed to burn fat, if you are consistently consuming too much food, your body will burn the fat you're eating, not necessarily what's stored!

If you're hitting all your targets and you're still not losing weight after about three months, the problem probably isn't food—you may need to address hormones, stress, or thyroid concerns.

While eating keto, be sure to include foods rich in these nutrients:

- **Vitamin A (retinol):** liver, eel; grass-fed butter, clarified butter or ghee (page 336); egg yolks

- **B vitamins:** organ meats, red meat, seafood (including shellfish and mollusks); cheese, nutritional yeast

- **Vitamin C:** broccoli, Brussels sprouts, cauliflower, collard greens, daikon radishes, garlic, kale, mustard greens, parsley, spinach; lemons, limes, strawberries

- **Carnitine:** red meat (darker meat has more)

- **Chromium:** liver; cheese, nutritional yeast

- **Conjugated linoleic acid (CLA):** Grass-fed beef and lamb

- **Vitamin D:** cold-water fish, such as salmon, herring, and mackerel; grass-fed butter or ghee (page 336)

- **Magnesium:** kale, other green leafy vegetables; pumpkin seeds (pepitas)

- **Manganese:** beet greens, turnip greens; pecans, walnuts; cinnamon, cloves, thyme, turmeric

- **Omega-3 fats:** cold-water fish, such as salmon, herring, and mackerel; pecans, walnuts, chia seeds, flax seeds

- **Probiotics:** fermented vegetables, such as cabbage (sauerkraut/kimchi), carrots, beets; low-sugar kombucha (fermented tea)

Heart Health

If you have a diagnosed heart condition, please consult a well-informed physician—one who's knowledgeable about keto—before making dietary changes. That said, all markers of heart health improve in nearly everyone who undertakes a healthy ketogenic diet. Decreasing carbohydrates almost always results in less LDL ("bad") cholesterol and lower triglycerides. You should also see improvements in HDL ("good") cholesterol, fasting blood glucose, and blood pressure. (If you're concerned about cholesterol in particular, be sure to read the discussion on pages 29 to 31, which talks extensively about what cholesterol is, what high cholesterol means, and the role diet plays in cholesterol levels.)

If heart health is your primary concern, your system needs several targeted nutrients for support.

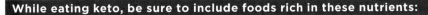

While eating keto, be sure to include foods rich in these nutrients:

- **Alpha lipoic acid (ALA):** red meat, organ meats

- **B vitamins:** organ meats, red meat, seafood (including shellfish and mollusks); cheese, nutritional yeast

- **Vitamin C:** broccoli, Brussels sprouts, cauliflower, collard greens, daikon radishes, garlic, kale, mustard greens, parsley, spinach; lemons, limes, strawberries

- **Calcium:** dairy, dark leafy greens, sardines with bones

- **Cholesterol:** egg yolks; seafood/shellfish; red meat, liver

- **Vitamin D:** cold-water fish, such as salmon, herring, and mackerel; grass-fed butter or ghee (page 336)

- **Magnesium:** kale, other green leafy vegetables; pumpkin seeds (pepitas)

- **Omega-3 fats:** cold-water fish, such as salmon, herring, and mackerel; pecans, walnuts, chia seeds, flax seeds

- **Potassium:** asparagus, avocados, spinach, Swiss chard

- **Probiotics:** fermented vegetables, such as cabbage (sauerkraut/kimchi), carrots; low-sugar kombucha (fermented tea)

- **Selenium:** eggs; garlic, red Swiss chard; Brazil nuts

- **Sodium:** unrefined, mineral-rich sea salt

- **Zinc:** oysters, shellfish; lamb, red meat, pumpkin seeds (pepitas)

Hypothyroidism

There is a lot of talk about whether someone with hypothyroidism should try eating keto. Fundamentally, there is no reason why eating keto would be problematic for those with well-managed hypothyroidism, assuming they are taking appropriate exogenous thyroid hormone to bring their thyroid levels into balance.

That said, it's very common for people to undereat on keto because the diet is so highly satiating, and a hypocaloric state—one in which you're burning more calories than you're consuming—can trigger low thyroid as a normal response to low energy input. In other words, if you are undereating on keto, you may inadvertently downregulate your body's metabolism as a self-preservation mechanism. Calorie (energy) balance is a delicate thing, and while reducing overall caloric intake is necessary for fat loss, the truth is that if you lower calories too much and too quickly, your metabolism (which is regulated largely by your thyroid) can take that as a sign to slow down. This is why I recommended making calculations regarding a healthy overall caloric intake earlier in this chapter—you don't want to overeat or undereat!

If you have hypothyroidism, here's how I recommend approaching keto:

- Talk to a keto-knowledgeable endocrinologist about your desire to try eating this way to be sure she's on board.

- Be sure that your thyroid medication is properly balanced before you attempt to change your diet. Have blood work done ahead of time to be sure your thyroid hormone is within a healthy range.

- Track your food intake using one of the Daily Trackers on pages 120 to 123 to be sure you aren't undereating.

- If you are trying to lose body fat, do not reduce your calories until you're at least four to six weeks into keto. This gives your body time to adapt to burning fat for fuel, which will then make it easier to eat at just a slight calorie deficit over time to support fat loss.

- Pay close attention to how you feel, eat when you're hungry, and note any symptoms of low thyroid (such as fatigue, weight gain, thinning hair, low body temperature, joint and muscle aches, slowed heart rate) that may crop up.

It's possible that while eating keto, your cells will become more sensitized to the presence of thyroid hormone (specifically, T3), so you need less of it. As your body adjusts to keto, please consult your endocrinologist to be sure your medication dosage is still correct; you may need a lower dosage than you did before.

If thyroid health is your primary concern, your system needs several targeted nutrients for support.

While eating keto, be sure to include foods rich in these nutrients:

- **Alpha lipoic acid (ALA):** red meat, organ meats

- **Vitamin A (retinol):** liver, eel; clarified butter or ghee (page 336); egg yolks

- **B vitamins:** organ meats, red meat; seafood (including shellfish and mollusks); cheese, nutritional yeast

- **Vitamin C:** broccoli, Brussels sprouts, cauliflower, collard greens, daikon radishes, garlic, kale, mustard greens, parsley, spinach; lemons, limes, strawberries

- **Choline:** eggs; organ meats; fish roe/caviar, cod; cauliflower

- **Chromium:** liver; cheese, nutritional yeast

- **Magnesium:** kale, other green leafy vegetables; pumpkin seeds (pepitas)

- **Iodine:** wild fish; seaweed, kelp, dulse

- **Vitamin D:** cold-water fish, such as salmon, herring, and mackerel; grass-fed butter or ghee (page 336)

- **Vitamin E:** avocados, broccoli, Brussels sprouts, spinach; extra-virgin olive oil, pecans

- **Manganese:** beet greens, turnip greens; pecans, walnuts; cinnamon, cloves, thyme, turmeric

- **Omega-3 fats:** cold-water fish, such as salmon, herring, and mackerel; pecans, walnuts, chia seeds, flax seeds

- **Probiotics:** fermented vegetables, such as cabbage (sauerkraut/kimchi), carrots; low-sugar kombucha (fermented tea)

- **Selenium:** eggs; garlic, red Swiss chard; Brazil nuts

- **Zinc:** oysters, shellfish; lamb, red meat; pumpkin seeds (pepitas)

Liver Health

If you're looking to optimize your liver detoxification processes, eating a healthy keto diet can absolutely be helpful. When your blood sugar is better controlled, you alleviate the burden on your liver to constantly monitor your metabolism, allowing more capacity for improved detoxification.

If you have been diagnosed with liver disease or condition, please consult with a well-informed physician before making dietary changes.

Whether your liver is healthy or you have a diagnosed liver condition, it's critical to eat a diet that supports optimal detoxification as well as balanced gut health (since most of the removed toxins are eliminated through our bowel movements). This means including plenty of foods rich in the following nutrients: B vitamins, vitamin C, choline, vitamin E, fiber, glutathione, glycine, magnesium, superoxide dismutase, selenium, and zinc.

While eating keto, be sure to include foods rich in these nutrients:

- **B vitamins:** organ meats, red meat; seafood (including shellfish and mollusks); cheese, nutritional yeast

- **Vitamin C:** broccoli, Brussels sprouts, cauliflower, collard greens, daikon radishes, garlic, kale, mustard greens, parsley, spinach; lemons, limes, strawberries

- **Choline:** eggs; organ meats, fish roe/caviar, cod; cauliflower

- **Vitamin E:** avocados, broccoli, Brussels sprouts, spinach; extra-virgin olive oil, pecans

- **Glutathione:** asparagus, avocados, broccoli; garlic, ginger, cumin, turmeric

- **Glycine:** bone broth (page 220), collagen peptides, gelatin (see page 160)

- **Magnesium:** kale, other green leafy vegetables; pumpkin seeds (pepitas)

- **Selenium:** eggs; garlic, red Swiss chard; Brazil nuts

- **Zinc:** oysters, shellfish; lamb, red meat; pumpkin seeds (pepitas)

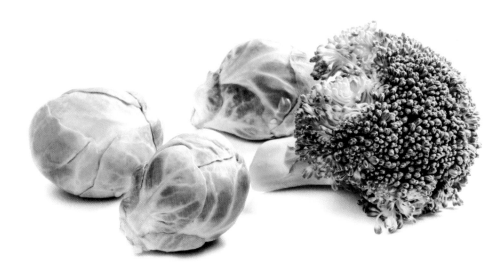

Neurological Health

Whether you have a diagnosed neurological condition, have sustained a traumatic brain injury, or are looking for neuroprotective benefits as a preventative measure, a keto diet is an excellent choice. While all of the mechanisms by which a keto diet can help these conditions are not yet fully understood, it's believed that it helps improve the life span of neurons.

There is some research that shows that ketones themselves (particularly beta hydroxybutyrate) may be neuroprotective in that they decrease free-radical damage and provide the brain with a fuel source that's more efficient than glucose. In addition, they may improve the production of energy (ATP) in mitochondria, the powerhouses of the cell, and that could improve brain function overall.*

If neurological health is your primary concern, your system needs several targeted nutrients for support.

While eating keto, be sure to include foods rich in these nutrients:

- **Alpha lipoic acid (ALA):** red meat, organ meats

- **B vitamins:** organ meats, red meat; seafood (including shellfish and mollusks); cheese, nutritional yeast

- **Vitamin C:** broccoli, Brussels sprouts, cauliflower, collard greens, daikon radishes, garlic, kale, mustard greens, parsley, spinach; lemons, limes, strawberries

- **Vitamin D:** cold-water fish, such as salmon, herring, and mackerel; grass-fed butter or ghee (page 336)

- **Choline:** eggs; organ meats, fish roe/caviar, cod; cauliflower

- **Vitamin E:** avocados, broccoli, Brussels sprouts, spinach; extra-virgin olive oil, pecans

- **Glutathione:** asparagus, avocados, broccoli; garlic, ginger, cumin, turmeric

- **Magnesium:** kale, other green leafy vegetables; pumpkin seeds (pepitas)

- **Omega-3 fats:** cold-water fish, such as salmon, herring, and mackerel; pecans, walnuts, chia seeds, flax seeds

- **Potassium:** avocados, spinach, Swiss chard

- **Probiotics:** fermented vegetables, such as cabbage (sauerkraut/kimchi), carrots; low-sugar kombucha (fermented tea)

- **Selenium:** eggs; garlic, red Swiss chard; Brazil nuts

- **Zinc:** oysters, shellfish; lamb, red meat; pumpkin seeds (pepitas)

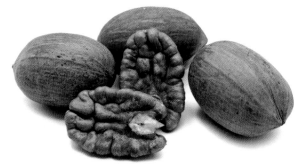

---

* Maciej Gasior, Michael A. Rogawski, and Adam L. Hartman, "Neuroprotective and Disease-Modifying Effects of the Ketogenic Diet," Behavioural Pharmacology 17, nos. 5–6 (Sept. 2006): 431–439; R. L. Veech et al., "Ketone Bodies, Potential Therapeutic Uses," IUBMB Life 51, no. 4 (April 2001): 241–247.

Systemic Inflammation

Keto can help lower inflammation in your body, but only when you eat real, whole foods and avoid inflammatory oils—which means eating a *healthy* keto diet. Don't fall into the trap of eating too many keto convenience foods like bars and packaged treats made with processed ingredients, or adding vegetable oil–based dressings or mayonnaise as your fat source when dining out, or eating large quantities of fattier cuts of meat that are not high quality and can be high in inflammatory omega-6 fats.

In other words, to lower inflammation while eating keto, food quality matters a lot. I've seen people plateau on keto after six months to a year, and I believe that eating inflammatory keto foods is a big part of the problem.

Furthermore, when you consider several of the diet-related causes of systemic inflammation—dysregulated blood sugar, digestive problems, and inflammatory foods (refined carbs, sugar, and vegetable oils)—you can see how eating an overall healthy ketogenic diet can lower inflammation simply because it doesn't include foods that aggravate these issues. Your blood sugar levels will self-regulate when you drop your carbs, your digestive problems will calm down when you stop feeding sugar to your gut bacteria (keep feeding it the good stuff, though, in fiber-rich vegetables!), and your inflammation will fall when you eat fewer inflammatory foods.

If lowering overall inflammation is your primary concern, your system needs several targeted nutrients for support.

While eating keto, be sure to include foods rich in these nutrients:

- **Vitamin C:** broccoli, Brussels sprouts, cauliflower, collard greens, daikon radishes, garlic, kale, mustard greens, parsley, spinach; lemons, limes, strawberries

- **Vitamin E:** avocados, broccoli, Brussels sprouts, spinach; extra-virgin olive oil, pecans

- **Omega-3 fats:** cold-water fish, such as salmon, herring, and mackerel; pecans, walnuts, chia seeds, flax seeds

Type 1 Diabetes

Maintaining a mostly keto way of eating over the long term is a great lifestyle strategy for managing type 1 diabetes, but it's not without risks, and it requires self-awareness and very regular testing of ketone levels and blood glucose.

If you feel confident that you can closely monitor and manage your blood glucose, ketones, and insulin dosing, then you can approach keto safely. However, since diabetic ketoacidosis—a condition in which you simultaneously have high ketone levels and high blood glucose (see page 37)—is a real potential problem for you, a couple of missed insulin doses or skipped readings could put you at risk, so it may not be worth attempting a keto diet.

I recommend that you speak with your endocrinologist or a medical professional who is well versed in ketogenic diets about your desire to change your diet and the implications it may have for you. With the lower carbs of a keto diet, you will likely need to reduce the amount of insulin you are taking quite drastically. The reduced need for insulin will save you money and reduce overall systemic stress over time because the constant, often imperfect management of insulin dosing is inflammatory. A continuous insulin delivery pump can mitigate this potential to a large degree, but reducing your overall need for the exogenous insulin is still a good idea.

The most important thing to know about eating keto with type 1 diabetes is that you need to decide that you are *committed* to it; otherwise, it may be dangerous. Since your body doesn't naturally produce insulin, once you're adapted to using fat for fuel, you can't suddenly flood your body with a lot of carbs one day—this is a recipe for developing diabetic ketoacidosis. This is a dangerous situation to be in, so I don't recommend dabbling.

If you feel unsure about whether or not you can truly commit to keto, try taking more of a low-carb approach, eating around 50 to 100 grams of carbs per day. That's high enough that you'll avoid ketosis, but it's low enough to keep your blood glucose in a healthy range. You'll require more insulin than you'd need on keto, but it does not put you at risk for diabetic ketoacidosis.

Signs of ketoacidosis include dry mouth, frequent urination, consistently high blood sugar levels, nausea, fruity breath, and difficulty breathing. It's very serious and requires a trip to the hospital, so it's not something to toy around with!

The Therapeutic Keto Eater plan on page 89 will show you how to balance your macros to maintain your keto diet properly with type 1 diabetes. But again, please work closely with your doctor or medical professional when approaching keto with type 1 diabetes.

If blood sugar regulation is your primary concern, your system needs several targeted nutrients for support.

While eating keto, be sure to include foods rich in these nutrients:

- **Vitamin A (retinol):** liver, eel; grass-fed butter, clarified butter or ghee (page 336), egg yolks

- **B vitamins:** organ meats, red meat; seafood (including shellfish and mollusks); cheese, nutritional yeast

- **Butyric acid:** grass-fed butter, clarified butter or ghee (page 336)

- **Vitamin C:** broccoli, Brussels sprouts, cauliflower, collard greens, daikon radishes, garlic, kale, mustard greens, parsley, spinach; lemons, limes, strawberries

- **Vitamin D:** cold-water fish, such as salmon, herring, and mackerel; grass-fed butter or ghee (page 336)

- **Vitamin E:** avocados, broccoli, Brussels sprouts, spinach; extra-virgin olive oil, pecans

- **Glycine:** bone broth (page 220), collagen peptides, gelatin (see page 160)

- **Omega-3 fats:** cold-water fish, such as salmon, herring, and mackerel; pecans, walnuts, chia seeds, flax seeds

- **Probiotics:** fermented vegetables, such as cabbage (sauerkraut/kimchi), carrots, beets; low-sugar kombucha (fermented tea)

- **Selenium:** eggs; garlic, red Swiss chard; Brazil nuts

- **Soluble fiber:** artichokes, asparagus, onions; shirataki noodles; chia and flax seeds

- **Zinc:** oysters, shellfish; lamb, red meat; pumpkin seeds (pepitas)

Insulin Resistance and Type 2 Diabetes

Insulin resistance is the precursor to type 2 diabetes. If your blood sugar levels are consistently elevated after meals, causing large amounts of insulin to be released into your bloodstream every time you eat, over time you can become insulin resistant. Just as you stop noticing a bad smell in a room after a while, your body begins to lose its ability to sense the insulin that your pancreas has released, so glucose isn't moved out of the bloodstream and into cells. Your body responds by making more insulin, which will keep blood sugar in the normal range for a while, but over time, this can lead to type 2 diabetes.

Not only is a ketogenic diet safe for type 2 diabetes and insulin resistance, but it works fairly quickly to improve and often even reverse these diseases. Many people find that they are able to reduce or eliminate the need for blood sugar–managing medications within a few days to a few weeks of eating keto. While this may not be the result for everyone, it is a very common and expected outcome.

Insulin resistance and type 2 diabetes are diseases of diet and lifestyle, so changing your diet and lifestyle will have the biggest impact on managing and even reversing it. Your success with keto may depend on how long you've had these conditions as well as other possible complications. If you have been diagnosed with insulin resistance or prediabetes, don't wait until you get the full-blown diagnosis of type 2 diabetes—start now!

The Therapeutic Keto Eater plan on page 89 will show you how to balance your macros to maintain your keto diet properly with type 2 diabetes. However, make sure you speak with your endocrinologist or a medical professional who is well versed in ketogenic diets about your desire to change your diet and the implications it may have for you. If you are taking medication for your diabetes, you'll likely need to adjust your dosage to avoid serious hypoglycemia, and you *must* do this in consultation with a health-care practitioner.

If you have type 2 diabetes, I highly recommend having blood work done before you begin eating keto and then three months after. This will help you track your triglycerides and HbA1c, important markers to measure for longer-term glucose management, so you can have quantitative data on how keto is affecting you beyond your daily blood glucose readings.

If blood sugar regulation is your primary concern, your system needs several targeted nutrients for support. For a list of these nutrients and the foods they're found in, see the list under "Type 1 Diabetes" at left.

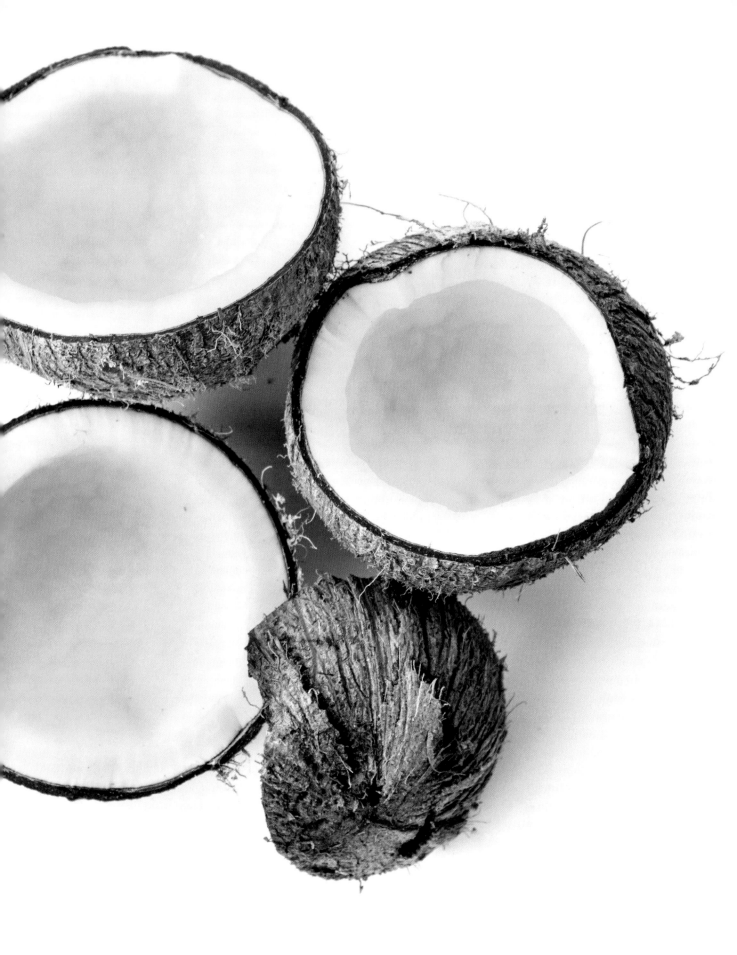

CHAPTER 8

Fine-Tuning Your Keto Diet

During the four weeks of your Keto Quick Start, the only macronutrient you need to count is carbs. You can see some great benefits just with that! In fact, it's fine to keep going indefinitely just counting your carb intake. But if you decide to focus more closely on your macros and count fat and protein, too, you may see better results, especially if you have a goal like fat loss or if your energy levels just aren't bouncing back as expected.

Fine-tuning your keto diet means tracking and adjusting your intake of fat and protein as well as carbs, and paying close attention to how you feel with every change you make. Keep in mind that I highly recommend staying on the Quick Start for at least four weeks before you begin tweaking your diet, so that your body has had a chance to adjust to your new way of eating.

START USING THE DAILY TRACKER

After at least four weeks on keto, you should be feeling comfortable with carb counts and have a sense for what you can eat in a day while staying within your target range. Now, to be more effective in reaching your goals, you can focus on hitting your protein and fat numbers, as calculated according to the instructions on page 90. The SAVVY Keto Daily Trackers (pages 120 to 123) are designed to make it easy to count all your food, as well as document your workouts and how you're feeling.

With the Daily Tracker, you will cross off servings of protein, fat, and carbs as you eat throughout the day. Over time, this will help you to know what portions consistently work best for you. The Daily Tracker is a fantastic starting point, and I recommend you use it to adhere to your target macros for at least one solid week. After one week, however, you can start to adjust what and how much you're eating based on how you're feeling. You are not stuck with one set of numbers if they don't feel good to you!

While your protein and fat targets will be based on your needs and calorie intake, continue to do your best to hit 30 grams of net carbs for the day. But if you end up closer to 50 in a day, do not stress—especially if it was from vegetables! In the grand scheme of this dietary change, a few grams here or there will not make or break you. In fact, it's nearly impossible to know the exact grams of carbohydrates or fiber in every single bite of food we eat. Nutritional science is not precise to that level, so attempting to micromanage your carb intake too intensely can be a futile effort, while hitting in the general area within a narrow margin will be just fine.

As you spend more time tracking your food intake, you'll really find your sweet spot: you'll know if you need to add more carbs to your plate on a daily or near-daily basis (after a workout, for instance) or on a weekly basis (one day per week when you are not counting—maybe a time when you attend a party or have a special holiday meal).

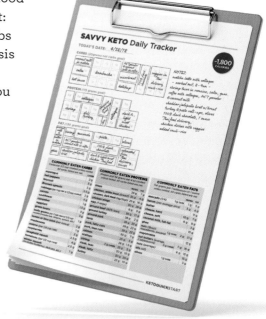

PAY ATTENTION TO HOW YOU FEEL

Tweaking your macros isn't just about tracking your food. It's also about tracking how you feel—which is the most important part! Keep journaling about your sleep, workouts, challenges, and more, using the template on page 79 if you like.

Your body may still be adjusting to eating keto, but as time goes on, it will start to thrive on the new fuel you're giving it, and you can expect your energy to be more even throughout the day. You may find that you're sleeping better, that aches and pains you used to feel have subsided, and that any skin irritations are beginning to subside.

You may find that you're sleeping better, that aches and pains you used to feel have subsided, and that any skin irritations are beginning to subside.

If you are struggling with your digestion at all, consider increasing your dietary fiber intake. (Yes, this means eating more carb foods, but remember that your net carb intake will not increase much!) You may also want to try a digestive enzyme supplement (I recommend one that includes a wide variety of enzymes as well as ox bile), a food-based fiber supplement, like ground flax seeds, that you can add to a smoothie, or probiotics, whether in foods like sauerkraut or in a supplement.

AND DON'T FORGET . . .

Remember, a big part of the SAVVY Keto approach is variety, so as you continue on your keto journey, take a chance on exploring some new foods. Even if you aren't interested in trying new protein sources or that wouldn't be budget-friendly, new herbs and spices can really change things up! Mix up some new spice blends (you'll find some recipes on pages 330 to 331) and watch your food transform.

And remember the importance of staying hydrated! If you're not taking electrolyte supplements and you're feeling off in your workouts or have persistent headaches, muscle cramps, or trouble sleeping, consider adding electrolytes (see page 76 for more). If you are taking electrolyte supplements, you may want to consider upping the amount if you're still feeling any of the aforementioned symptoms.

MOVING FORWARD

Once you've been tracking your fat and protein along with your carbs for a few weeks, you may find that you've hit your stride and you don't need to make many additional tweaks from week to week. But I recommend that you continue to journal and closely tune in to your body's signals of satiety (fullness). As time goes on, you may find that your appetite decreases slightly while you're adjusting to burning more ketones and body fat for fuel. So instead of continuing to serve yourself the same size portions as you did previously, pay attention to whether or not you truly need as much food. You may find that you do, and you may find that you don't.

Now, I'm not advising this because decreasing the amount of food you eat is always the goal—that certainly isn't the case! But it's often easy to overconsume healthy, delicious food just because, well, it tastes good. And when you truly know what portions work best for you to eat to satiety and not beyond, it's a really great place to be.

Once you've been eating keto for about three months, it's a good time to reassess.

Once you've been eating keto for about three months, it's a good time to reassess. If you're feeling great and want to continue, then go ahead! If you're feeling like maybe keto is a great reset for you but you don't want to maintain it year-round, consider using it as a reset tool once per year. There's no hard-and-fast rule that once you eat keto, you must always do so. My hope for you is that you learn how your body feels while eating this way and that it's a useful tool, and should you need it for specific health challenges, you'll have it in your diet-and-lifestyle arsenal moving forward.

Now that you know how to eat keto, if you ever want or need to again in the future, you're well equipped!

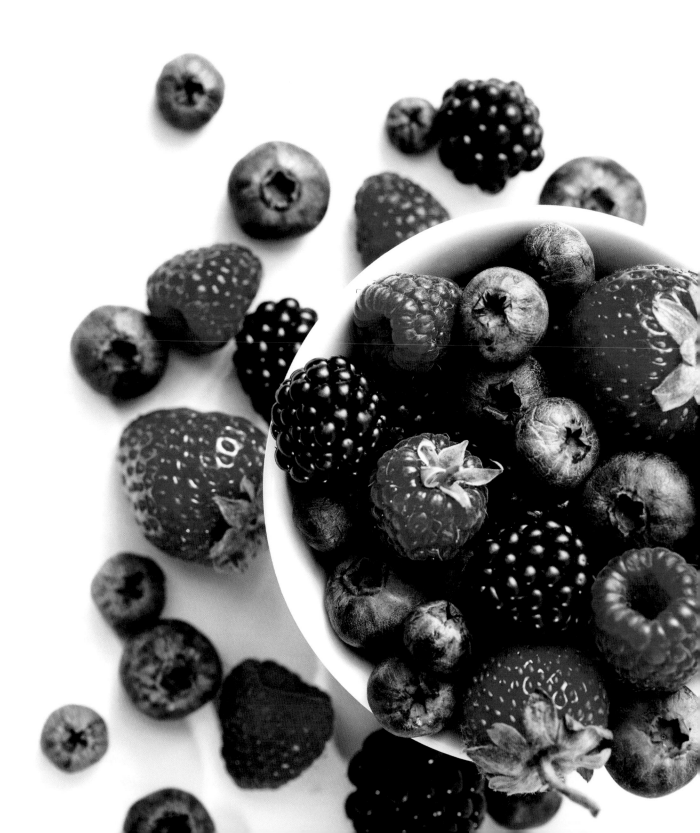

HOW TO USE
THE SAVVY KETO DAILY TRACKER

After you've gone through at least four weeks on keto without tracking your fat and protein, if you find you still have some fine-tuning to do, the SAVVY Keto Daily Tracker may be just what you need.

On the pages that follow, you'll find four templates for tracking what you eat, each for a different daily calorie goal. Each tracker is designed for a diet that's 60%–70% fat, 25%–33% protein, and 5%–8% carbs—the suggested balance for Everyday Fat Burners. (Remember that, while you're counting net carbs, and that's what you should stick to in tracking, the carb percentage is calculated based on total carbs.) If your total calorie target is higher or lower, or if you're a Fat-Fueled Athlete or a Therapeutic Keto Eater and therefore have a slightly different balance of macros, then visit balancedbites.com/ketoquickstart for a wide variety of other tracker templates.

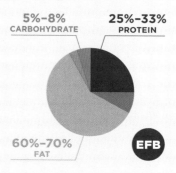

5%–8% CARBOHYDRATE

25%–33% PROTEIN

60%–70% FAT

EFB

HOW TO USE THE TRACKER

Simply cross off the squares representing the grams of each macronutrient that you've eaten. You may choose to do so as shown in the example at right, by outlining the boxes for each item you're eating and writing the food within that space, or you can use any open space on the page to keep notes about foods you've eaten.

The list of foods at the bottom of the page gives the amount of carbs, fat, and protein per serving. You can also print a blank template from the URL above and write in the foods you eat most often for easy reference.

For the most part, foods that come in packages, like breakfast sausages, sauces, and other specialty items, are not included in the lists of foods. If you find you're eating the same breakfast sausages each week, for example, you may want to write their nutrient information on your tracker page and photocopy it so you always have that information handy.

I recommend printing a week's worth of these templates at a time so that you can see how you like to use them, then print later weeks as needed. Once you're comfortable with using the tracker and the breakdown of calories and macronutrients is working well for you, then that's a good tracker to stick with for at least eight weeks.

If you find that the tracker you're using feels like far too much food for your appetite, then select a tracker with a lower calorie target. On the other hand, if you find that you are starving despite eating all of the food on the tracker each day, then pick the next one up in calories.

A FEW THINGS TO KEEP IN MIND

- **You will very likely find that you easily hit your carb and fat intake goals for the day but that protein is a bit challenging.** If you're still hungry at the end of the day, you'll likely find that you have more protein left to eat in your overall daily intake—and eating the rest of your protein allotment is better than eating more fat that you don't need, especially if you're trying to actively burn stored body fat. (Read more about why protein is important on page 47.)

- **Calorie amounts will always be an approximate!** There is no way to know for sure the exact number of calories in a food, even when you weigh or measure it. So, while finishing your day as close as possible to what's on your tracker is great, if you're still hungry at the end of the day, eat a bit of additional protein and some fat. The purpose of the tracker isn't to leave you hungry but to help you avoid overconsuming calories, which many find easy to do when eating a high-fat diet.

- **Note that calories are calculated using total carbs, but net carbs are tracked here.** If you prefer to track total carbs, you can visit balancedbites.com/ketoquickstart for a different version of this template with total carbs listed.

SAVVY KETO Daily Tracker

TODAY'S DATE: _4/28/18_

CARBS (30grams net carbs goal)

coconut milk in matcha	1g	1g	1g	MCT powder & coconut milk in coffee	1g	veggies im Thai delivery	1g 1g
salsa	kombucha			sauerkraut	100% dark chocolate	cauli - rice	
hot sauce	1g	1g	1g	ketchup	1g	1g	1g

PROTEIN (115 grams goal)

5g	5g	collagen	5g	5g cheddar jalapeño brat	5g	5g	5g
5g	5g shrimp	5g deli turkey	5g		5g collagen	5g dark & light meat chicken	5g
5g	5g	5g	5g	choc.		5g	5g

FAT (130 grams goal)

coconut milk & cacao butter in matcha	shrimp	guacamole	5g pesto	5g	olives
	MCT powder & coconut milk in coffee		100% dark chocolate		estimated from Thai delivery sauces
ghee	cheddar jalapeño brat		dark & light meat chicken Thai food	5g	

NOTES:
matcha latte with collagen
– worked out, 8 – 9am –
shrimp tacos in romaine, salsa, guac.
coffee with collagen, MCT powder
& coconut milk
cheddar jalapeño brat w/kraut
turkey & pesto roll-ups, olives
100% dark chocolate, 1 ounce
Thai food delivery,
chicken dishes with veggies
added cauli – rice

COMMONLY EATEN CARBS
Carbs per 1/2 cup cooked unless noted. All carbs listed are net.

	CARBS
asparagus	2 g
bell peppers	3 g
broccoli	3 g
Brussels sprouts	3.5 g
cabbage *(per 1 cup raw or 1/2 cup cooked)*	2 g
carrots	4 g
cauliflower	1 g
cucumber	1.5 g
eggplant	3 g
green beans	3 g
leafy greens *per 1 cup raw or 1/2 cup cooked (includes kale, lettuces, spinach, etc.)*	1 g
lemon or lime juice *(per ounce)*	2 g
mushrooms	1 g
onions *(per 1/4 cup raw)*	3 g
raspberries	3.5 g
spaghetti squash	4 g
tomatoes *(per 1/2 cup raw)*	2.5 g
winter squash *(includes butternut, delicata, etc.)*	7 g

COMMONLY EATEN PROTEINS
Protein and fat grams per 4 oz cooked unless noted. All carbs listed are net.

		PROTEIN	FAT
bison		28 g	7 g
chicken, dark meat *(leg/thigh)*		25 g	16 g
chicken, white meat *(breast)*		35 g	4 g
chicken wings		30 g	28 g
egg *(1 large)*		6 g	5 g
ground beef *(85% lean)*		30 g	17 g
ground pork		28 g	23 g
ground turkey		28 g	2 g
lamb		28 g	22 g
pork, fatty cuts		28 g	23 g
pork, lean cuts		30 g	7 g
salmon		25 g	5 g
scallops		26 g	1.5 g
shrimp	2 g CARBS	25 g	2 g
steak, fatty		30 g	20 g
steak, lean		30 g	10 g
turkey		28 g	2 g

COMMONLY EATEN FATS
Fat grams per 1 tablespoon or 1 ounce unless noted. All carbs listed are net.

		PROTEIN	FAT
avocado *(1/4)*	1 g CARB	1 g	5 g
bacon *(per average slice)*		3 g	4 g
butter			11 g
cheese, hard		10 g	7 g
cheese, soft		6 g	8 g
coconut milk, full-fat			3 g
ghee			15 g
mayonnaise			12 g
nut butters *(average, 2 tablespoons)*	3 g CARBS	7 g	16 g
nuts *(average)*		6 g	15 g
nuts *(Brazil, macadamia, pecans)*	1 g CARB	2 g	21 g
oils *(all)*			15 g
olives	1 g CARB		3 g

SAVVY KETO Daily Tracker

~1,800 CALORIES

TODAY'S DATE: _____

CARBS (30 grams net carbs goal)

1g	1g	1g	1g	1g	1g	1g	1g	1g	1g
1g	1g	1g	1g	1g	1g	1g	1g	1g	1g
1g	1g	1g	1g	1g	1g	1g	1g	1g	1g

PROTEIN (115 grams goal)

5g	5g	5g	5g	5g	5g	5g	
5g	5g	5g	5g	5g	5g	5g	5g
5g	5g	5g	5g	5g	5g	5g	5g

FAT (130 grams goal)

5g	5g	5g	5g	5g	5g	5g	5g	
5g	5g	5g	5g	5g	5g	5g	5g	5g
5g	5g	5g	5g	5g	5g	5g	5g	5g

COMMONLY EATEN CARBS

Carbs per 1/2 cup cooked unless noted. All carbs listed are net.

	CARBS
asparagus	2 g
bell peppers	3 g
broccoli	3 g
Brussels sprouts	3.5 g
cabbage *(per 1 cup raw or 1/2 cup cooked)*	2 g
carrots	4 g
cauliflower	1 g
cucumber	1.5 g
eggplant	3 g
green beans	3 g
leafy greens *per 1 cup raw or 1/2 cup cooked (includes kale, lettuces, spinach, etc.)*	1 g
lemon or lime juice *(per ounce)*	2 g
mushrooms	1 g
onions *(per 1/4 cup raw)*	3 g
raspberries	3.5 g
spaghetti squash	4 g
tomatoes *(per 1/2 cup raw)*	2.5 g
winter squash *(includes butternut, delicata, etc.)*	7 g

COMMONLY EATEN PROTEINS

Protein and fat grams per 4 oz cooked unless noted. All carbs listed are net.

	PROTEIN	FAT
bison	28 g	7 g
chicken, dark meat *(leg/thigh)*	25 g	16 g
chicken, white meat *(breast)*	35 g	4 g
chicken wings	30 g	28 g
egg *(1 large)*	6 g	5 g
ground beef *(85% lean)*	30 g	17 g
ground pork	28 g	23 g
ground turkey	28 g	2 g
lamb	28 g	22 g
pork, fatty cuts	28 g	23 g
pork, lean cuts	30 g	7 g
salmon	25 g	5 g
scallops	26 g	1.5 g
shrimp *2 g CARBS*	25 g	2 g
steak, fatty	30 g	20 g
steak, lean	30 g	10 g
turkey	28 g	2 g

COMMONLY EATEN FATS

Fat grams per 1 tablespoon or 1 ounce unless noted. All carbs listed are net.

	PROTEIN	FAT
avocado *(1/4)* 1 g CARB	1 g	5 g
bacon *(per average slice)*	3 g	4 g
butter		11 g
cheese, hard	10 g	7 g
cheese, soft	6 g	8 g
coconut milk, full-fat		3 g
ghee		15 g
mayonnaise		12 g
nut butters *(average, 2 tablespoons)* 3 g CARBS	7 g	16 g
nuts *(average)*	6 g	15 g
nuts *(Brazil, macadamia, pecans)* 1 g CARB	2 g	21 g
oils *(all)*		15 g
olives 1 g CARB		3 g

SAVVY KETO Daily Tracker

TODAY'S DATE:_____

~2,000 CALORIES

CARBS (30 grams net carbs goal)

1g	1g	1g	1g	1g	1g	1g	1g	1g	1g
1g	1g	1g	1g	1g	1g	1g	1g	1g	1g
1g	1g	1g	1g	1g	1g	1g	1g	1g	1g

PROTEIN (130 grams goal)

5g	5g	5g	5g	5g	5g	5g	5g
5g	5g	5g	5g	5g	5g	5g	5g	5g
5g	5g	5g	5g	5g	5g	5g	5g	5g

FAT (150 grams goal)

5g	5g	5g	5g	5g	5g	5g	5g	5g	5g
5g	5g	5g	5g	5g	5g	5g	5g	5g	5g
5g	5g	5g	5g	5g	5g	5g	5g	5g	5g

COMMONLY EATEN CARBS

*Carbs per 1/2 cup cooked unless noted.
All carbs listed are net.*

	CARBS
asparagus	2 g
bell peppers	3 g
broccoli	3 g
Brussels sprouts	3.5 g
cabbage *(per 1 cup raw or 1/2 cup cooked)*	2 g
carrots	4 g
cauliflower	1 g
cucumber	1.5 g
eggplant	3 g
green beans	3 g
leafy greens *per 1 cup raw or 1/2 cup cooked (includes kale, lettuces, spinach, etc.)*	1 g
lemon or lime juice *(per ounce)*	2 g
mushrooms	1 g
onions *(per 1/4 cup raw)*	3 g
raspberries	3.5 g
spaghetti squash	4 g
tomatoes *(per 1/2 cup raw)*	2.5 g
winter squash *(includes butternut, delicata, etc.)*	7 g

COMMONLY EATEN PROTEINS

*Protein and fat grams per 4 oz cooked
unless noted. All carbs listed are net.*

	PROTEIN	FAT
bison	28 g	7 g
chicken, dark meat *(leg/thigh)*	25 g	16 g
chicken, white meat *(breast)*	35 g	4 g
chicken wings	30 g	28 g
egg *(1 large)*	6 g	5 g
ground beef *(85% lean)*	30 g	17 g
ground pork	28 g	23 g
ground turkey	28 g	2 g
lamb	28 g	22 g
pork, fatty cuts	28 g	23 g
pork, lean cuts	30 g	7 g
salmon	25 g	5 g
scallops	26 g	1.5 g
shrimp 2 g CARBS	25 g	2 g
steak, fatty	30 g	20 g
steak, lean	30 g	10 g
turkey	28 g	2 g

COMMONLY EATEN FATS

*Fat grams per 1 tablespoon or 1 ounce
unless noted. All carbs listed are net.*

	PROTEIN	FAT
avocado *(1/4)* 1 g CARB	1 g	5 g
bacon *(per average slice)*	3 g	4 g
butter		11 g
cheese, hard	10 g	7 g
cheese, soft	6 g	8 g
coconut milk, full-fat		3 g
ghee		15 g
mayonnaise		12 g
nut butters *(average, 2 tablespoons)* 3 g CARBS	7 g	16 g
nuts *(average)*	6 g	15 g
nuts *(Brazil, macadamia, pecans)* 1 g CARB	2 g	21 g
oils *(all)*		15 g
olives 1 g CARB		3 g

KETO**QUICK**START

SAVVY KETO Daily Tracker

~2,500 CALORIES

TODAY'S DATE: _____

CARBS (30 grams net carbs goal)

1g	1g	1g	1g	1g	1g	1g	1g	1g	1g
1g	1g	1g	1g	1g	1g	1g	1g	1g	1g
1g	1g	1g	1g	1g	1g	1g	1g	1g	

PROTEIN (165 grams goal)

5g	5g	5g	5g	5g	5g	5g	5g	5g	5g	5g
5g	5g	5g	5g	5g	5g	5g	5g	5g	5g	5g
5g	5g	5g	5g	5g	5g	5g	5g	5g	5g	5g

FAT (190 grams goal)

5g	5g	5g	5g	5g	5g	5g	5g	5g	5g	5g	5g
5g	5g	5g	5g	5g	5g	5g	5g	5g	5g	5g	5g
5g	5g	5g	5g	5g	5g	5g	5g	5g	5g	5g	5g

COMMONLY EATEN CARBS

Carbs per 1/2 cup cooked unless noted. All carbs listed are net.

	CARBS
asparagus	2 g
bell peppers	3 g
broccoli	3 g
Brussels sprouts	3.5 g
cabbage *(per 1 cup raw or 1/2 cup cooked)*	2 g
carrots	4 g
cauliflower	1 g
cucumber	1.5 g
eggplant	3 g
green beans	3 g
leafy greens *per 1 cup raw or 1/2 cup cooked (includes kale, lettuces, spinach, etc.)*	1 g
lemon or lime juice *(per ounce)*	2 g
mushrooms	1 g
onions *(per 1/4 cup raw)*	3 g
raspberries	3.5 g
spaghetti squash	4 g
tomatoes *(per 1/2 cup raw)*	2.5 g
winter squash *(includes butternut, delicata, etc.)*	7 g

COMMONLY EATEN PROTEINS

Protein and fat grams per 4 oz cooked unless noted. All carbs listed are net.

	PROTEIN	FAT
bison	28 g	7 g
chicken, dark meat *(leg/thigh)*	25 g	16 g
chicken, white meat *(breast)*	35 g	4 g
chicken wings	30 g	28 g
egg *(1 large)*	6 g	5 g
ground beef *(85% lean)*	30 g	17 g
ground pork	28 g	23 g
ground turkey	28 g	2 g
lamb	28 g	22 g
pork, fatty cuts	28 g	23 g
pork, lean cuts	30 g	7 g
salmon	25 g	5 g
scallops	26 g	1.5 g
shrimp *2 g CARBS*	25 g	2 g
steak, fatty	30 g	20 g
steak, lean	30 g	10 g
turkey	28 g	2 g

COMMONLY EATEN FATS

Fat grams per 1 tablespoon or 1 ounce unless noted. All carbs listed are net.

	PROTEIN	FAT
avocado *(1/4)* 1 g CARB	1 g	5 g
bacon *(per average slice)*	3 g	4 g
butter		11 g
cheese, hard	10 g	7 g
cheese, soft	6 g	8 g
coconut milk, full-fat		3 g
ghee		15 g
mayonnaise		12 g
nut butters *(average, 2 tablespoons)* 3 g CARBS	7 g	16 g
nuts *(average)*	6 g	15 g
nuts *(Brazil, macadamia, pecans)* 1 g CARB	2 g	21 g
oils *(all)*		15 g
olives 1 g CARB		3 g

SAVVY KETO Daily Tracker

TODAY'S DATE:_____

~3,000 CALORIES

CARBS (30 grams net carbs goal)

1g	1g	1g	1g	1g	1g	1g	1g	1g	1g
1g	1g	1g	1g	1g	1g	1g	1g	1g	1g
1g	1g	1g	1g	1g	1g	1g	1g	1g	1g

PROTEIN (185 grams goal)

5g	5g	5g	5g	5g	5g	5g	5g	5g	5g	5g	5g
5g	5g	5g	5g	5g	5g	5g	5g	5g	5g	5g	5g
5g	5g	5g	5g	5g	5g	5g	5g	5g	5g	5g	5g

FAT (230 grams goal)

5g	5g	5g	5g	5g	5g	5g	5g	5g	5g	5g	5g	5g	5g	5g
5g	5g	5g	5g	5g	5g	5g	5g	5g	5g	5g	5g	5g	5g	
5g	5g	5g	5g	5g	5g	5g	5g	5g	5g	5g	5g	5g	5g	5g

COMMONLY EATEN CARBS

Carbs per 1/2 cup cooked unless noted. All carbs listed are net.

	CARBS
asparagus	2 g
bell peppers	3 g
broccoli	3 g
Brussels sprouts	3.5 g
cabbage *(per 1 cup raw or 1/2 cup cooked)*	2 g
carrots	4 g
cauliflower	1 g
cucumber	1.5 g
eggplant	3 g
green beans	3 g
leafy greens *per 1 cup raw or 1/2 cup cooked (includes kale, lettuces, spinach, etc.)*	1 g
lemon or lime juice *(per ounce)*	2 g
mushrooms	1 g
onions *(per 1/4 cup raw)*	3 g
raspberries	3.5 g
spaghetti squash	4 g
tomatoes *(per 1/2 cup raw)*	2.5 g
winter squash *(includes butternut, delicata, etc.)*	7 g

COMMONLY EATEN PROTEINS

Protein and fat grams per 4 oz cooked unless noted. All carbs listed are net.

	PROTEIN	FAT
bison	28 g	7 g
chicken, dark meat *(leg/thigh)*	25 g	16 g
chicken, white meat *(breast)*	35 g	4 g
chicken wings	30 g	28 g
egg *(1 large)*	6 g	5 g
ground beef *(85% lean)*	30 g	17 g
ground pork	28 g	23 g
ground turkey	28 g	2 g
lamb	28 g	22 g
pork, fatty cuts	28 g	23 g
pork, lean cuts	30 g	7 g
salmon	25 g	5 g
scallops	26 g	1.5 g
shrimp 2 g CARBS	25 g	2 g
steak, fatty	30 g	20 g
steak, lean	30 g	10 g
turkey	28 g	2 g

COMMONLY EATEN FATS

Fat grams per 1 tablespoon or 1 ounce unless noted. All carbs listed are net.

	PROTEIN	FAT
avocado *(1/4)* 1 g CARB	1 g	5 g
bacon *(per average slice)*	3 g	4 g
butter		11 g
cheese, hard	10 g	7 g
cheese, soft	6 g	8 g
coconut milk, full-fat		3 g
ghee		15 g
mayonnaise		12 g
nut butters *(average, 2 tablespoons)* 3 g CARBS	7 g	16 g
nuts *(average)*	6 g	15 g
nuts *(Brazil, macadamia, pecans)* 1 g CARB	2 g	21 g
oils *(all)*		15 g
olives 1 g CARB		3 g

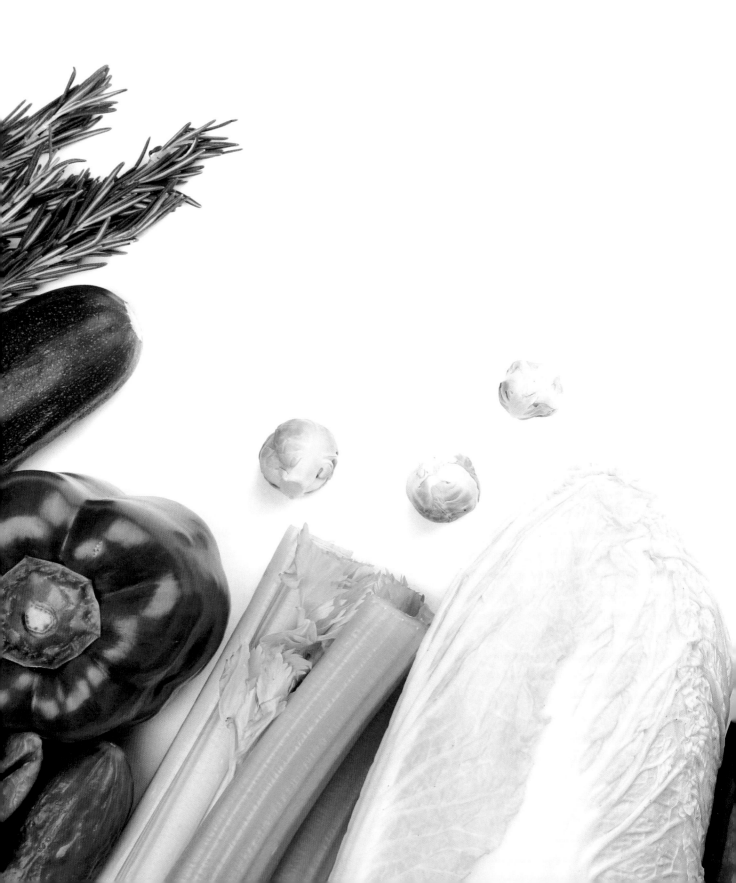

CHAPTER 9

FAQs

KETO BASICS

Q: *What is the line between fat-adaptation and keto-adaptation? Do I always need to be in ketosis to be "keto"?*

A: Technically, the presence of a certain level of ketones in your blood is the single indicator that you are in ketosis. However, being in ketosis isn't the only way to have *metabolically* beneficial effects—in other words, it's not the only way to burn fat for fuel.

If generally optimized health and fat loss are your goals, then I'd argue that being in ketosis twenty-four/seven isn't critical. If you have a diagnosed neurological condition, are healing from a traumatic brain injury, or are battling certain types of cancer, the need to stay in ketosis may be more imperative. (See page 89 for my recommendations for these conditions.)

Q: *Can I eat more carbs some days and still get the benefits of ketosis?*

A: It depends. If you aren't athletic, eating more carbs on some days will likely take you temporarily out of ketosis. That said, since you'll be pretty well adapted to burning fat for fuel, you'll likely get right back into ketosis within a day or so. As a general rule, having an "off keto" day now and then, about once a week or so, can be a great way to give yourself a mental break while continuing your keto diet as a longer-term lifestyle.

If you are athletic and you're using up glycogen in high-intensity exercise or training that pushes your heart rate very high, then there may be a benefit to consuming some small amounts of carbohydrate before a workout, to the tune of 5 to 15 grams (not very much!), and you may find that you feel best when you replenish carbs after a very intense workout to the tune of 20 to 50 grams. That said, most people who exercise (rather than train very intensely) do not need this carbohydrate replenishment physiologically—it's more of a mental break from eating keto all the time.

During the first four weeks of eating keto, I find that keeping carbs as low as possible is ideal.

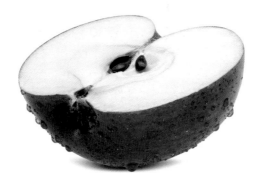

Q: *Is a Cyclical Ketogenic Diet or Targeted Ketogenic Diet better than consistently sticking to very low carbs?*

A: One isn't better per se, but if cycling some carbs into your diet means that you can remain mostly in ketosis in the long term, then it's worth doing. (More reasons for adding carbs occasionally are discussed in chapter 7.) I recommend remaining in ketosis or eating to promote ketosis as best you can for at least three to four solid weeks before introducing more carbs. After that point, cycling carbs according to the plan you're following (see pages 88 to 89) is a good idea if it helps you. Track how you feel and adjust accordingly. I also recommend not limiting non-starchy veggies. If you want to, you can test your ketone level to be sure they aren't kicking you out of ketosis, but I think you'd be hard-pressed to find someone for whom an extra cup of kale did that. Extra carbs from sugary sources very likely will, however.

Q: *Can I balance occasional non-keto meals with keto and still lose weight? Or is it all or nothing?*

A: Since you can lose weight eating a variety of ways, it's not essential to eat keto to lose weight, and it's not essential that you remain in ketosis to lose weight. There are two main benefits of eating keto when it comes to weight loss: first, you're more easily satiated, so you may eat fewer calories overall, and second, your body is primed to burn body fat, which makes fat loss easier for some people. Furthermore, keto offers the potential benefits of increased mental clarity, more energy, and better hormonal balance, which also can make it easier to adhere to keto long-term.

But if you want to eat a higher-carb meal now and then or eat more carbs for one day each week, it won't necessarily mean you won't be able to lose weight; it may just kick you out of ketosis for a day or two. But the goal is long-term success, not short-term weight loss. So if enjoying a higher-carb meal now and then or a higher-carb day once a week makes staying on keto more manageable in the long term for you, then over time, you'll reap the benefits of fat-burning and keto more than you would if you stuck to it strictly for a short period. Ultimately, you have to try it and see how you feel!

Q: *What if I'm eating keto and my cholesterol is high even after adjusting my lifestyle habits per the notes on page 29?*

A: If your total cholesterol is very high (well over 300), it may be time to see your doctor and get tested for a genetic disorder called familial hypercholesterolemia. People often think, "High cholesterol runs in my family," when in fact the problem is poor diet and lifestyle choices, not a true genetic disorder. But if you have familial cholesterolemia, diet and lifestyle changes won't lower your cholesterol. In addition, if your LDL cholesterol measures high (over 200 on more than one test), it's a good idea to get your thyroid tested. LDL readings over 200 may indicate hypothyroidism (low thyroid). In either case, consult your physician.

Q: *Can I eat keto without measuring or tracking macros?*

A: Yes, you can simply pay attention to any carb-rich foods you're eating (see the foods list on pages 56 to 57) and limit those to 30 grams net carbs per day while freely eating protein and fat until you feel full.

That said, if your goal is to lose body fat and you don't see progress within about sixty days, you'll need to start monitoring your overall caloric intake—the Everyday Fat Burner plan on page 88 and information on keto for fat loss on page 104 may be especially helpful. At that point, knowing how much you're eating and whether it's enough or too many calories overall will be important. Both significantly undereating or overeating can be a cause of stalled fat loss on keto (or any way of eating!).

Q: *How long should I eat keto?*

A: You can eat keto for as little as a few months or for as long as you like. The real benefits don't begin to kick in for at least a few weeks, and deciding whether or not you truly feel better eating keto is likely to take at least eight to twelve weeks. If you don't want to continue eating keto because it doesn't feel good for you, you don't enjoy it, or it isn't working well for your life, you can try increasing your carbs by around 25 grams every few days until you get to a point that feels good for you. Remember to scale back your fat intake at the same time as you up your carb intake, so that your daily calories remain unchanged.

Keep in mind that you may be able to eat more than the standard 30 grams of net carbs per day and remain in ketosis! You can play with what you're eating to see what your personal carb threshold is. It's particularly easy to add more fiber-rich vegetables while staying in ketosis. I encourage you to eat as many healthy, whole, low-carb veggies (see the list on page 56) as you can while staying in ketosis.

Q: *How do I determine my personal carb threshold?*

A: You can either test your ketones day after day to determine how many carbs you can eat while remaining in ketosis, or you can use qualitative data like how you feel, your digestion, your sleep, energy, mood, appetite, mental clarity, and so on. Keeping a daily journal is invaluable for tracking this data (see page 79).

Q: *Do I have to be keto for life?*

A: No. As with any way of eating, get what you want from it, experiment, see how you feel, and decide how you want to move forward from there. It would be very seasonally appropriate to eat keto for three to four months, from around November through February, each year if you are so inclined—since local fruit and vegetables are mostly out of season this time of year, it's natural to eat very low-carb.

KETO EATING

Q: *How can I get enough fiber and stay in ketosis?*

A: If you're counting net carbs, which I recommend, you'll subtract fiber from the total carbs you eat each day. With a goal of 30 grams of net carbs each day, you can eat a relatively large quantity of non-starchy fibrous vegetables while staying in ketosis. For example, if you wanted to eat 4 cups of cooked broccoli in a day, that's about 21 grams of fiber and only 24 grams of net carbs. And it's a lot of broccoli!

You can also easily add fiber by adding 2 to 4 tablespoons of ground flax seeds or chia seeds to your smoothies. As a last resort, if you really find you need a lot more fiber, you can add about 1/2 to 1 teaspoon of psyllium husk to a smoothie.

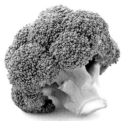

Alternatively, you may find that adding a digestive enzyme to larger meals (taken midway through the meal) helps you to digest food better—it may turn out that you don't need more fiber, simply improved digestion overall!

Q: *How low-carb does a recipe have to be to qualify as keto?*

A: Technically, a recipe isn't "keto" or "non-keto," since ketosis is a metabolic state, not a set of dietary rules. Furthermore, there are no keto police, so while I would tell you not to eat something like Splenda, for example, simply due to its potentially toxic nature, someone else may say it's "keto" because it has no carbs. First and foremost, you really need to decide what your personal standards are when it comes to food. In addition—and I know this seems confusing—the reality is that depending on your body's unique metabolism, it's possible that you could eat a meal with a significant amount of carbohydrates in it and remain in ketosis!

To more directly answer the question, I'd generally consider a meal that has up to 50 grams of total carbs or 30 grams of net carbs to be keto-friendly, since you could easily eat zero or next to zero carbs in your two other meals (and any snacks) that day.

But ideally, a keto meal would more likely have somewhere between 8 and 15 grams of net carbs, assuming that some of your meals are zero or nearly zero carb. For example, I'd consider eggs, bacon, and leafy greens for breakfast to be a nearly zero-carb meal since it might just have 1 gram of carbs from the leafy greens, which I'd consider negligible in terms of impact on your blood sugar.

Q: *How do I measure or calculate carbs in a meal or recipe?*

A: If you're not using the SAVVY Keto Daily Tracker, then use any of the websites listed below to figure out roughly how many carbs are in a recipe or meal. You can enter the carbohydrate elements and the portion amount or approximate amount you're eating.

- Recipe nutrition calculators include NutritionData.com, LiveStrong.com, and Recipal.com, and there are several keto tracking apps as well, such as CarbManager.

- Meal trackers include FitDay.com, MyFitnessPal.com, and many apps, including CarbManager. I used FitDay.com for many years and found it easy and reliable, but it may not be the most up-to-date in terms of functionality.

Q: *How can I eat keto if I can't eat dairy or eggs?*

A: Without eggs or dairy, keto is definitely a bit tricky, but it isn't impossible!

For dairy-free keto, lean on avocados, coconut, nuts and seeds, healthy fats and oils (both for cooking and added to meals as in salad dressing), and fattier cuts of meat and eggs for your daily fat intake and to replace cheese and milk in a dish. When I first ate keto, I was dairy-free for the first year and a half! It's very possible; just stay focused on what you can eat, not what you can't!

For egg-free keto, breakfast is usually the hardest meal to figure out. Lean on traditional breakfast meats like sausages and bacon (pre-cook or prep these ahead of time for quick reheating if your time is limited in the mornings), as well as cauliflower hash and avocado. Try some sausage and avocado over arugula, for instance, or smoothies (see pages 188 and 190) or dinner leftovers.

When it comes to baked goods, if they don't call for many eggs, you can often replace them with a "flax egg." A quick online search will reveal many ways to replace eggs in recipes—vegan websites often have tons of information on this!

All of the recipes in this book (and my previous books!) note when they contain eggs, so you can avoid them if you need to. My previous books are all dairy-free and many are also keto-friendly, so that's another resource for recipes.

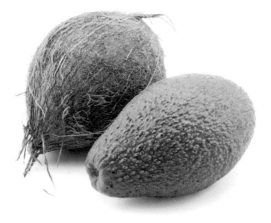

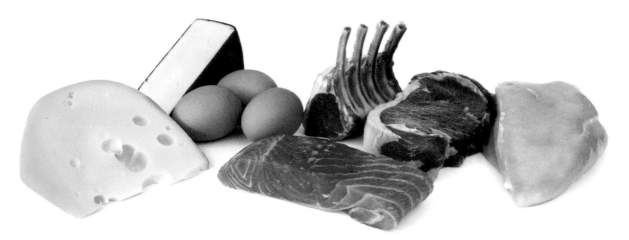

Q: *What is the carnivore diet? Is it the same as keto?*

A: The carnivore diet is an all-animal-foods way of eating that many people try after eating keto for a period of time to see if they feel better or see health improvements. It is not synonymous with keto. If you still struggle with digestion after three to six months eating keto (particularly if you find digesting vegetables difficult), you may find that eating carnivore and avoiding plant foods feels better for your system for a week or two.

Alternatively, you could look into some longer-term fasting—from twenty-four hours up to a week—to see if that helps. (*The Complete Guide to Fasting*, by Dr. Jason Fung and Jimmy Moore, has some excellent advice on longer-term fasting.) As a general approach, I do think that as humans, we do best in the longer term on a mixed, omnivorous diet, but there are a variety of approaches that can help in the shorter term.

Q: *Should I avoid alcohol while eating keto or during my Keto Quick Start?*

A: Yes. Here's the bottom line: when you drink alcohol, your liver's primary focus becomes detoxifying that alcohol. When you're trying to lose body fat, regulate blood sugar levels, or improve health in any way, you don't want to distract your liver from metabolic or detoxification processes. When you interfere with optimal liver function, you're setting yourself up for a longer journey and less-than-optimal results from your Keto Quick Start—meaning any fat loss or improved health will either be stalled, take longer, or not happen at all.

Now, whether or not your body will remain in ketosis when drinking alcohol varies from person to person. There are absolutely lower-carb options for drinks, but I wouldn't take the approach of consuming low-carb alcohol when you're on a health journey. If you've lost the body fat you set out to lose, are managing blood sugar levels well, and all other health markers seem optimal or close to optimal, then that's where enjoying a low-carb or keto-friendly alcoholic beverage once in a while may come into play. I recommend *Keto Happy Hour* by Kyndra D. Holley as a resource for low-carb beverages.

KETO TROUBLESHOOTING

Q: *Why am I gaining weight on keto?*

A: I know it can be confusing to be on a "fat-burning diet" and then gain weight! The truth of the matter is that any way of eating can result in weight gain if you overconsume food. And when you're eating high-fat in particular, this is easy to do, especially in the beginning, before you're familiar with what portion sizes will be satiating for you. If you simply add fat to everything or eat all high-fat meats without noting your portion sizes, your total calories will increase very quickly. A tablespoon of oil or an ounce of cheese is 120 calories, so a few heavy-handed pours per day or an extra ounce of cheese on your salad can add up quickly.

A few words of advice if you're gaining weight on keto:

1. Weigh, measure, and track your food intake for a few days to see what exactly you're eating! If you don't know where you're starting, you can't know how to adjust.

2. If you haven't been using the SAVVY Keto Daily Tracker, start using it according to your current caloric needs.

3. If you are still gaining weight while using the Daily Tracker, then lower your daily intake by about 250 calories for two to three weeks and see where you are. If you find that you've reduced calories as far as you can without feeling like you're hungry all the time, then you may have hit a point where, unfortunately, this is not about the food! Sometimes there are other factors at play, like poor hormonal balance caused by stress, lack of sleep, or other reasons that adjusting your food can't help, or a gut imbalance that requires the direct assistance of a health-care practitioner.

4. If you are struggling with what feels like a sluggish metabolism—you feel as if you've hit a plateau, or as if you should be losing weight because you're not overeating now whereas you probably did before keto—add exercise to your daily routine. At a minimum, walk for sixty minutes, but if you can add weight training, that will yield even better results because having more muscle mass increases your body's ability to burn fat at rest.

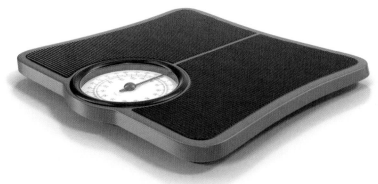

Q: *Why am I losing more weight than I want to on keto?*

A: This is often a result of spontaneously undereating. In other words, you didn't intend to drop your caloric intake, but you've dropped your carb consumption without correspondingly increasing protein and fat, so you're consuming fewer calories overall. It can take a little time to figure out how to add protein and fat to replace carbs, and during that time, you may lose weight unintentionally.

A few words of advice if you're losing weight you didn't want to lose on keto:

1. Weigh, measure, and track your food intake for a few days to see what exactly you're eating! If you don't know where you're starting, you can't know how to adjust.

2. If you haven't been using the SAVVY Keto Daily Tracker, start using it according to your current caloric needs.

3. If you are still losing weight while using the Daily Tracker, then increase your daily intake by about 250 calories for a week and see where you are. If you need to, increase by 250 calories again for one week. Repeat as needed until you either gain back what you lost or your weight is stable at a place where you feel good.

4. If you are exercising for more than sixty minutes per day, especially cardio activity, then be sure to add even more food to your daily intake, or scale your exercise back!

Q: *How can I help my body handle and absorb an increased intake of fat?*

A: Some signs that you aren't digesting and absorbing fat properly include loose stools or eliminations that are lighter or greenish in color; dry hair, skin, and nails; indigestion; and an overly full feeling after meals containing fats.

To help your body out, first, try not to increase your fat intake too rapidly. So if you currently eat relatively low-fat, don't suddenly jump into a high-fat diet out of the gate. Work your way up to your target amount of fat over the course of your first week. If this means you need to gradually lower your carb intake so there isn't an overall reduction in calories, instead of immediately cutting it to 30 net carbs per day, then so be it.

Second, take a digestive enzyme that includes lipase and ox bile. There are many on the market, and you can even find store-brand options at health food stores like Whole Foods that contain a variety of enzymes to help you break down all of your food. Take digestive enzymes when you're halfway through a meal. If you are eating a snack or lighter meal, you can often break an enzyme pill in half and take less at a time.

And finally, go easy on the MCT oil or powder (pure fat!) if you want to introduce it. Take it slowly to avoid urgent trips to the bathroom.

Q: *I'm experiencing muscle cramps / fatigue / dizziness. Why? And what should I do?*

A: Assuming you're consuming enough calories and getting enough sleep, muscle cramps, fatigue, and dizziness are likely signs that you need more electrolytes: sodium, chloride, potassium, and magnesium. It's a good idea to increase your intake of electrolytes from whole-food sources, which the meal plans in this book will help you to do—think dark leafy greens for magnesium, dairy foods for calcium, avocado for potassium, and salt for sodium. That said, if you're still having symptoms of electrolyte imbalance, you can try taking a supplement. Pay close attention to how you feel after supplementation. You may find that you didn't truly need a supplement but rather to simply tweak what you're eating slightly to balance yourself out. (See page 76 for more information on electrolyte-rich foods and supplements.)

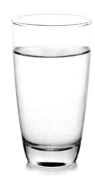

Q: *I'm very thirsty. Is this normal?*

A: Yes, this is normal. Along with potentially needing to up your electrolyte intake, as discussed above, you may find you want to increase your water intake. I recommend sparkling or flat mineral water to get the best of both worlds—hydration with mineral electrolytes!

Q: *How do I know if keto isn't right for me?*

A: If you do not feel well after eating keto for three months and you've tried the troubleshooting tips above, then keto may not be an ideal approach for you.

There is no one way of eating that feels best for everyone. It's not always a matter of "doing it right." While a ketogenic diet will generally "work" for everyone in the sense that your body will physically be able to get into ketosis (once you've adjusted and tweaked your diet as needed), that doesn't mean it feels good for everyone, or that it will work in terms of your lifestyle and/or training and exercise habits.

You may be eating perfectly according to the keto "rules" and seeing the expected blood ketone measurements, but if you don't feel well, then keto isn't working for you. Ultimately, while quantitative data is relevant and important, it should never replace the most important question: "How do you feel?"

Furthermore, I consider a way of eating to work for you when you enjoy it and find it relatively easy to adhere to (after the first month or two; it's always difficult to change your nutrition at first!), and you also reap health benefits from it.

If you are someone who is prone to undereating, or you end up undereating on keto, and you experience any signs of ill health, then I don't think keto is best for you. It can be hard to know if you're undereating, so try tracking a day's worth of food now and then to see where you're at. Signs of ill health include low energy, poor mood, poor sleep, brain fog, skin issues, hair loss, low body temperature, and hormonal imbalances. If you experience any of these after about three months of eating a well-balanced keto diet, then it's not right for you.

DINING OUT & TRAVEL TIPS

Eating keto while dining out is not difficult, but it does require some forethought and planning. Some cuisines and restaurants make it more challenging, but it's really never impossible. Below are some guiding principles and tips for navigating dining out, followed by dishes to choose or avoid at different restaurants. I've also noted when bringing something with you will make your life much easier, like some extra-virgin olive oil or your own healthy mayonnaise. Preparation is key!

KNOW BEFORE YOU GO

- **Avoid starches:** bread, pasta, rice, beans, quinoa, potatoes, tortillas, baked goods (bagels, croissants, muffins, cakes, and cookies), breakfast cereals/granolas.

- **Avoid premade salad dressings,** which typically contain added sugar (premade sugar-free dressings are made with unhealthy ingredients).

- **Find the protein and fat on the menu:** meat, eggs, seafood, avocado, olive oil, hollandaise sauce (ask your server to confirm that it's made without flour).

- **If you know you'll be dining out often, traveling for work, or on a longer vacation, prepare a few keto-friendly items to take with you.**

PREPARE AND PREVIEW

- **Don't arrive starving.** Before you head out the door, eat a small snack of some nuts, nut butter, a few bites of avocado, or some leftover meat.

- **Preview the restaurant's menu online** before you go. Call ahead if you need to ask about specific menu items or ingredients.

- **Check out reviews** from other diners on a site like Yelp or TripAdvisor. (This is especially helpful when traveling.)

AT PARTIES

- **Before you go,** ask the host what they plan on serving, so you know what to expect.

- **Bring a dish or two** that you know you can enjoy and that will satisfy your hunger. The host will be happy to have the contribution, and you'll be glad to know that you won't be hungry all night if they're serving only foods that you aren't eating.

- **If necessary, eat a meal or snack before you go!**

AT THE RESTAURANT

- **Pass on the bread basket**—ask the server not to bring it to the table at all if you can to keep temptation away! Ask for sliced veggies or olives instead.

- **For an appetizer,** choose items like meatballs, chicken wings, charcuterie (meats and cheeses), or vegetable-based items, or opt for a salad starter.

- **Add a side salad** with olive oil and vinegar or lemon wedges, or any non-starchy green vegetables, like spinach, green beans or snap peas (not plain peas), asparagus, or Brussels sprouts, with butter or olive oil. This adds fiber, volume, and of course more vitamins and minerals to your meal, which helps you feel more satiated and keeps your digestion on track!

- **Entrées are easy.** While finger food is often breaded, fried, or otherwise carb-loaded, it's easy to find entrées that are made of simpler, healthier ingredients.

- **Look for grilled, broiled, or baked options.** These typically aren't breaded, so they'll be safer bets. But ask the server for details on how things are prepared to avoid flours and sugars. Don't worry, they're used to questions! Be polite, but get the answers you need. If you end up ordering a leaner cut of meat, be sure to ask for butter, olive oil, bacon, an egg, or avocado to add some fat to the meal.

- **Make substitutions as necessary.** If a meal comes with french fries, bread, or pasta, ask that the kitchen either leave it off of the plate or substitute some vegetables.

KETO DINING BY CUISINE TYPE

🇺🇸 AMERICAN

✔ **CHOOSE:** Bunless or lettuce-wrapped burgers and salads with lemon wedges or vinegar and olive oil. Entrées with grilled, steamed, or baked proteins and vegetables without sauces. Ask for olive oil, butter, vinegar, and lemon for seasoning. If you go somewhere that only sells sandwiches, ask for an "un-wich"—all of the fixings on top of lettuce on a plate—or look for any type of green salad and load it up with toppings like meat, cheese, olive oil, and vinegar. Avoid premade salad dressings, which typically contain added sugar.

➕ **BRING:** Packets or a travel-sized bottle of extra-virgin olive oil or your own homemade dressing; packets of healthy mayonnaise.

✖ **AVOID:** Fried foods, anything breaded, sandwiches, wraps, and premade dressings.

🇮🇳 INDIAN

✔ **CHOOSE:** Most Indian food is easy to enjoy if you can eat dairy. If you can't eat dairy, ask your server what items you can enjoy. Tandoori meats are often marinated in yogurt, so they're good if you can eat dairy.

✖ **AVOID:** Skip the naan (bread), samosas, rice, sweet chutney sauces, lentils, beans, and chickpeas. Ask about sugar and flour in sauces and spice rubs. A main staple flour in Indian cuisine is chickpea (garbanzo bean) flour, and while it's gluten-free and higher in protein, it's also high-carb and best to avoid for your Keto Quick Start.

A STRONG CAUTION ABOUT FAST FOOD: *While you may be able to find keto-friendly fast-food options in the sense that they're high-fat and low-carb, I strongly advise against leaning on fast food for regular meals. Fast-food restaurants use poor-quality oils and meats that are highly inflammatory, and in the longer term they will not yield the results you seek.*

☯ CHINESE

✔ **CHOOSE:** Steamed chicken, shrimp, or fish along with steamed vegetables. Request that no MSG be added to your food.

➕ **BRING:** Coconut aminos or gluten-free tamari*; travel bottle of sesame oil blended with coconut aminos.

✖ **AVOID:** Rice, sauces, spring rolls, dumplings, wontons, and fried or battered items. If it's a local restaurant you dine at often and you feel comfortable, you can request no MSG and sauces without sugar. But if you're not comfortable making that request, it's best to avoid Chinese food. Many of the sauces contain hidden sweeteners and soy, which, while not specifically "not keto," is often inflammatory for many people, and I recommend avoiding it when possible.

I don't typically recommend soy-based foods or products as a regular part of a healthy diet, but in small amounts here or there or when dining out, gluten-free tamari is an okay choice.

🇮🇹 ITALIAN FOOD & PIZZA

✔ **CHOOSE:** Broiled chicken, fish, shrimp, or other protein with red sauce and veggies or salad on the side. Meat or fish cooked with butter or olive oil and capers, anchovies, garlic, etc. Antipasto dishes of meat, cheeses, roasted vegetables, and olives are great (like a Caprese salad). Ask for olive oil and vinegar or lemon wedges on the side, along with grated cheese to add flavor to a dish. Many restaurants now offer zucchini noodles or spaghetti squash as a noodle option, which is perfect if you can get it!

➕ **BRING:** Packets or a travel-sized bottle of extra-virgin olive oil.

✖ **AVOID:** Bread (including bruschetta and croutons), pasta, and breaded meats, eggplant, and cheese. Ask about sauces and how items are prepared (meatballs often contain breadcrumbs).

JAPANESE & SUSHI

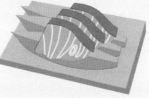

✔ **CHOOSE:** Sashimi or broiled fish; ask what sauces are used and avoid soy sauce. Ask for a side of sliced cucumber and/or daikon radish to eat with your fish. Add avocado to anything you order for additional fat.

➕ **BRING:** Coconut aminos or gluten-free tamari*; travel bottle of sesame oil blended with coconut aminos.

✖ **AVOID:** Rice, anything fried or tempura-battered, imitation crab, and most sauces. Miso soup has about 8 grams of carbs per cup, so I'd avoid it unless you've eaten almost no carbs all day.

MEXICAN

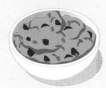

✔ **CHOOSE:** Meat, salsa, and guacamole—often you can ask for these ingredients to be placed over a salad or vegetables. Ask for raw celery or carrots to dip into guacamole and salsa. Ask for a side of vegetables to add to your entrée. Fajitas *without* the tortillas are a good option— enjoy as is or over greens. If an entrée can be prepared without flour or any starchy ingredients, add avocado, guacamole, sour cream, and/or cheese for additional fat.

✖ **AVOID:** Tortillas, tortilla chips, beans, and rice—which means avoiding enchiladas, tacos, quesadillas, fajitas, etc.

MEDITERRANEAN

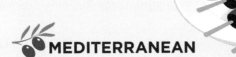

✔ **CHOOSE:** Kofta kebabs, grilled meats and seafood, tomato and cucumber salad, feta or other cheese, hmiss (red pepper dip), tzatziki (yogurt dip), zaalouk or baba ghanoush (made with eggplant). Ask for cucumbers or other vegetables to enjoy with any dip or salad.

➕ **BRING:** Packets or a travel-sized bottle of extra-virgin olive oil.

✖ **AVOID:** Bread, pita, couscous, tabbouleh, hummus, and falafel (made from chickpeas); premade salad dressings.

THAI

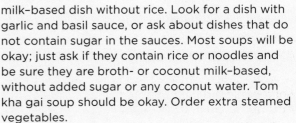

✔ **CHOOSE:** Chicken satay or a curry dish or other coconut milk–based dish without rice. Look for a dish with garlic and basil sauce, or ask about dishes that do not contain sugar in the sauces. Most soups will be okay; just ask if they contain rice or noodles and be sure they are broth- or coconut milk–based, without added sugar or any coconut water. Tom kha gai soup should be okay. Order extra steamed vegetables.

✖ **AVOID:** Sauces that contain sugar (ask about ingredients). Also avoid rice, noodles, Thai iced tea (typically presweetened), and desserts. Avoid tom yum soup (typically prepared with a coconut water base instead of broth).

25 TIPS FOR MAKING KETO EASIER WITH A FAMILY

SHOPPING / PLANNING

1. Plan ahead! Open up all of your favorite cookbooks and pick recipes in advance so you can prepare your shopping list ahead of time.

2. Buy chopped, shredded, riced, or noodled veggies! There's absolutely no shame in that game. Save time, effort, and cleanup!

3. Buy clean premade salad dressings and sauces to save time. But if you're looking to save money, making them with the recipes on pages 344 to 347 will be your best bet!

4. Find clean rotisserie chickens at grocery stores near you. Many these days can be found totally "naked," with nothing added or with just salt and pepper or other spices. Avoid MSG, maltodextrin, and all other additives that aren't spices or seasonings you recognize. Use shredded chicken in recipes or atop salads.

5. Frozen veggies are A-OK. Grab frozen riced cauliflower, peppers, and more. Keep them on hand for quick meals.

6. Buy the largest spaghetti squash you can find, or two smaller ones! It's the same amount of effort to cook it, so you might as well get more than you need. Store the extra cooked squash in the fridge or even the freezer and just reheat it when you're ready!

7. Shop in bulk at places like Costco and avoid smaller specialty stores if you need larger quantities and want to save money.

8. Try new recipes slowly, two to three per week, tops. For the rest of your meals, just make small swaps for yourself. As your family becomes more accustomed to new recipes (and maybe votes for them to be repeats!), more of your healthy favorites can enter the regular rotation. You'll be surprised at how many *Keto Quick Start* recipes will be family favorites and crowd-pleasers—no bland "diet food" here!

PREP

9. Meal prep or "mini prep" on the weekends— either cook full meals to store in the refrigerator or freezer, or prep proteins and a few sides to mix and match here and there. Some favorites to prep ahead are Marinated Onions (page 290), Spicy Citrus Slaw (page 280), and Weeknight Roasted Chicken (page 212).

10. When you bring home veggies that need prepping, wash and prep them before you put them away. This makes them easy to grab and eat or grab and cook without extra prep. For example, rinse, stem, and chop kale, then place it in an airtight container before putting it away.

11. Keep on hand fresh salad greens like arugula (which doesn't wilt too quickly) or mixed baby greens so you can add a quick side salad to any protein you cook for dinner, or pair them with hard-boiled eggs, precooked protein, or tuna salad made at the last minute.

12. If you can, buy an extra refrigerator (or keep your old one when you replace it, assuming it still works) or freezer to keep in your garage or storage area. Craigslist is a great resource for older/used appliances, and low-end models are often on sale at very deep discounts at stores like Best Buy, Target, and Walmart. Having the extra storage space will save you money in the long run!

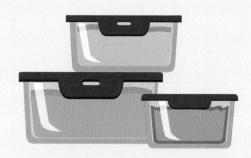

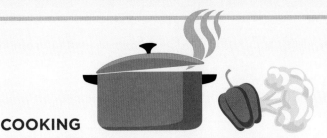

COOKING

13. Get comfortable with roasting *lots* of things—and on multiple trays at once! Be sure you own more than one baking sheet and roasting pan; have at least two of each, but up to four is a good idea. Similarly, when it's grilling season, load up your grill and get tons of protein prepped at once while enjoying time outside. The Best-Tasting Chicken (page 204) is an excellent easy recipe that always delivers on flavor and is never dried out.

14. Cook one meal with a small variation for yourself or let family members leave one item off their plates and don't make a big fuss about it. For instance, make zoodles with meat sauce for yourself and boil some pasta noodles for them, or make their portions half noodles and half zoodles. Leave the bun off your burger or use lettuce or a portobello mushroom bun while the rest of your family has a refined-grain bun.

15. Always cook more protein than you need, whether you're roasting, grilling, or browning in a skillet. If 1 pound feeds your family for a night, always cook at least 2 pounds at a time and immediately put half into a storage container to keep for later (instead of leaving it up for grabs for seconds).

16. Season simply, or separately. Either use a simple seasoning blend like Trifecta Spice Blend (page 330) for everyone, or split a tray of baked chicken thighs, for example, and season half with Taco & Fajita Spice Blend (page 331) and the other half with Greek Spice Blend (page 330) to allow for variety with zero extra effort. Find more seasoning recipes on pages 330 to 331.

17. Batch-cook soups, stews, and chilies! Make a double batch in a slow cooker and freeze half for another day when things are busy and all you have time to do is defrost and eat.

18. Bake. Your. Bacon. This is a massive time-saver, and your bacon grease will be less filled with debris to strain off after the fact. Bake at 375°F for about 20 to 30 minutes, or until done to your liking. You can reheat bacon in the microwave for just 20 seconds or so if you have some prepped ahead.

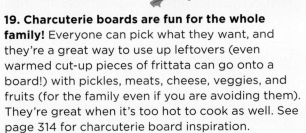

RECIPE, MEAL & SNACK IDEAS

19. Charcuterie boards are fun for the whole family! Everyone can pick what they want, and they're a great way to use up leftovers (even warmed cut-up pieces of frittata can go onto a board!) with pickles, meats, cheese, veggies, and fruits (for the family even if you are avoiding them). They're great when it's too hot to cook as well. See page 314 for charcuterie board inspiration.

20. Find some go-to sheet pan dinners your family loves so you can chop, season, and set it all in the oven without much attention. Try searching Pinterest or the web for "keto sheet pan dinners" to find options and ideas.

21. Cook extra-large frittatas that can feed the family with leftovers. For a family of four or more, I recommend using a 12-inch cast-iron skillet with at least a dozen eggs. For two to four people, I recommend using a 10-inch skillet with eight to ten eggs. (Plus the veggies, cheese, and seasonings, of course.) See pages 176 and 178 for some delicious frittata ideas.

22. Always keep a dozen hard-boiled eggs in the fridge as a quick protein and fat source for you and the whole family. You can eat them alone, put them on a salad, eat them with tomato slices, or use them to quickly whip up egg salad to eat in lettuce wraps.

23. Keep easy proteins like deli meats on hand and buy some healthy low-carb crackers like Flackers to pair with salami and cheese.

24. Breakfast for dinner keeps things quick, easy, and family-friendly. Throw your own eggs and bacon over salad for a breakfast salad for dinner—or make Poachies Breakfast Salad with Hollandaise Sauce (page 170), another tasty option.

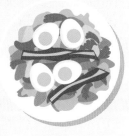

25. Keep only healthy foods (and *healthy* treat options) in the house. It may cause an uprising at first, but in the longer term it's well worth it. Reserve less-healthy treats for trips out of the house, dinner at a special restaurant, and special occasions.

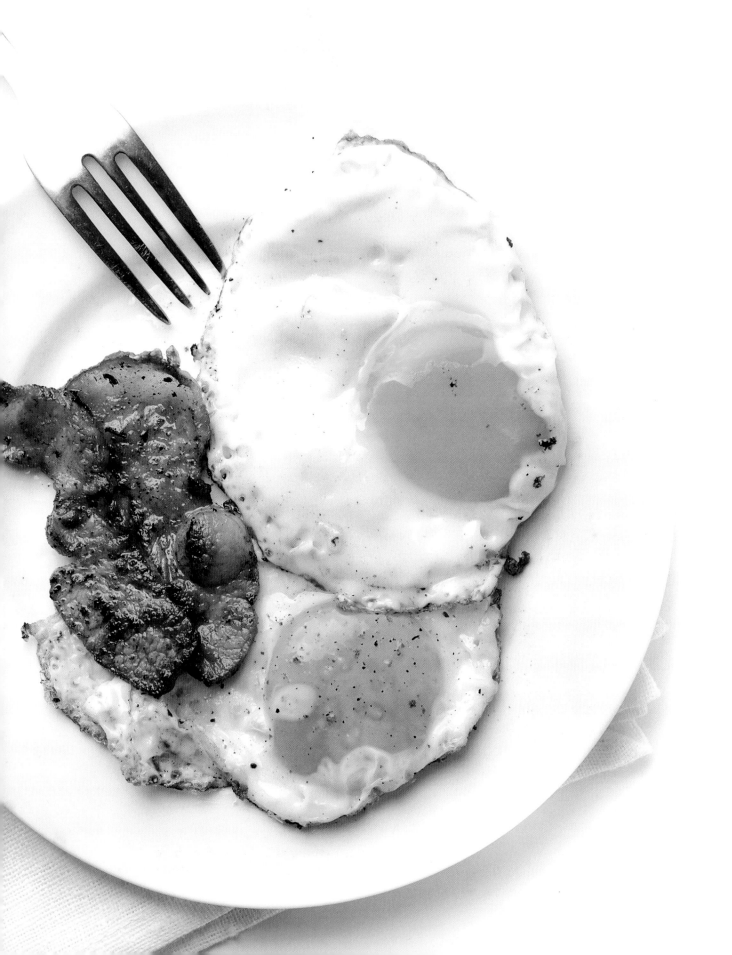

CHAPTER 10

Meal Plans

In the following pages you'll find four meal plans, each for one week. They can be used in any order, at any time—there's no need to use them sequentially! If you are looking for nightshade-free options, plan 4 is designed especially for you.

While there is a fair amount of cooking involved, I created these plans to maximize your productivity in the kitchen and limit your time there as much as possible. They mimic how I typically cook and will help you become more comfortable in the kitchen long-term. Leftovers are anything but dull in my mind, and I love to get creative in making recipes work together easily, without compromising flavor. You're welcome to mix and match these plans with the Easy Keto Meal Ideas on pages 154 to 155; just be sure you adjust your shopping list accordingly.

Shopping lists for all the meal plans are on pages 150 to 153. Before you head to the store, check your refrigerator and pantry to see what items you already have on hand.

Each day in the plans includes meals for breakfast, lunch, and dinner. Each day also highlights what you'll need to cook—some days have more cooking and meal prep, while others have none at all. Before each week begins, a day is set aside for prepping some items for the week (like hard-boiling eggs, making spice blends, or cooking some dishes for day 1). This "day 0" is likely to be the last day of the previous week, so if you start day 1 on Monday, the prep day will be the Sunday before.

Keep in mind that these plans are designed for two people, and leftovers are used accordingly—if a meal makes four servings, its leftovers may be used on another day. So if you're cooking for more than two people, adjust the portions accordingly. All portion sizes are based on the number of people I believe each recipe will feed, but always use your best judgment when shopping—if a recipe seems to make a lot of food for what you and your family normally eat, perhaps adjust down elsewhere in your shopping to account for that.

The net carbs listed in the meal plans are all for one person. They're calculated assuming you eat one serving per recipe, or the exact amount of food noted in a meal that doesn't have a recipe. On days when your net carbs don't add up to the amount you're aiming for, you can add some snacks or treats from the book.

Lastly, remember that these meal plans are entirely optional! You don't need to follow them to have success on your Keto Quick Start. These plans are simply here to help you if you're feeling like you don't know how to map out your week and you want a bit of support—I've got you covered!

MEAL PLAN 1

DAY 0 — COOK/PREP

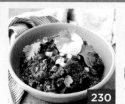
230
Make **Sloppy Joe Chili** for day 1

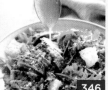
346
Make **Caesar Dressing** for day 1

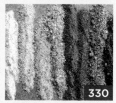
212
Make **Weeknight Roasted Chicken** for days 1 and 2 using 4 pounds chicken and 1/3 cup spice blend

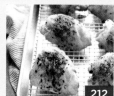
330
Make spice blends for the week: **Super Garlic, Taco & Fajita**, spice blend of choice

Hard-boil **6 eggs** (per person) for days 2, 4, and 6

DAY 1 — 30 g DAILY NET CARBS

BREAKFAST	LUNCH	DINNER

BREAKFAST — 2 g NET CARBS

Per person: 2 eggs any style with 2 breakfast sausages or 2 slices of bacon, **served over fresh arugula,** romaine, or kale/baby kale with dressing of choice. Egg-free? Add extra sausage or bacon.

LUNCH — 13 g NET CARBS

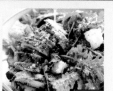
202
Baby Kale Caesar Salad with Grilled Chicken

DINNER — 15 g NET CARBS

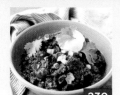
230
Sloppy Joe Chili

DAY 2 — 15 g DAILY NET CARBS

BREAKFAST	LUNCH	DINNER

BREAKFAST — 8 g NET CARBS

188
Chocolate Raspberry Smoothie + 2 hard-boiled eggs per person

LUNCH — Deli Meat Roll-Ups — 3 g NET CARBS

Per person: On each of 2 leaves of lettuce, layer 2 slices bacon; 2 slices deli meat; 2 slices tomato; 1/2 avocado, sliced; and 1 teaspoon each of mayo & mustard

DINNER — 4 g NET CARBS

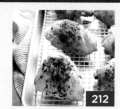
212
Weeknight Roasted Chicken + 4 cups roasted broccoli*

EASY COOK

*Roast **broccoli**: Toss with 1/4 cup cooking fat, spread on a baking sheet, and roast at 350°F until browned and crispy; sprinkle with salt before serving.

DAY 3 — 29 g DAILY NET CARBS

BREAKFAST	LUNCH	DINNER

BREAKFAST — 1 g NET CARBS

Per person: 3 eggs fried with spice blend of choice + 2 sausages or 3 slices bacon **or prosciutto,** topped with chopped fresh chives or green onions

LUNCH — 13 g NET CARBS

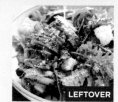
LEFTOVER
Baby Kale Caesar Salad with Grilled Chicken

DINNER — 15 g NET CARBS

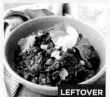
LEFTOVER
Sloppy Joe Chili

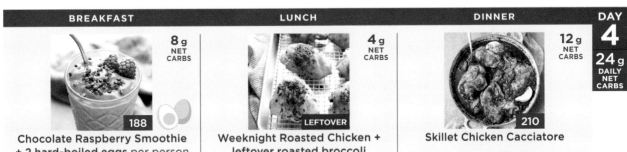

BREAKFAST	LUNCH	DINNER	DAY **4**

8 g NET CARBS — 188

4 g NET CARBS — LEFTOVER

12 g NET CARBS — 210

24 g DAILY NET CARBS

Chocolate Raspberry Smoothie + 2 hard-boiled eggs per person

Weeknight Roasted Chicken + leftover roasted broccoli

Skillet Chicken Cacciatore

COOK/PREP

Make **Skillet Chicken Cacciatore** (page 210)

Make **Super Garlic Stir-Fry Bowl** (page 248) for day 5

Make **Marinated Onions** (page 290) for fish tacos, day 6

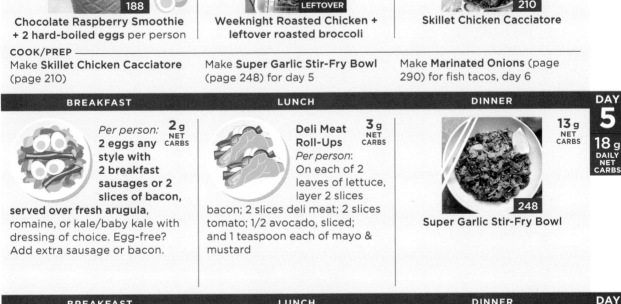

BREAKFAST	LUNCH	DINNER	DAY **5**

2 g NET CARBS

3 g NET CARBS

13 g NET CARBS — 248

18 g DAILY NET CARBS

Per person: 2 eggs any style with 2 breakfast sausages or 2 slices of bacon, served over fresh arugula, romaine, or kale/baby kale with dressing of choice. Egg-free? Add extra sausage or bacon.

Deli Meat Roll-Ups
Per person: On each of 2 leaves of lettuce, layer 2 slices bacon; 2 slices deli meat; 2 slices tomato; 1/2 avocado, sliced; and 1 teaspoon each of mayo & mustard

Super Garlic Stir-Fry Bowl

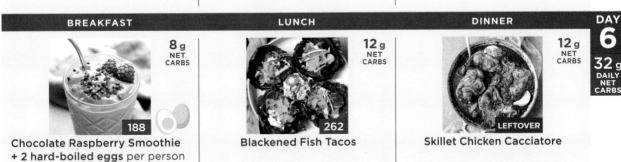

BREAKFAST	LUNCH	DINNER	DAY **6**

8 g NET CARBS — 188

12 g NET CARBS — 262

12 g NET CARBS — LEFTOVER

32 g DAILY NET CARBS

Chocolate Raspberry Smoothie + 2 hard-boiled eggs per person

Blackened Fish Tacos

Skillet Chicken Cacciatore

EASY COOK

Make **Blackened Fish Tacos** (page 262)

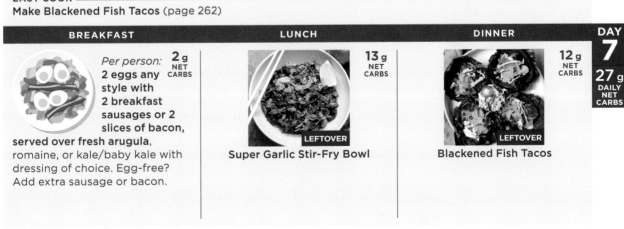

BREAKFAST	LUNCH	DINNER	DAY **7**

2 g NET CARBS

13 g NET CARBS — LEFTOVER

12 g NET CARBS — LEFTOVER

27 g DAILY NET CARBS

Per person: 2 eggs any style with 2 breakfast sausages or 2 slices of bacon, served over fresh arugula, romaine, or kale/baby kale with dressing of choice. Egg-free? Add extra sausage or bacon.

Super Garlic Stir-Fry Bowl

Blackened Fish Tacos

MEAL PLAN 2

DAY 0 — COOK/PREP

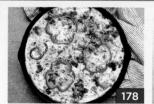
178

Make **Italian Sausage, Peppers & Spinach Frittata** for day 1

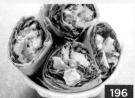
196

Make chicken salad for **Chicken Salad Collard Wraps** for day 1

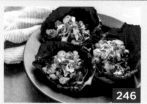
246

Marinate meat for **Tacos al Pastor** for day 1

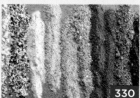
330

Make spice blends for the week: **Super Garlic, Chorizo, Greek, Italian**

DAY 1 — 27 g DAILY NET CARBS

BREAKFAST

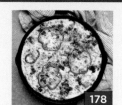
6 g NET CARBS
178

Italian Sausage, Peppers & Spinach Frittata

LUNCH

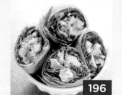
4 g NET CARBS
196

Chicken Salad Collard Wraps

DINNER

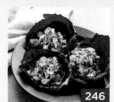
17 g NET CARBS
246

Tacos al Pastor

EASY COOK —————

Assemble **wraps** in a.m.   Make **Tacos al Pastor** (page 246)

DAY 2 — 22 g DAILY NET CARBS

BREAKFAST

2 g NET CARBS

Per person: **2 eggs any style with 2 breakfast sausages or 2 slices of bacon,** served over fresh arugula, romaine, or kale/baby kale with dressing of choice. Egg-free? Add extra sausage or bacon.

LUNCH

3 g NET CARBS

Deli Meat Roll-Ups
Per person:
On each of 2 leaves of lettuce, layer 2 slices bacon; 2 slices deli meat; 2 slices tomato; 1/2 avocado, sliced; and 1 teaspoon each of mayo & mustard

DINNER

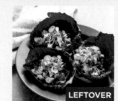
17 g NET CARBS
LEFTOVER

Tacos al Pastor

DAY 3 — 18 g DAILY NET CARBS

BREAKFAST

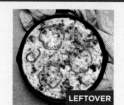
6 g NET CARBS
LEFTOVER

Italian Sausage, Peppers & Spinach Frittata

LUNCH

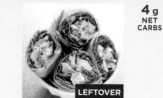
4 g NET CARBS
LEFTOVER

Chicken Salad Collard Wraps

DINNER

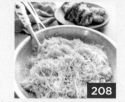
8 g NET CARBS
208

Cacio e Pepe Spaghetti Squash with Grilled Chicken Thighs

EASY COOK —————

Assemble **wraps** in a.m.   Make **Cacio e Pepe Spaghetti Squash with Grilled Chicken Thighs** (page 208). Roast the spaghetti squash and chicken thighs at the same time. While the chicken is finishing cooking, finish the cacio e pepe spaghetti squash.

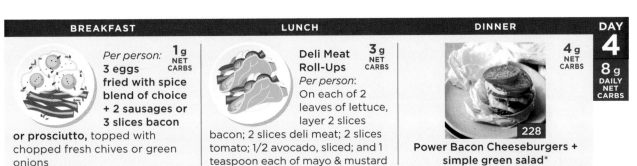

BREAKFAST	LUNCH	DINNER	DAY 4

BREAKFAST — **1 g NET CARBS**
Per person: 3 eggs fried with spice blend of choice + 2 sausages or 3 slices bacon or prosciutto, topped with chopped fresh chives or green onions

LUNCH — Deli Meat Roll-Ups — **3 g NET CARBS**
Per person: On each of 2 leaves of lettuce, layer 2 slices bacon; 2 slices deli meat; 2 slices tomato; 1/2 avocado, sliced; and 1 teaspoon each of mayo & mustard

DINNER — **4 g NET CARBS** — 228
Power Bacon Cheeseburgers + simple green salad*

DAY 4 — **8 g DAILY NET CARBS**

COOK/PREP
Make **Power Bacon Cheeseburgers** (page 228). If using Bacon-y Caramelized Onions, start those early!

Make **Chunky Cobb-Style Egg Salad** (page 174) for day 5

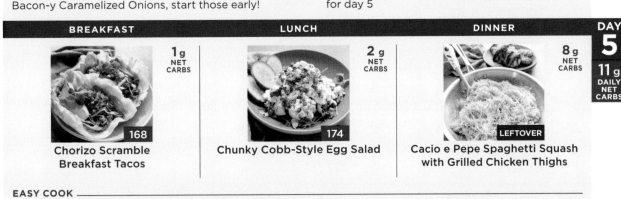

BREAKFAST	LUNCH	DINNER	DAY 5

BREAKFAST — **1 g NET CARBS** — 168
Chorizo Scramble Breakfast Tacos

LUNCH — **2 g NET CARBS** — 174
Chunky Cobb-Style Egg Salad

DINNER — **8 g NET CARBS** — LEFTOVER
Cacio e Pepe Spaghetti Squash with Grilled Chicken Thighs

DAY 5 — **11 g DAILY NET CARBS**

EASY COOK
Make **Chorizo Scramble Breakfast Tacos** (page 168)

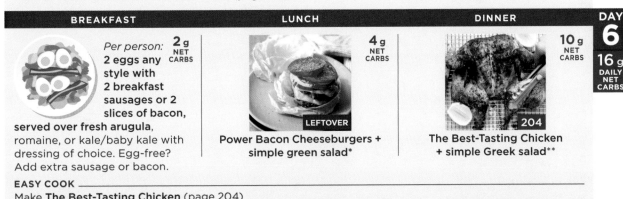

BREAKFAST	LUNCH	DINNER	DAY 6

BREAKFAST — **2 g NET CARBS**
Per person: 2 eggs any style with 2 breakfast sausages or 2 slices of bacon, served over fresh arugula, romaine, or kale/baby kale with dressing of choice. Egg-free? Add extra sausage or bacon.

LUNCH — **4 g NET CARBS** — LEFTOVER
Power Bacon Cheeseburgers + simple green salad*

DINNER — **10 g NET CARBS** — 204
The Best-Tasting Chicken + simple Greek salad**

DAY 6 — **16 g DAILY NET CARBS**

EASY COOK
Make **The Best-Tasting Chicken** (page 204)

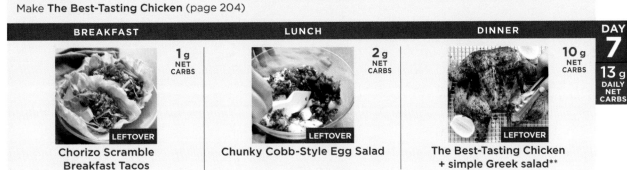

BREAKFAST	LUNCH	DINNER	DAY 7

BREAKFAST — **1 g NET CARBS** — LEFTOVER
Chorizo Scramble Breakfast Tacos

LUNCH — **2 g NET CARBS** — LEFTOVER
Chunky Cobb-Style Egg Salad

DINNER — **10 g NET CARBS** — LEFTOVER
The Best-Tasting Chicken + simple Greek salad**

DAY 7 — **13 g DAILY NET CARBS**

* **Simple green salad:** *Per person:* Toss 2 cups lettuce with 2 tablespoons dressing of choice.
** **Simple Greek salad:** *Per person:* Toss 1/2 cup chopped tomatoes, 1/2 cup chopped cucumbers, 1/8 cup chopped red onions, and 2 tablespoons Kalamata olives with 1 tablespoon lemon juice, 1 tablespoon olive oil, and salt and pepper to taste; add 1 ounce of feta cheese if desired.

MEAL PLAN 3

DAY 0 — COOK/PREP

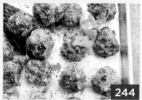

Make **Thai Meatballs** for day 1
244

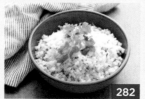

Make **Cilantro Cauli-Rice** for day 1
282

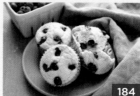

Make **Lemon Blueberry Keto Muffins** for day 1
184

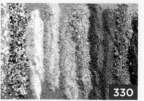

Make spice blends for the week: **Italian, Trifecta, spice blend of choice**
330

DAY 1 — 23 g DAILY NET CARBS

BREAKFAST
15 g NET CARBS

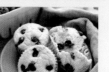

Lemon Blueberry Keto Muffin + 2 breakfast sausages
184

LUNCH
3 g NET CARBS

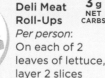

Deli Meat Roll-Ups
Per person: On each of 2 leaves of lettuce, layer 2 slices bacon; 2 slices deli meat; 2 slices tomato; 1/2 avocado, sliced; and 1 teaspoon each of mayo & mustard

DINNER
5 g NET CARBS

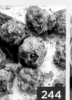

Thai Meatballs
244

Cilantro Cauli-Rice
282

DAY 2 — 18 g DAILY NET CARBS

BREAKFAST
2 g NET CARBS

Per person: 2 eggs any style with 2 breakfast sausages or 2 slices of bacon, served over fresh arugula, romaine, or kale/baby kale with dressing of choice. Egg-free? Add extra sausage or bacon.

LUNCH
5 g NET CARBS

LEFTOVER Thai Meatballs

LEFTOVER Cilantro Cauli-Rice

DINNER
11 g NET CARBS

1 grilled 8-ounce steak *per person* + simple tomato salad*

EASY COOK
Grill **2 (8-ounce) steaks** per person. Save 1 steak per person for day 3.

DAY 3 — 32 g DAILY NET CARBS

BREAKFAST
15 g NET CARBS

LEFTOVER

Lemon Blueberry Keto Muffin + 2 breakfast sausages

LUNCH
11 g NET CARBS

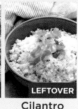

LEFTOVER steak + simple tomato salad*

This day looks like a lot, but these are easy recipes!

DINNER
6 g NET CARBS

You can top everything with crumbled feta cheese if you like; just add 1 net carb to your total.

Weeknight Roasted Chicken
212

Caponata Dip
326

Blistered Shishito Peppers
288

COOK/PREP

Make **Weeknight Roasted Chicken** (page 212)

Make **Caponata Dip** (page 326)

Make **Blistered Shishito Peppers** (page 288)

Make **Meat & Greens Bowl** (page 236) for day 4

* Simple tomato salad: *Per person:* Toss 3 small tomatoes, chopped, with 2 tablespoons chopped fresh basil, 1 tablespoon extra-virgin olive oil, 1 tablespoon lemon juice, and salt and pepper; add 1 ounce crumbled feta if desired.

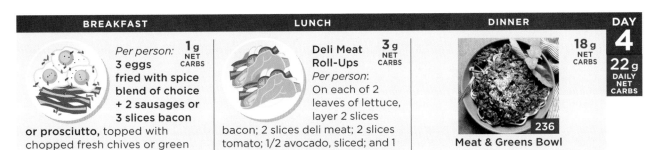

BREAKFAST	LUNCH	DINNER	DAY 4

BREAKFAST — *Per person:* **1 g NET CARBS** — 3 eggs fried with spice blend of choice + 2 sausages or 3 slices bacon or prosciutto, topped with chopped fresh chives or green onions

LUNCH — **Deli Meat Roll-Ups** **3 g NET CARBS** — *Per person:* On each of 2 leaves of lettuce, layer 2 slices bacon; 2 slices deli meat; 2 slices tomato; 1/2 avocado, sliced; and 1 teaspoon each of mayo & mustard

DINNER — **18 g NET CARBS** — Meat & Greens Bowl *(236)*

DAY 4 — **22 g DAILY NET CARBS**

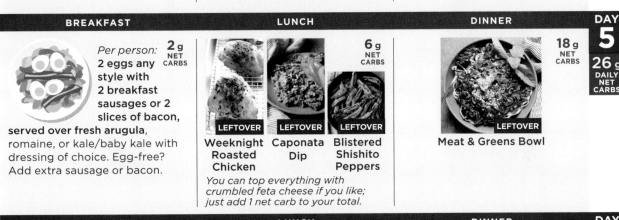

BREAKFAST	LUNCH	DINNER	DAY 5

BREAKFAST — *Per person:* **2 g NET CARBS** — 2 eggs any style with 2 breakfast sausages or 2 slices of bacon, served over fresh arugula, romaine, or kale/baby kale with dressing of choice. Egg-free? Add extra sausage or bacon.

LUNCH — **6 g NET CARBS** — LEFTOVER Weeknight Roasted Chicken · LEFTOVER Caponata Dip · LEFTOVER Blistered Shishito Peppers

You can top everything with crumbled feta cheese if you like; just add 1 net carb to your total.

DINNER — **18 g NET CARBS** — LEFTOVER Meat & Greens Bowl

DAY 5 — **26 g DAILY NET CARBS**

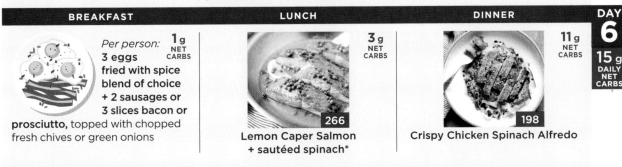

BREAKFAST	LUNCH	DINNER	DAY 6

BREAKFAST — *Per person:* **1 g NET CARBS** — 3 eggs fried with spice blend of choice + 2 sausages or 3 slices bacon or prosciutto, topped with chopped fresh chives or green onions

LUNCH — **3 g NET CARBS** — Lemon Caper Salmon + sautéed spinach* *(266)*

DINNER — **11 g NET CARBS** — Crispy Chicken Spinach Alfredo *(198)*

DAY 6 — **15 g DAILY NET CARBS**

EASY COOK ——
Make **Lemon Caper Salmon** (page 266)   Make **Crispy Chicken Spinach Alfredo** (page 198)

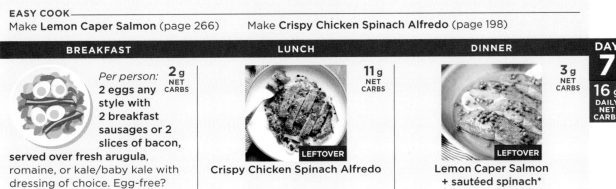

BREAKFAST	LUNCH	DINNER	DAY 7

BREAKFAST — *Per person:* **2 g NET CARBS** — 2 eggs any style with 2 breakfast sausages or 2 slices of bacon, served over fresh arugula, romaine, or kale/baby kale with dressing of choice. Egg-free? Add extra sausage or bacon.

LUNCH — **11 g NET CARBS** — LEFTOVER Crispy Chicken Spinach Alfredo

DINNER — **3 g NET CARBS** — LEFTOVER Lemon Caper Salmon + sautéed spinach*

DAY 7 — **16 g DAILY NET CARBS**

* Sautéed spinach: *Per person*: Sauté 2 cups spinach in 1 teaspoon of olive oil, then season with salt and pepper.

MEAL PLAN 4 Nightshade-Free Options

DAY 0

COOK/PREP

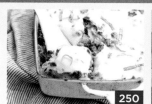
250

Make **Spaghetti Bolognese Bake** for day 1 (use canned pumpkin instead of tomato paste if nightshade-free)

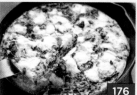
176

Make **Kale, Bacon & Goat Cheese Frittata** for day 1

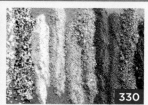
330

Make spice blends for the week: **Ranch, Greek, Trifecta**

Hard-boil **4 eggs** (per person) for days 2 and 5

DAY 1

17 g DAILY NET CARBS

BREAKFAST

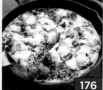
176

4 g NET CARBS

Kale, Bacon & Goat Cheese Frittata

LUNCH

Deli Meat Roll-Ups
3 g NET CARBS

Per person: On each of 2 leaves of lettuce, layer 2 slices bacon; 2 slices deli meat; 2 slices tomato (omit if nightshade-free); 1/2 avocado, sliced; and 1 teaspoon each mayo & mustard

DINNER

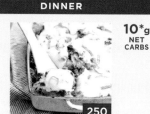
250

10*g NET CARBS

Spaghetti Bolognese Bake (use canned pumpkin instead of tomato paste if nightshade-free)

Nutrition facts are based on using tomato paste in Spaghetti Bolognese Bake. If using pumpkin, the net carbs for this recipe = 9.

DAY 2

24 g DAILY NET CARBS

BREAKFAST

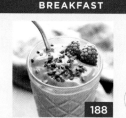
188

8 g NET CARBS

Chocolate Raspberry Smoothie + 2 hard-boiled eggs per person

LUNCH

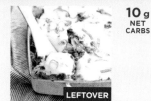
LEFTOVER

10 g NET CARBS

Spaghetti Bolognese Bake

DINNER

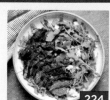
224

6 g NET CARBS

Umami Steak & Arugula Salad

EASY COOK ————————————————
Make **Umami Steak & Arugula Salad** (page 224)

DAY 3

16 g DAILY NET CARBS

BREAKFAST

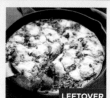
LEFTOVER

4 g NET CARBS

Kale, Bacon & Goat Cheese Frittata

LUNCH

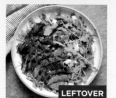
LEFTOVER

6 g NET CARBS

Umami Steak & Arugula Salad

DINNER

200 292

6 g NET CARBS

Hidden Veggie Ranch Burgers + Spicy Roasted Asparagus with Lemon

COOK/PREP

Make **White Chicken Chili** (page 214) for day 4 (omit the jalapeño if nightshade-free)

Make **Hidden Veggie Ranch Burgers** (page 200) (omit the tomato if nightshade-free)

Make **Spicy Roasted Asparagus with Lemon** (page 292; omit the red pepper flakes if nightshade-free)

BREAKFAST	LUNCH	DINNER	DAY **4**

 Per person: **2 eggs any style with 2 breakfast sausages or 2 slices of bacon,** **2 g** NET CARBS **served over fresh arugula,** romaine, or kale/baby kale with dressing of choice. Egg-free? Add extra sausage or bacon.

 Deli Meat Roll-Ups **3 g** NET CARBS *Per person:* On each of 2 leaves of lettuce, layer 2 slices bacon; 2 slices deli meat; 2 slices tomato (omit if nightshade-free); 1/2 avocado, sliced; and 1 teaspoon each of mayo & mustard

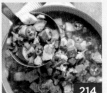 **9 g** NET CARBS 214 **White Chicken Chili** (omit the jalapeño if nightshade-free)

14 g DAILY NET CARBS

BREAKFAST	LUNCH	DINNER	DAY **5**

 8 g NET CARBS 188 **Chocolate Raspberry Smoothie + 2 hard-boiled eggs** per person

 9 g NET CARBS LEFTOVER **White Chicken Chili**

 4 g NET CARBS 284 **1 grilled 8-ounce steak** *per person +* **Creamy Cauliflower Purée**

21 g DAILY NET CARBS

EASY COOK ⎯⎯
Grill 1 (8-ounce) **steak** per person   Make **Creamy Cauliflower Purée** (page 284)

BREAKFAST	LUNCH	DINNER	DAY **6**

 Per person: **2 eggs any style with 2 breakfast sausages or 2 slices of bacon, served over fresh arugula,** romaine, or kale/baby kale with dressing of choice. Egg-free? Add extra sausage or bacon. **2 g** NET CARBS

LEFTOVER **Hidden Veggie Ranch Burgers**   LEFTOVER **Spicy Roasted Asparagus with Lemon**   **6 g** NET CARBS

234   282   **20 g** NET CARBS **Beef Satay Skewers** (omit the red pepper flakes) **+ Cilantro Cauli-Rice**

28 g DAILY NET CARBS

COOK/PREP ⎯⎯
Make **Beef Satay Skewers** (page 234; omit the red pepper flakes from marinade & satay sauce)
Make **Cilantro Cauli-Rice** (page 282)

BREAKFAST	LUNCH	DINNER	DAY **7**

 Per person: **3 eggs fried with spice blend of choice + 2 sausages or 3 slices bacon or prosciutto,** topped with chopped fresh chives or green onions **1 g** NET CARBS

 Deli Meat Roll-Ups **3 g** NET CARBS *Per person:* On each of 2 leaves of lettuce, layer 2 slices bacon; 2 slices deli meat; 2 slices tomato (omit if nightshade-free); 1/2 avocado, sliced; and 1 teaspoon each of mayo & mustard

 LEFTOVER **Beef Satay Skewers**   LEFTOVER **Cilantro Cauli-Rice**   **20 g** NET CARBS

24 g DAILY NET CARBS

SHOPPING LISTS

Meal Plan 1

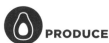 **PRODUCE**

arugula, 1/2 pound

avocados, 3 medium

baby kale, 8 cups

broccoli florets, 4 cups

cabbage, 1 head

chives

cilantro, 1 bunch

garlic, 1 head

green bell pepper, 1 medium

green onions, 1 bunch

lemon, 1

lettuce, 1 head

limes, 3

portobello mushrooms, 4

red bell peppers, 3

red cabbage, 1 head

red onions, 2 small + 2 medium

tomatoes, 2 medium

yellow onions, 2 medium + 1 large

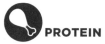 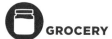 **PROTEIN**

bacon, 8 slices

bacon, thick-cut, 2 slices

breakfast sausages, 1 dozen

chicken legs, bone-in, skin-on, 4 (about 2 pounds)

chicken thighs, bone-in, skin-on, 6 pounds

deli meat, 8 slices

eggs, 30 large

ground beef, 85% lean, 2 pounds

ground pork, 2 pounds

salmon, 4 (6-ounce) fillets, boneless, skin-on

sausages, 4

 GROCERY

cacao powder, 1/4 cup + 2 tablespoons

chopped tomatoes, 1 (26.46-ounce) box

coconut aminos, 1/4 cup + 3 tablespoons

coconut milk, full-fat, 3/4 cup

cooking fat of choice, 1/4 cup + 2 tablespoons

diced tomatoes, 1 (28-ounce) can

frozen raspberries, 3 packed cups

grass-fed collagen peptides, 6 scoops

ground chia or flax seeds, 1/4 cup + 2 tablespoons

hard cheese, 2 ounces

sesame seeds

 CHECK YOUR KITCHEN FOR THESE STAPLES

apple cider vinegar

balsamic vinegar

Dijon mustard

dried oregano leaves

extra-virgin olive oil

fish sauce

garlic powder

ginger powder

granulated garlic

granulated onion

ground cinnamon

ketchup, homemade (page 340) or store-bought

mayonnaise, homemade (page 335) or store-bought

prepared yellow mustard

pure vanilla extract

red wine vinegar

smoked paprika

SPICE BLENDS, DRESSINGS & SAUCES FROM THE BOOK

Avocado Crema (page 342)

Caesar Dressing (page 346)

Pesto (page 343)

spice blend of choice

Super Garlic Spice Blend (page 330)

Taco & Fajita Spice Blend (page 331)

Heads up! Spice blends from this book are available for purchase ready-made, all organic at **balancedbites.com/spices.**

Shopping lists do not include optional items.

When more than one option is given on a single line in the ingredients list, the shopping list includes only the first option.

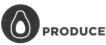

Meal Plan 2

PRODUCE

arugula, 1/2 pound

avocados, 3 medium

Boston/butter lettuce, 1 head

celery, 2 stalks

chives, 1 bunch

cilantro, 1 bunch

coleslaw mix, 1 (16-ounce) bag

collard greens, 1 head

cucumber, 1 medium

dill, 1 bunch

garlic, 8 cloves

iceberg lettuce, 1 head

jalapeño pepper, 1

lemons, 3

lettuce, 1 head

limes, 5

microgreens, 4 cups

red bell pepper, 1

red onions, 2 medium

shallots, 2 large

spaghetti squash, 1 medium (about 3 pounds)

tomatoes, 4 medium

yellow onion, 1 small + 1 medium

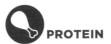PROTEIN

bacon, 28 slices

breakfast sausages, 8

chicken, 1 whole (3 1/2 to 4 pounds)

chicken breast, 2 pounds

chicken livers, 1/4 pound

chicken thighs, bone-in, skin-on, 2 pounds

deli meat, 8 slices

eggs, 42 large

ground beef, 85% lean, 1 1/4 pounds

ground pork, 2 pounds

pork leg roast, boneless, 2 pounds

sausages, 4

GROCERY

butter, 1/4 cup (1/2 stick)

chipotle peppers in adobo sauce, 1 (7-ounce) can

coconut milk, full-fat, 1/4 cup

cooking fat of choice, 1/4 cup

frozen chopped spinach, 1 (9-ounce) package

hard cheese, 4 ounces

Kalamata olives, 1/2 cup

pico de gallo

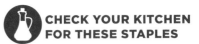CHECK YOUR KITCHEN FOR THESE STAPLES

apple cider vinegar

dried oregano leaves

extra-virgin olive oil

granulated garlic

granulated onion

ground cumin

ketchup, homemade (page 340) or store-bought

mayonnaise, homemade (page 335) or store-bought

paprika

prepared yellow mustard

SPICE BLENDS, DRESSINGS & SAUCES FROM THE BOOK

Chorizo Spice Blend (page 331)

dressing of choice

Greek Spice Blend (page 330)

Italian Spice Blend (page 330)

Quick Salsa (page 306)

spice blend of choice

Super Garlic Spice Blend (page 330)

Shopping lists do not include optional items.

When more than one option is given on a single line in the ingredients list, the shopping list includes only the first option.

Heads up! Spice blends from this book are available for purchase ready-made, all organic at **balancedbites.com/spices.**

SHOPPING LISTS

Meal Plan 3

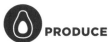 **PRODUCE**

arugula, 1/2 pound

avocados, 2 medium

basil, 1 bunch

blueberries, 1/2 cup

cauliflower, 1 medium head

chives, 1 bunch

cilantro, 1 bunch

eggplant, 1 large (about 1 1/4 pounds)

garlic, 6 cloves

green onion, 1

Italian kale, 1 bunch

lemons, 7

lettuce, 1 head

lime, 1

shishito peppers, 12 ounces

spinach, 5 (5-ounce) bags (about 13 cups)

tomatoes, 3 medium + 12 small

yellow onion, 1 large

zucchini, 4 large + 4 medium

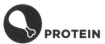 **PROTEIN**

bacon, 8 slices

breakfast sausages, 20

chicken thighs, bone-in, skin-on, 3 pounds

chicken thighs, boneless, skinless, 1 1/2 pounds

deli meat, 8 slices

eggs, 28 large

ground beef, 85% lean, 2 pounds

ground chicken, 1 pound

ground pork, 1 pound

sausages, 8

steaks, 4 (8-ounce)

wild salmon, 4 (6-ounce) fillets

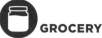 **GROCERY**

almond flour, 1 cup

capers, 1/2 cup

cashew flour, 1 1/4 packed cups

coconut aminos, 2 tablespoons

coconut flour, 1/4 cup

coconut milk, full-fat, 1/2 cup

cooking fat of choice, 1/4 cup + 2 tablespoons + 2 teaspoons

cream cheese, full-fat, 1/2 cup

hard cheese, 2 ounces

pine nuts, for garnish

red curry paste , 1 tablespoon

red pepper flakes, for garnish

sugar-free pasta sauce, 1 (24-ounce) jar

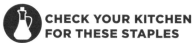 **CHECK YOUR KITCHEN FOR THESE STAPLES**

baking soda

butter

coarse sea salt

dried dill weed

extra-virgin olive oil

fish sauce

ginger powder

granulated garlic

ground cumin

mayonnaise, homemade (page 335) or store-bought

prepared yellow mustard

pure vanilla extract

 SPICE BLENDS, DRESSINGS & SAUCES FROM THE BOOK

dressing of choice

Italian Spice Blend (page 330)

spice blend of choice

Trifecta Spice Blend (page 330)

Shopping lists do not include optional items.

When more than one option is given on a single line in the ingredients list, the shopping list includes only the first option.

Heads up! Spice blends from this book are available for purchase ready-made, all organic at **balancedbites.com/spices.**

Meal Plan 4

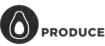

PRODUCE

arugula, 1 1/2 pounds

asparagus, 1 pound

avocados, 5 medium

button mushrooms, 10 ounces

carrots, 2 medium

cauliflower, 2 medium heads

celery, 1 stalk

chives, 1 bunch

cilantro, 1 bunch

garlic, 1 head

green onions, 2

iceberg lettuce, 1 head

kale, 2 cups

lemons, 3

lettuce, 1 1/4 pounds

limes, 2

parsley, 1 bunch

red onion, 1 medium

spaghetti squash, 1 medium
(about 3 pounds)

tomatoes, 2 medium

yellow onions, 1/2 small +
2 medium

zucchini, 5 medium

Shopping lists do not include
optional items.

When more than one option
is given on a single line in the
ingredients list, the shopping
list includes only the first
option.

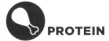

PROTEIN

bacon, 1 3/4 pounds

breakfast sausages, 8

chicken thighs, boneless,
skinless, 1 1/2 pounds

deli meat, 12 slices

eggs, 30 large

ground chicken thigh, 2 pounds

ground pork, 1 pound

ground veal or beef, 1 pound

rib-eye steak, 2 pounds

sausages, 4

sirloin steak, 2 pounds

steaks, 2 (8-ounce)

GROCERY

blue cheese, 4 ounces

butter, 1/4 cup (1/2 stick)

cacao powder, 1/2 cup

canned pumpkin, 6 ounces

chicken broth, homemade (page
220) or store-bought, 2 to 3 cups

coconut aminos, 3/4 cup +
2 tablespoons

coconut milk, full-fat, 2 1/4 cups

cooking fat of choice,
2 tablespoons

fish sauce, 4 to 6 dashes

frozen raspberries, 2 packed cups

grass-fed collagen peptides,
8 scoops

ground chia or flax seeds, 1/2 cup

mozzarella, 16 ounces

peanut butter, unsweetened,
1/2 cup

pumpkin seeds, 1/4 cup

toasted sesame seeds,
1/2 teaspoon

CHECK YOUR KITCHEN FOR THESE STAPLES

coarse sea salt

dried oregano leaves

extra-virgin olive oil

granulated garlic

ground coriander

ground cumin

ground ginger

mayonnaise, homemade
(page 335) or store-bought

prepared yellow mustard

pure vanilla extract

rice vinegar

SPICE BLENDS, DRESSINGS & SAUCES FROM THE BOOK

Balsamic Vinaigrette (page 344)

dressing of choice

Greek Spice Blend (page 330)

Ranch Dressing (page 347)

Ranch Spice Blend (page 331)

spice blend of choice

Trifecta Spice Blend (page 330)

Heads up! Spice blends
from this book are available
for purchase ready-made,
all organic at
balancedbites.com/spices.

EASY KETO MEAL IDEAS FOR YOUR INSPIRATION

These two pages are filled with ideas for you to build quick-fix meals and inspiration for combinations of meat and veggies to try. Of course, salads are one of the easiest quick meals because they don't require much cooking! Get in those greens!

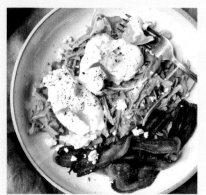

Arugula salad with poached eggs, bacon, and goat cheese

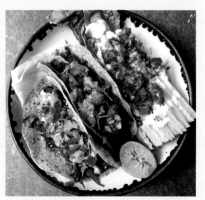

Grain-free tortillas, taco-seasoned salmon, red cabbage slaw, salsa, cilantro, and sour cream; romaine lettuce, lime

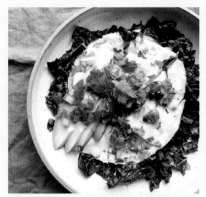

Fried eggs over kale cooked with bacon fat and lemon juice; salsa, avocado, and cilantro

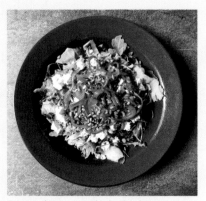

Butter lettuce salad, chicken, blue cheese, sunflower seeds, Marinated Onions (page 290)

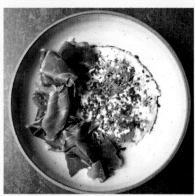

Fried eggs with goat cheese, chives, and seasonings; prosciutto

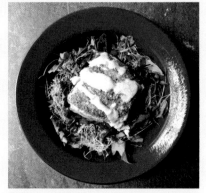

Salmon with Ranch Dressing (page 347) over greens, microgreens, and red cabbage slaw

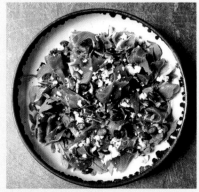

Arugula salad with prosciutto, pumpkin seeds, goat cheese, and Balsamic Vinaigrette (page 344)

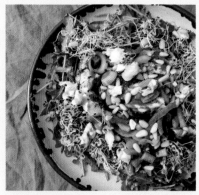

Marinated Onions (page 290) over salad with goat cheese and pine nuts

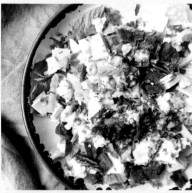

Romaine, deli turkey, bacon, chives, Ranch Dressing (page 347)

For more meal ideas and inspiration, check out the **#ketoquickstart** tag on Instagram or follow me **@dianesanfilippo.**

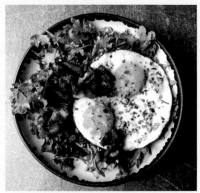

Fried eggs over baby kale salad with crisped bacon and seasonings; Balsamic Vinaigrette (page 344)

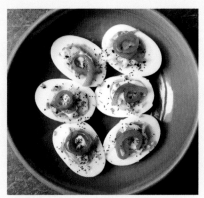

8-minute boiled eggs with mayonnaise, Bagel Spice Blend (page 330), and Marinated Onions (page 290)

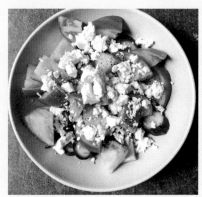

Greek village salad: tomatoes, cucumber, feta, olive oil, and lemon juice; oregano and sea salt

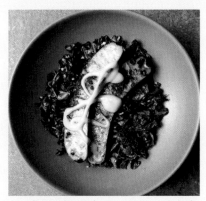

A split pork apple sausage over kale cooked with bacon fat and lemon juice; mustard

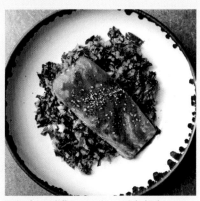

Fried cauliflower rice with kale; salmon with a coconut aminos reduction and sesame seeds

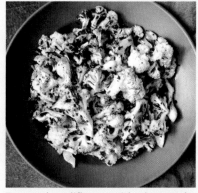

Roasted cauliflower with ghee and Greek Spice Blend (page 330) (pairs with any grilled or roasted protein!)

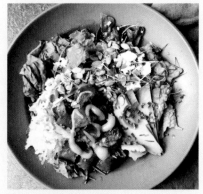

Romaine salad with goat cheese, pumpkin seeds, sausage, and sauerkraut; mustard

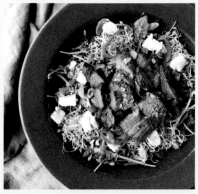

Mixed greens and broccoli sprouts with blue cheese, steak, Marinated Onions (page 290), and Balsamic Vinaigrette (page 344)

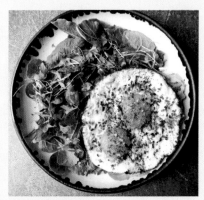

Baby kale with microgreens, Balsamic Vinaigrette (page 344), fried eggs with Super Garlic Spice Blend (page 330) and red pepper flakes

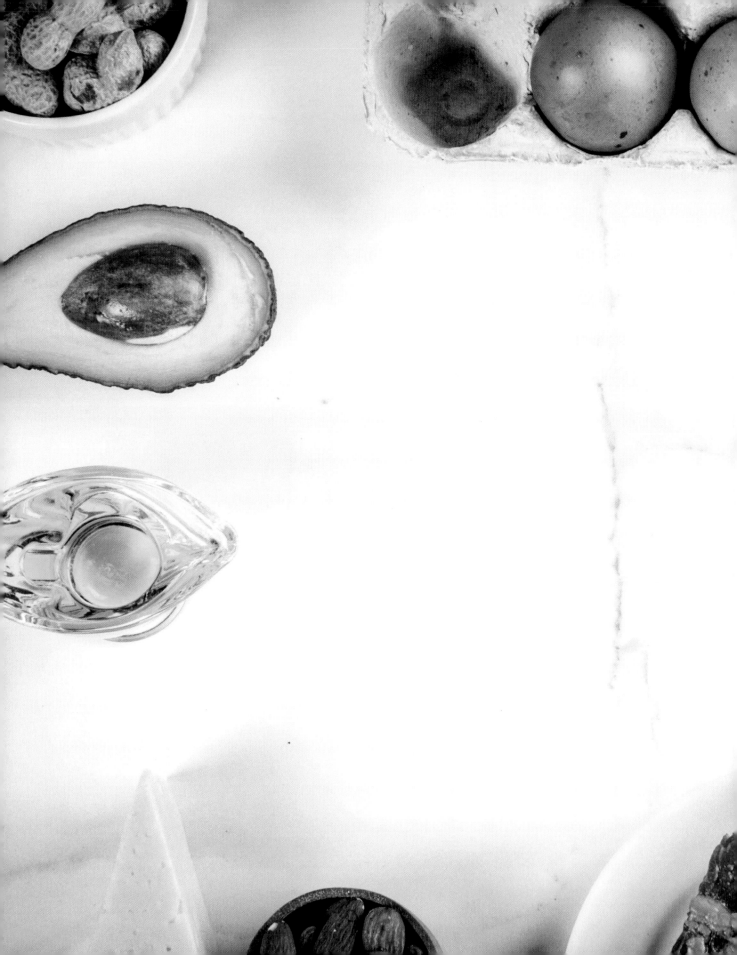

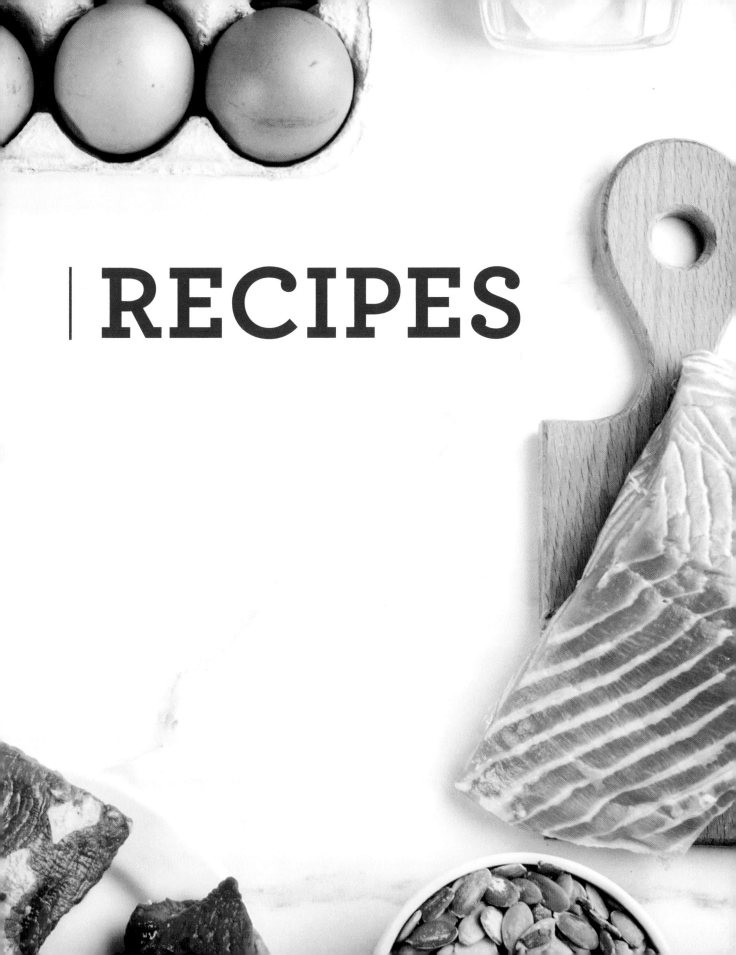

RECIPES

NOTES ABOUT THE RECIPES AND INGREDIENTS

While most of the information on the recipe pages is straightforward, including ingredients, you may come across some details or items that are new to you. In this section, I'll give you a heads-up on some of what you'll find on the recipe pages, from the allergen information to the calorie and macronutrient counts to the ingredients. You'll learn what some of the special ingredients are and where to find them locally or online. I highly recommend planning ahead for meals you want to make, so that if you can't find an ingredient locally, you'll have time for it to arrive from an online order.

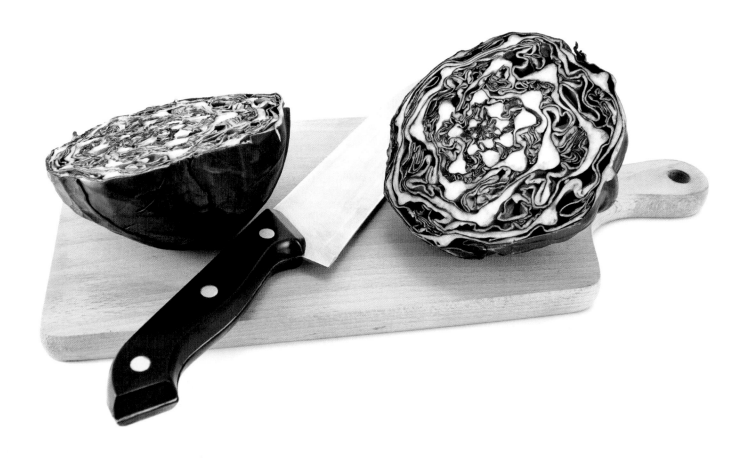

Allergen and Special Diet Indicators

On each recipe page is a list of common allergens or ingredients that may be problematic for some people. When an item appears in bold, it means that the recipe contains that item.

When an allergen can be omitted or swapped out for a different ingredient without drastically altering the final dish, this is noted on the recipe page.

NUTS	The recipe contains almonds, Brazil nuts, cashews, peanuts, walnuts, pecans, hazelnuts, or pistachios. (Does not indicate if a recipe contains coconut, as coconut is not considered a traditional nut for allergy purposes.)
EGGS	The recipe contains eggs.
NIGHTSHADES	The recipe contains nightshade vegetables: tomatoes, potatoes, eggplant, or peppers. (Does not indicate if a recipe contains black pepper, which is not a nightshade.)
FODMAPS	The recipe contains high-FODMAP ingredients, primarily avocado, coconut, onions, garlic, bell peppers, and tomatoes. Most other high-FODMAP foods—grains, sweet fruits, and sweeteners, for example—are not particularly keto-friendly, so you'll naturally avoid them for the most part.
DAIRY	The recipe contains dairy: milk, cheese, sour cream, yogurt. (Does not indicate if a recipe contains eggs, as eggs are not a dairy food. Also does not indicate if a recipe contains ghee, since the milk proteins have been removed.)
21DSD-FRIENDLY	The recipe is okay to eat on the 21-Day Sugar Detox (21DSD), a three-week program in which participants avoid sweetened foods, eat limited fruit, and limit other carb-rich foods. Many people find that completing the 21DSD before easing into keto makes the transition easier. Furthermore, many people find that the 21DSD is even more effective than keto at breaking sugar cravings or addictions because sweet foods (even carb-free ones) are not allowed. If you are struggling at all with carb cravings, even after your Keto Quick Start, you may want to try the 21DSD and then come back to keto after your palate has been reset so you don't crave sweet flavors.

Calorie and Macronutrient Counts

The calorie and macronutrient information for each recipe includes any ingredients listed as optional. For example, if cheese is listed as optional, it is included and counted in the nutrition facts. However, ingredients that are "for serving" or "for garnish" are not included in the nutrition facts.

Each recipe indicates the number of servings it makes, but this is only a guideline—if you are using a SAVVY Keto Daily Tracker (pages 120 to 123), your portion sizes may vary, so adjust what you put on your plate accordingly.

Ingredients

Some ingredients in the recipes may be new to you or a bit confusing. The following notes will help clarify how to use and select ingredients. For more recommended products and brands, visit **balancedbites.com/ketoquickstart**.

BACON, SAUSAGE & CURED MEATS

I recommend looking for high-quality, organic versions of these meats, from animals raised in their natural environments whenever possible. Avoid any with additives like BHA or BHT. See page 66 for more on choosing high-quality meats.

CACAO or COCOA POWDER

Look for unsweetened varieties; many on the grocery store shelves are presweetened. The first choice should be cacao powder, which is in a raw form and contains more beneficial antioxidants. If you can't find cacao, then cocoa powder will still work in the recipes flavor-wise; it simply won't have as many nutritional benefits.

COCONUT AMINOS

This is a soy-free and gluten-free replacement for traditional soy sauce. Coconut Secret and Trader Joe's brands tend to be sweeter than soy sauce, while Big Tree brand is more similar to traditional soy sauce in that it's saltier and more concentrated. I recommend tasting the product before using it in your recipe to see if it seems strong or slightly sweet, and adjusting how much you use accordingly. In sauces that are reduced, I recommend using the sweeter coconut aminos, whereas in a stir-fry or fried rice, I recommend using the stronger, more traditional-tasting version.

COCONUT CREAM & COCONUT MILK

You can buy coconut cream or you can get it from coconut milk. To get the cream from a can of full-fat coconut milk, chill it for at least eight hours, then open the can and scoop out the thick cream on the top.

In recipes, when I call for coconut milk, I recommend full-fat coconut milk, though you may choose to use a lite version for smoothies if you prefer the texture. You may also substitute dairy milk, almond milk, cashew milk, or any other nut milk for coconut milk. I highly recommend using organic nut or coconut milk or grass-fed dairy milk. Calorie information in recipes containing milk is calculated assuming full-fat coconut milk is used.

COLLAGEN PEPTIDES & GELATIN

Collagen peptides are a type of protein powder made from collagen-rich parts of animals, mainly connective tissue and tendons. They are colorless and tasteless and mix easily into many liquids, like coffee, tea, and smoothies, and can even be added to soups and stews. The amino acids provided by collagen, including glycine, proline, and hydroxyproline, support healthy joints, hair, skin, and nails. You may use other forms of protein in a protein shake if you prefer them, but I recommend collagen to round out the amino acids you're already eating. You can also eat gelatin-containing foods to obtain these amino acids, as collagen peptides are simply a more broken-down version of gelatin. Collagen peptides will not "gel" or become semisolid in recipes, while gelatin will.

COOKING FAT

When a recipe calls for "cooking fat of choice," you may choose any cooking fat featured in the Guide to Healthy Fats & Oils (page 69). I generally recommend either ghee (page 336) or coconut oil as a primary cooking fat. Olive oil may also be used over low to medium heat, but take care not to allow it to burn or smoke in your pan.

HOT SAUCE

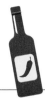

When looking for a keto-friendly hot sauce, check ingredient labels for any forms of added sugar. While an organic hot sauce is ideal, a favorite in many recipes is Frank's Red Hot for its classic Buffalo-style flavor. Other brands of hot sauces that are free of sugar or sweeteners are Tabasco and Arizona Gunslinger / Arizona Pepper's Organic Harvest Foods. Always read labels, though, as ingredients may change over time!

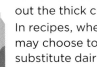

MATCHA

Matcha is a specially grown, finely ground green tea powder and is available in three different grades: ceremonial, premium, and culinary. Ceremonial grade is the most expensive and has the best flavor, but for everyday use, premium grade is a perfect quality. For recipes that are not traditional beverages, like the Matcha Chia N'Oatmeal on page 182, culinary grade works just fine, but it may taste slightly bitter if used for drinking.

MICROGREENS & SPROUTS

Most grocery stores carry some form of microgreens or sprouts, which are new growth from the seeds of foods like broccoli, arugula, peas, radishes, kale, cilantro, and more. They generally range from 1 to 4 inches in length, and they are very nutrient-dense and may contain more vitamins and minerals, ounce for ounce, than their fully grown counterparts.

MILK

When more than one kind of milk is listed in the ingredients list, use any milk you like, but avoid skim or low-fat. Keto-friendly recipes are designed to include plenty of healthy fats, and the lack of fat would change the texture of the resulting dish. Recipes using milk have calories calculated assuming full-fat coconut milk is used. *See also:* coconut cream & coconut milk.

NUT & SEED BUTTERS

In any recipe in this book, you can choose the nut or seed butter that you prefer; just be sure you're using an unsweetened variety. Whichever nut or seed butter is listed first in the ingredients list is what I recommend for the recipe and what is used to calculate the nutritional info for that recipe, but if you have an allergy to it or don't have it on hand, any others will work. Raw nut butters were used in the recipes, with the exception of peanut butter. Choosing raw or roasted nut butter is up to you; it will change the flavor profile of the dish but will not be problematic.

NUTRITIONAL YEAST

This is a slightly cheesy-flavored deactivated yeast (it will not work in baking recipes to leaven anything). It's used in place of a grated cheese topping or to add a cheesy flavor when you're avoiding dairy. Nutritional yeast contains B-complex vitamins and can be found either in bulk or with other dairy-free items at the grocery store. I recommend keeping it refrigerated once opened, though this isn't required. One popular, widely available brand of nutritional yeast is Bragg's.

RICED CAULIFLOWER

If a recipe calls for riced cauliflower, you can make it from a large head of raw cauliflower by pulsing coarsely chopped florets in a food processor until the texture is crumbly, or you can buy a package of riced cauliflower. Riced cauliflower is readily available both frozen and fresh at most grocery stores. Frozen will last longer, but fresh may cook slightly faster. When making cauliflower mash or polenta, it's best to use a fresh head of cauliflower because pre-riced cauliflower may be too dry to yield a smooth result.

SEA SALT & GROUND BLACK PEPPER

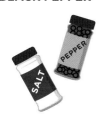

In general, I've used finely ground versions of both, though you may choose to finish a dish with some additional coarse or Maldon brand sea salt or freshly cracked black pepper. Always season as you cook, and taste your food (when the meat is no longer raw or, with a veggie-based dish, while cooking) to ensure you won't need to add much salt and/or pepper at the table. This will yield more flavorful food without making it salty or overly peppery.

"Season lightly" or a "few pinches" means to pinch the seasoning between your thumb and first two fingers and add it to your dish, while "season generously" or "season liberally" means to pinch the seasoning with all of your fingers and evenly coat the surface of whatever you are cooking (typically meat, potatoes, or other raw items that can handle a hearty amount of seasoning). Don't be shy with seasonings; doing so will result in bland food.

STEVIA, GREEN STEVIA, STEVIA EXTRACT & OTHER SWEETENERS

While eating keto, I generally recommend limiting sweeteners as much as possible. You will find that the less often you eat sweet foods, the less you'll crave them. That said, you will find that there are times when you want a hint of sweetness in a dish, and there are a few options for keto-friendly alternatives to sugar. For most people who are eating keto in an effort to feel optimally healthy or lose weight (as opposed to those with diabetes), I recommend using natural caloric sweeteners like honey and maple syrup (though still sparingly and infrequently) instead of more highly refined and potentially problematic sweeteners.

- **Green stevia:** The stevia plant looks a lot like other herbs, and when dried and ground, it closely resembles ground sage (visually, not in flavor). It is often featured in herbal teas to add natural sweetness, but it can have a bitter aftertaste for some people. Green stevia can't be used as a 1:1 sugar replacement, but a pinch here or there can add a bit of sweetness to smoothies or teas. I do not recommend using large amounts of green stevia in anything, only a pinch at a time.

- **Stevia extract (liquid or powder):** This is one of the most common forms of stevia, and a few drops of the liquid or a few shakes of the powder can sweeten a recipe quite easily. This does not replace sugar 1:1 in recipes, as its bulk/weight and texture (or lack thereof) don't act as sugar does. My favorite brand of stevia extract is NOW Foods Organic Better Stevia.

- **Blended granulated sweeteners** (typically stevia and sugar alcohols like erythritol): These are commonly used as 1:1 sugar replacements in keto recipes. You will not find these sweeteners used in this book; I do not use or recommend them as a regular part of your diet. That said, if you are diabetic or wish to use these sweeteners as an infrequent addition to your diet, you can make that choice. These stevia-blended sweeteners are still relatively new, so the data on how healthful they are isn't in yet.

- **Other keto-friendly sweeteners:** Some other commonly used sweeteners include monk fruit, sugar alcohols (erythritol, sorbitol, mannitol, xylitol, isomalt), and yacon syrup or other syrups high in soluble fiber. Some sweeteners marketed as low-carb or keto-friendly may be blends of any of the above. The taste of many of these sweeteners can be off-putting for some but palatable for others, and many of them can cause digestive upset and distress. Since I can't say how healthful any of these sweeteners are with certainty, because they are too new as "foods" for me to make a judgment, I recommend limiting them and not including them in your everyday life or consuming them in large quantities. Reserve these sweeteners for treats on special occasions, or for when you need an on-the-go option and the sweetener is found in an otherwise healthy protein bar.

TOMATO SAUCE (PASTA SAUCE/ MARINARA)

When looking for a keto-friendly tomato sauce, check ingredient labels for any forms of added sugar and avoid vegetable oils like soybean and canola oil. While an organic tomato sauce is ideal, one with "clean" ingredients is perfectly okay! Some brands I love, if you aren't making your own, are Yellow Barn Organic/Biodynamic and Rao's (not organic). Always read labels, though, as ingredients may change over time!

KITCHEN TOOLS

Your Keto Quick Start may require that you're in the kitchen a lot more than you used to be, and that's a good thing! I know not everyone feels warm fuzzies about being in the kitchen, but I promise that the single best way to improve your health is to eat food that you cook for yourself 80 to 90 percent of the time. It doesn't have to be difficult, and these tools will help a lot! I'm also noting some bonus items that are certainly not necessary but that will definitely make your life easier—I use them nearly every day.

COOKWARE & TOOLS

These tools assume you're using either a gas or electric cooktop, not induction.

Cast-iron skillet: I recommend having at least one 10-inch pan, but 8-inch and 12-inch pans are also very useful. A

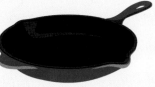

good cast-iron skillet is perfect for making frittatas and searing meats before finishing them in the oven, and for cooking anything that requires high, even heat, like ground meat or seared vegetables. Avoid cooking acidic ingredients, like tomatoes or dishes with a lot of lemon, in cast iron. Look for one that comes preseasoned. Lodge is an excellent brand, but any will do.

Cast-iron grill pan: If you don't have access to an outdoor grill, a grill pan is your best bet. These typically come in two types: a single burner and a double burner, which has one grooved side and one smooth, griddle-style side. A single-burner pan is plenty, but if you like to batch-grill a lot of protein, then a larger one may be a good idea.

Stainless-steel skillet: I recommend having at least one 10-inch pan, but a 12-inch one is also very useful. Stainless steel is perfect for searing and browning, including meat and vegetables, of course. It can be used like a cast-iron skillet but is a better choice for cooking anything with acidic ingredients, like tomatoes and lemons.

Stainless-steel sauté pan: I recommend having a 10-inch sauté pan. This is similar to a skillet but has high sides, so it's perfect for cooking dishes that need stirring, like meat sauces—the high sides keep everything in the pan without risking spills!

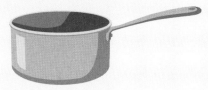

Nontoxic ceramic nonstick pan: I recommend having at least one 10-inch pan, but 8-inch and 12-inch pans are also very useful. GreenPan is one great brand of nontoxic nonstick cookware made from ceramic, perfect for cooking nearly anything. While it isn't as easy to brown food in a GreenPan as in a stainless-steel or cast-iron skillet, it's perfect for most stovetop recipes that require quick cooking and easy cleanup. This type of pan is essential for making pancakes or anything that sticks to surfaces easily. I don't recommend using Teflon-based or Calphalon nonstick pans.

Enameled cast-iron pot / Dutch oven: I recommend an 8-quart or larger pot. An enameled cast-iron pot is perfect for making soups and stews. It conducts and holds heat extremely well and can be transferred from the stovetop to the oven for slow braising. If you do not own a slow cooker, you can use this pot instead by setting your oven to 325°F and cooking the dish for around 4 to 6 hours.

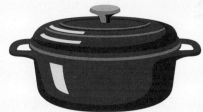

Rimmed baking sheets and wire baking rack: I recommend having at least two full-sized pans (11 by 14-inch or 12 by 16-inch or so) in your kitchen. While I prefer older, lighter-weight pans because they conduct heat better than newer, thicker ones, either kind will do. Stainless steel is a healthier option than anything with a Teflon coating. A wire baking rack that fits on your baking sheet is perfect when having room between the food and the pan is helpful, as when baking bacon or skin-on chicken. If you can buy a baking sheet that comes with an inset rack, that's ideal because they'll be the perfect size to use together.

Roasting pan: I recommend having one that's either as large as or slightly smaller than your baking sheets, either 11 by 14-inch or 16 by 13-inch. A roasting pan has high sides to keep ingredients snugly in place while they cook. Roasting pans are perfect for cooking a whole chicken and vegetables all together.

Cutting board: One large wooden cutting board is sufficient for any kitchen, but having two is very useful, especially when prepping a lot of food at once. To keep a wooden cutting board from slipping on your countertop, place either a damp cloth or paper towel under it. Voilà! No more sliding around!

Mixing bowls: Having a range of sizes is useful when you're prepping and mixing ingredients.

Measuring cups and spoons: Any kind will do, and I recommend having at least one set of cups and two sets of spoons. It's easy to lose a measuring spoon now and then, so having an extra set on hand is a good idea.

Spiral slicer: This is an essential kitchen tool for turning vegetables into noodles or thinly sliced pieces without the need for skilled knife work. I love the Inspiralizer brand because it both suctions to and clamps down on your countertop and has an easily adjustable four-blade dial. Some of my favorite vegetables to spiral slice are zucchini, cucumbers, cabbage, and onions.

★ BONUS ITEMS

Cookbook stand: Most cookbooks won't lay flat unless you break the binding, and you don't want to break the binding because then your book will fall apart! So for anyone who has cursed their cookbooks for closing in the middle of a recipe, a cookbook stand is indispensable. You can find them made of anything from wood to stainless steel and beyond. You can even just get a book stand from your local office supply store—it'll work great and be inexpensive.

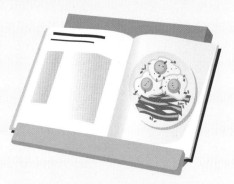

UTENSILS

Chef's knife: I recommend a 7- to 8-inch stainless-steel knife. This is the single most important utensil any home cook can have. You can use a chef's knife to cut almost anything you need to prepare for recipes. A paring knife may be a useful addition, but it isn't necessary. To properly hold a chef's knife, pinch the base of the blade with your thumb and index finger, then wrap your remaining three fingers around the handle. This gives you a "choked-up" grip (think of holding a baseball bat) on the knife that gives you more control and power than if you grip it with all fingers around the handle.

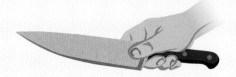

Silicone spatula, scraper, and spoonula: Made from a heat-resistant material, these are perfect for stirring and scraping because they won't scratch the surface of any type of pot or pan. I use a few full-sized versions of these as well as a mini version for scraping the last bits of sauces or dressings out of a jar. A flat slotted spatula is also great to have if you're going to be making my Pumpkin Spice Keto Pancakes (page 186).

Tongs: I love both straight-up stainless-steel tongs and silicone-tipped tongs for using in a GreenPan whose surface I don't want to destroy. Use tongs to flip meat and seafood or remove them from a pan.

Whisk: One good large whisk is a perfect tool for a lot of mixing jobs. While you can use a fork for scrambling a few eggs, cooking a large frittata is way easier with the help of a whisk!

Kitchen shears: One good pair of kitchen shears or scissors goes a long way toward making life easier! While you could slice packages of bacon open with a sharp chef's knife, it's much safer and easier to use shears. You'll also use the shears to help break down a whole chicken in the event that you decide to split it and remove the backbone (a technique called "spatchcocking").

Microplane grater: While this is perfect for hard cheeses, I also love to grate whole cloves of garlic or peeled pieces of ginger on a grater; it's an easy alternative to mincing.

APPLIANCES

Electric multicooker (with pressure cooker setting): For saving time when making broths, soups, stews, chilis, and cooking tougher cuts of meat into a tender result, an electric pressure cooker can't be beat. What would take 4 to 6 hours in a slow cooker takes 10 to 45 minutes in an electric pressure cooker. Broth that normally takes 24 hours in a slow cooker takes just 2 hours in an electric pressure cooker. (An Instant Pot is one example of a multicooker that can act as a pressure cooker, as well as a slow cooker, rice cooker, and more.)

Slow cooker: Perfect for cooking dishes like chili or larger cuts of meats that require time to become tender. I recommend having a 7-quart or larger slow cooker. Most slow cookers have a high and low setting; some also have a timer and a "keep warm" setting, and if you can, I recommend getting one with these features. But these days, many set-it-and-forget-it recipes are developed for an electric pressure cooker, and since a multicooker like an Instant Pot can work as both a pressure cooker and a slow cooker, you can kill two birds with one stone if you opt for one of those instead of a slow cooker.

Blender or high-powered blender: A blender will make life way easier when it comes to combining and whipping liquids smoothly. I love using a high-powered blender like a Blendtec or a Vitamix, but they can be costly and aren't absolutely necessary.

Food processor: As a general rule of thumb, blenders are for working with liquids or almost-liquids and food processors are for working with solids (including solids you're breaking down into semi-liquids/purées). A food processor is ideal for making puréed cauliflower and cauliflower mash, and even for shredding vegetables. You can also use a food processor for making homemade nut butters and sauces like pesto, where you start with solid, dry ingredients and add oil to blend it into a paste. A large processor usually has about a 10- to 12-cup capacity, but a small processor is useful in many kitchens and would hold about 4 to 6 cups.

Immersion blender (aka hand blender): For making homemade mayonnaise, an immersion blender is your absolute best tool. You can also use one to purée steamed cauliflower so that you don't need to transfer it to a food processor. Be sure you turn it on only when the blade is completely submerged in whatever you're blending.

Toaster oven: I find a toaster oven to be indispensable for daily cooking and reheating. Cooking in a toaster oven is quick, easy, and efficient in terms of both effort and energy requirements, since there is little to no preheating time and it won't warm your entire house.

Single-serving blender: If you're cooking for one or like to blend hot or cold drinks regularly, this is the easiest way! Mine lives on my countertop at all times, while my high-powered blender is only taken out for larger recipes. Ninja is one great brand.

Electric tea kettle: This is certainly not a necessary gadget, but I'll tell you, I use mine daily, not only for heating water for coffee or matcha but also for making the whole process of boiling water much faster! So if you're boiling a lot of eggs regularly, for instance, heating one to two batches of water in an electric kettle can make the process way faster. This is an especially helpful gadget if you've chosen not to keep a microwave in your home, and it's inexpensive.

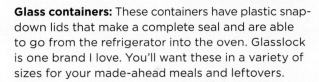

FOOD STORAGE

Glass containers: These containers have plastic snap-down lids that make a complete seal and are able to go from the refrigerator into the oven. Glasslock is one brand I love. You'll want these in a variety of sizes for your made-ahead meals and leftovers.

Glass storage/mason jars (with plastic lids): These are kitchen staples for anyone who cooks and needs to store liquids. Use them for sauces, dressings, and even smoothies or salads on the go. Unless you're going to use them for canning, I recommend getting the white plastic lids instead of the two-piece metal lids; the plastic lids make life way easier!

Used glass jars: Yes, you read that correctly! I recommend saving glass jars from all kinds of products, like nut butters, spices, and more, to wash and reuse. This will help you find just the right container for your leftovers and meal prep.

White labels and a black permanent marker: For labeling all of your meal prep. I typically use either Avery brand or generic round labels and adhere them to the plastic lids of my containers (it's much easier to remove them from the lids than from the glass).

A small funnel: For pouring your dressings, sauces, and even spice blends into bottles and jars, or for refilling your olive oil jar from a large 3-liter tin!

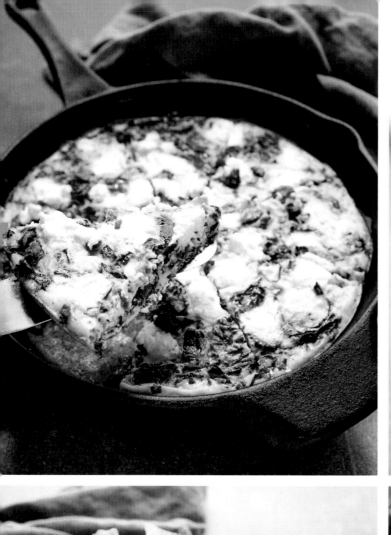

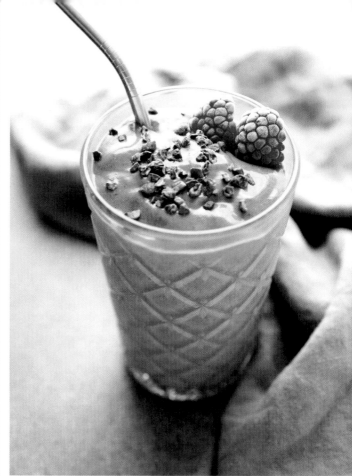

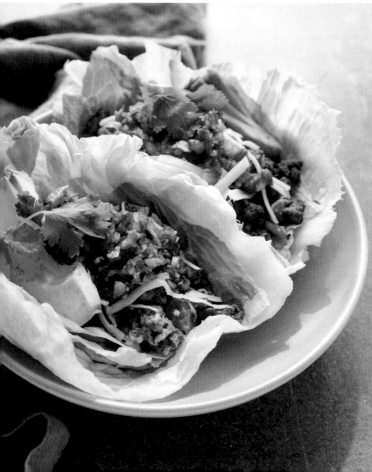

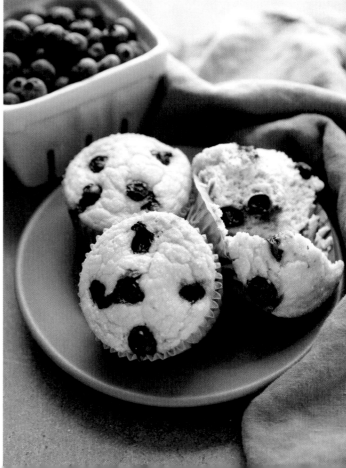

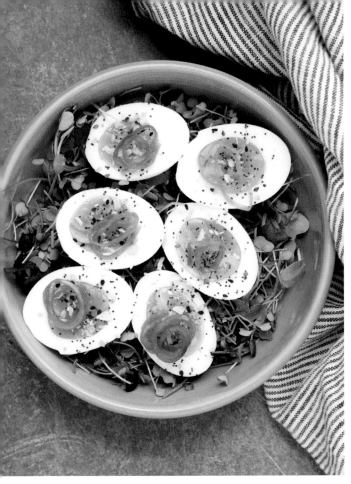

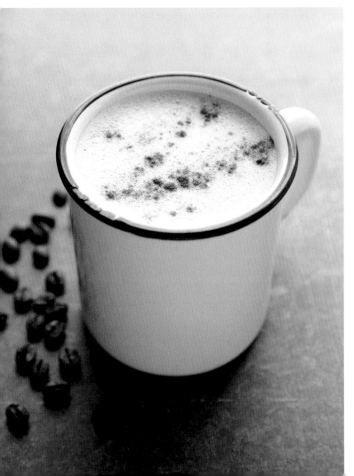

Breakfast

Chorizo Scramble Breakfast Tacos

PREP TIME: 5 minutes | COOK TIME: 10 to 15 minutes | YIELD: 8 tacos (2 per serving)

These tacos are a really quick way to enjoy a higher-protein breakfast that combines sausage and eggs. I also love using chorizo in place of Italian sausage in other recipes, so keep this chorizo recipe handy for just such an occasion. Have fun with the toppings and use whatever you have on hand!

FOR THE CHORIZO

1 pound ground pork, beef, turkey, or chicken

2 tablespoons Chorizo Spice Blend (page 331)

1 tablespoon apple cider vinegar

1 tablespoon cooking fat of choice

8 large eggs

FOR SERVING

1 head iceberg lettuce or butter lettuce, leaves separated

1/2 cup shredded cheese (optional)

1 medium avocado, sliced

1/2 cup Quick Salsa (page 306)

Fresh cilantro

Place the ground meat in a large skillet over medium heat and add the spice blend and vinegar. Cook for about 10 minutes, until the meat is cooked through, using a wooden spoon to break up the meat as it cooks.

Reduce the heat to low and make a hole in the center of the meat. Add the cooking fat, then crack the eggs directly into the hole and lightly scramble them. I recommend using a heat-resistant silicone spatula for this task. Stir the meat and eggs together until the eggs are cooked through, about 2 minutes.

To serve, divide the egg-and-meat mixture among 8 double-layered lettuce leaves and top with cheese (if desired), avocado, and salsa. Garnish with fresh cilantro.

EGG-FREE?
You can make breakfast tacos using this chorizo without eggs! They're delicious!

DAIRY-FREE?
Omit the cheese.

CALORIES: **467** | FAT: **37 g** | PROTEIN: **32 g** | CARBS: **1 g** | FIBER: **0 g** | NET CARBS: **1 g**

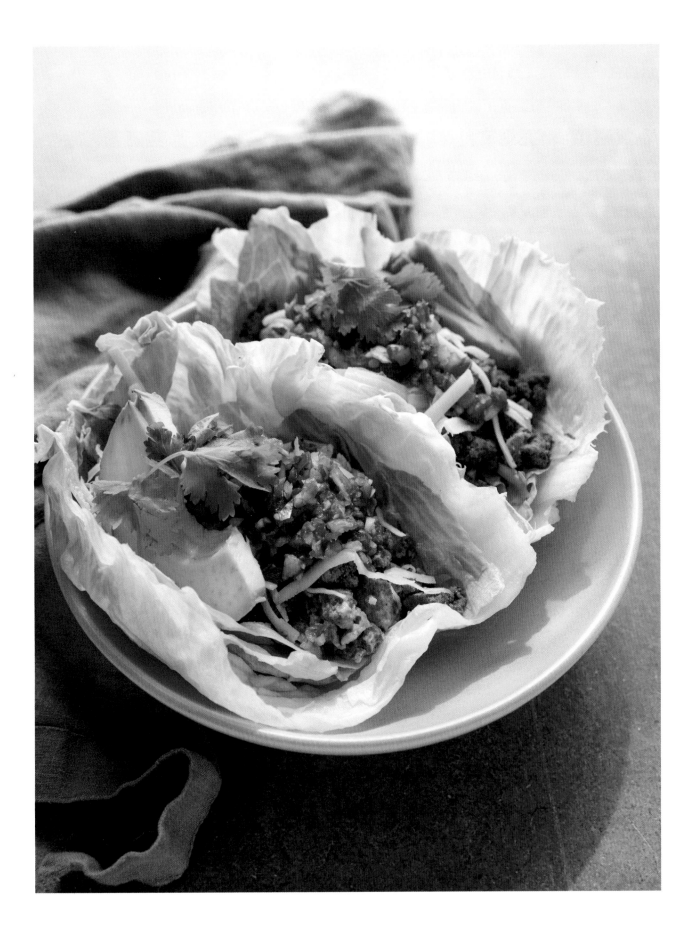

Poachies Breakfast Salad with Hollandaise Sauce

PREP TIME: **10 minutes** | COOK TIME: **5 minutes** | YIELD: **1 serving**

Salads for breakfast are so refreshing, especially when topped with a rich, delicious dressing. The hollandaise is delicious, but Balsamic Vinaigrette (page 344) would also work perfectly. Try this salad with soft-boiled eggs if poaching eggs intimidates you—but I promise, with a little practice, you'll be a poaching pro!

2 large eggs

1 tablespoon apple cider vinegar

3 slices bacon

1 cup baby arugula

2 or 3 pinches of Chorizo Spice Blend (page 331)

2 tablespoons Hollandaise Sauce (page 334)

Fill a 3-inch-deep sauté pan halfway with water. Bring to a simmering boil over medium-high heat.

Crack each egg into a separate ramekin. I typically poach two eggs at a time.

Add the apple cider vinegar to the boiling water, then slowly stir in a circular motion. Carefully add one egg to the center of the pan. After 10 to 15 seconds, gently stir the water again. Add the second egg. Cook for 3 minutes. Using a slotted spoon, gently remove the eggs from the water and place them on a paper towel–lined plate or cutting board to rest. Repeat this process with any remaining eggs.

While the eggs are cooking, cook the bacon in a separate skillet over medium heat.

Assemble the salad: Place the arugula on a plate and top with the eggs, then sprinkle with the spice blend and add the bacon. Drizzle with hollandaise sauce before serving.

CALORIES: **705** | FAT: **66 g** | PROTEIN: **24 g** | CARBS: **3 g** | FIBER: **0 g** | NET CARBS: **3 g**

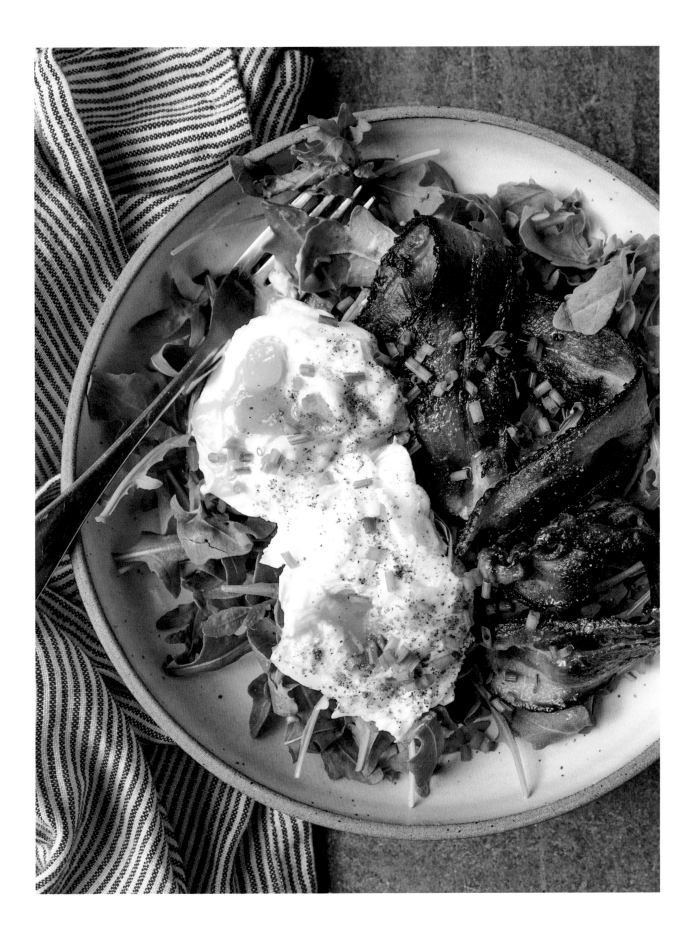

Easy Soft-Boiled Eggs

PREP TIME: **5 minutes** | COOK TIME: **7 minutes** | YIELD: **12 eggs (3 per serving)**

Want a runny yolk but don't want to fry or poach an egg? Enter soft-boiled eggs! These are probably my favorite way to enjoy eggs quickly. If you happen to have an electric kettle, use it to boil your water to save time—that's a favorite kitchen hack of mine.

1 dozen large eggs, room temperature

Fill a large bowl with ice water.

Fill a large saucepan about two-thirds full with water, cover, and bring to a boil over high heat. When the water comes to a boil, gently place the eggs in the pot using a slotted spoon. Boil for 7 minutes, then move the eggs to the ice bath and wait 1 minute before peeling the eggs. Serve warm.

Store peeled eggs in an airtight container in the refrigerator for up to 1 week. To reheat, place a few eggs in a bowl of hot tap water for about 5 minutes.

SERVING SUGGESTION

Try sprinkling with Bagel Spice Blend (page 330) and serving with Marinated Onions (page 290) and microgreens.

CALORIES: **214** | FAT: **15 g** | PROTEIN: **19 g** | CARBS: **1 g** | FIBER: **0 g** | NET CARBS: **1 g**

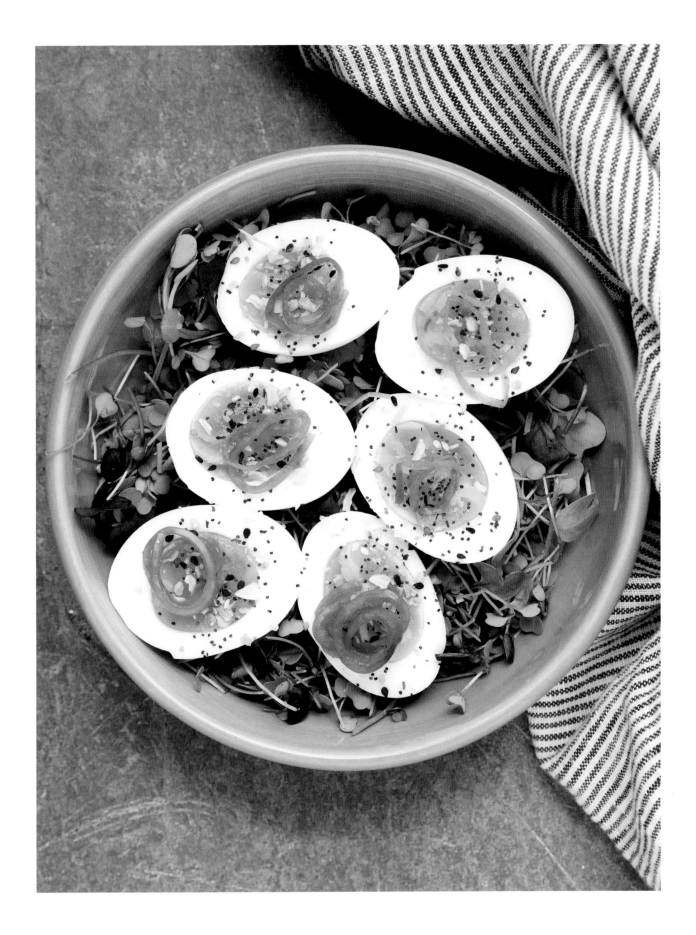

Chunky Cobb-Style Egg Salad

PREP TIME: **5 minutes, plus time to chill the eggs** | COOK TIME: **10 minutes** | YIELD: **6 servings**

Mix up your egg salad style by keeping the ingredients chunky and you'll have the best part of a Cobb salad: the toppings! Adding some blue cheese would take it to the next level. Enjoy this for any meal of the day, but I especially love it as a quick and easy breakfast, especially when made ahead.

8 cups water

1 dozen large eggs, room temperature

1/4 cup mayonnaise, homemade (page 335) or store-bought

2 tablespoons chopped fresh chives

2 tablespoons chopped fresh dill

2 tablespoons minced shallots or red onions

12 slices cooked bacon, chopped

Sea salt and ground black pepper

Microgreens, for serving

Sliced cucumbers, for serving (optional)

Fill a large pot with the water and bring to a boil. Fill a large bowl with ice water.

Place the eggs in the boiling water and cook for 10 minutes. Transfer the eggs to the ice water and chill for 10 minutes. This will keep them from turning green around the yolks.

Peel the eggs, place them in a large bowl, and mash them with a potato masher or large fork. Mix in the mayonnaise, chives, dill, and shallots. Stir in the bacon so it is evenly distributed.

Season with salt and pepper to taste and serve over microgreens and with sliced cucumbers on the side, if desired.

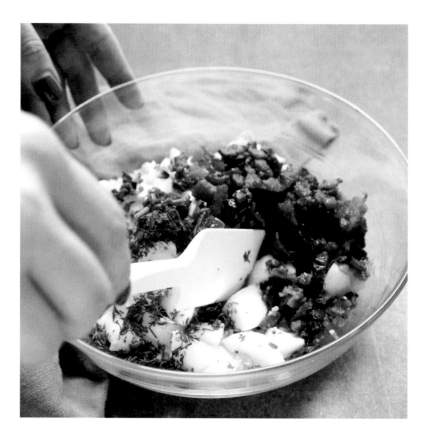

CALORIES: **498** | FAT: **46 g** | PROTEIN: **20 g** | CARBS: **2 g** | FIBER: **0 g** | NET CARBS: **2 g**

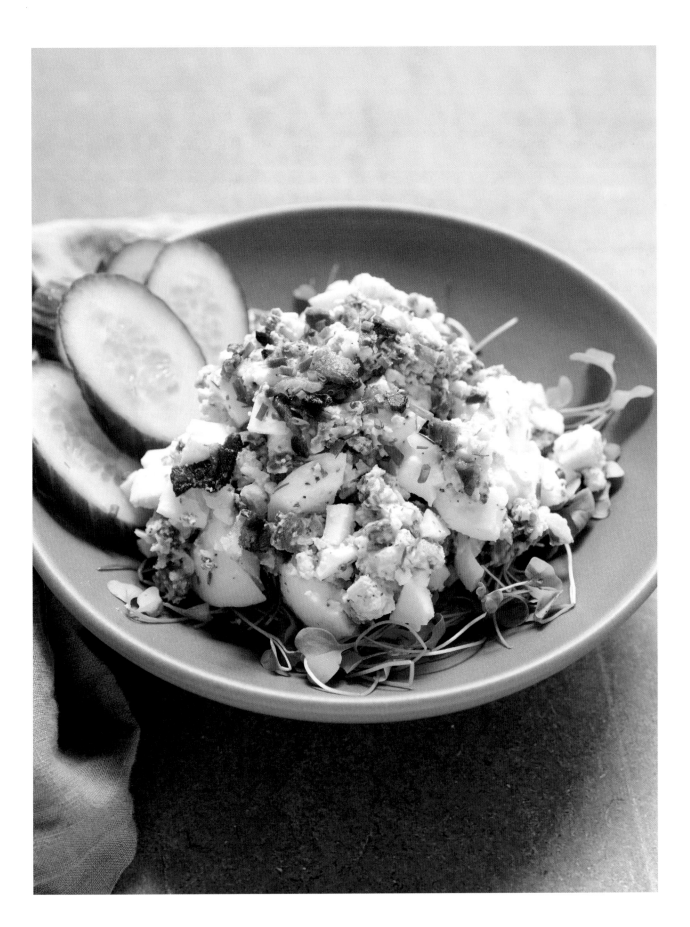

NUTS | **EGGS** | NIGHTSHADES | **FODMAPS** | **DAIRY** | **21DSD-FRIENDLY**

Kale, Bacon & Goat Cheese Frittata

PREP TIME: 15 minutes | COOK TIME: **45 minutes** | YIELD: **4 servings**

Frittatas are the perfect portable breakfast, and they're so easy to reheat in a toaster oven (my preference) or microwave. This combination packs tons of nutrient-dense kale with your eggs and gets amazing flavor from the bacon and goat cheese. It'll be an instant family favorite.

1/2 pound bacon, chopped

1 tablespoon cooking fat of choice (optional)

2 cups chopped fresh kale

8 large eggs

1/4 cup full-fat coconut, nut, or dairy milk

1/2 teaspoon sea salt

1/2 teaspoon ground black pepper

4 ounces goat cheese, crumbled

Preheat the oven to 375°F.

Heat an ovenproof 12-inch skillet over medium heat. Place the bacon in the pan and cook for 5 to 10 minutes, until crispy. Taste the cooked bacon—if it's fairly salty, use less salt later in the recipe. If the pan is looking a little dry, add the cooking fat.

Add the kale to the skillet and cook until softened, 3 to 4 minutes.

While the bacon and kale are cooking, in a large mixing bowl whisk together the eggs, coconut milk, salt, and pepper.

Pour the egg mixture into the skillet, over the bacon and kale. Top with the goat cheese (if using).

Transfer the skillet to the oven and bake for 25 to 30 minutes, until the eggs are no longer runny, the frittata puffs up a bit, and the edges are golden brown.

DAIRY-FREE?
Omit the cheese.

LOW-FODMAP?
Use almond or other nut milk or a lactose-free dairy milk; dairy and coconut both contain FODMAPs.

176   **BREAKFAST**   CALORIES: **549** | FAT: **48 g** | PROTEIN: **26 g** | CARBS: **5 g** | FIBER: **1 g** | NET CARBS: **4 g**

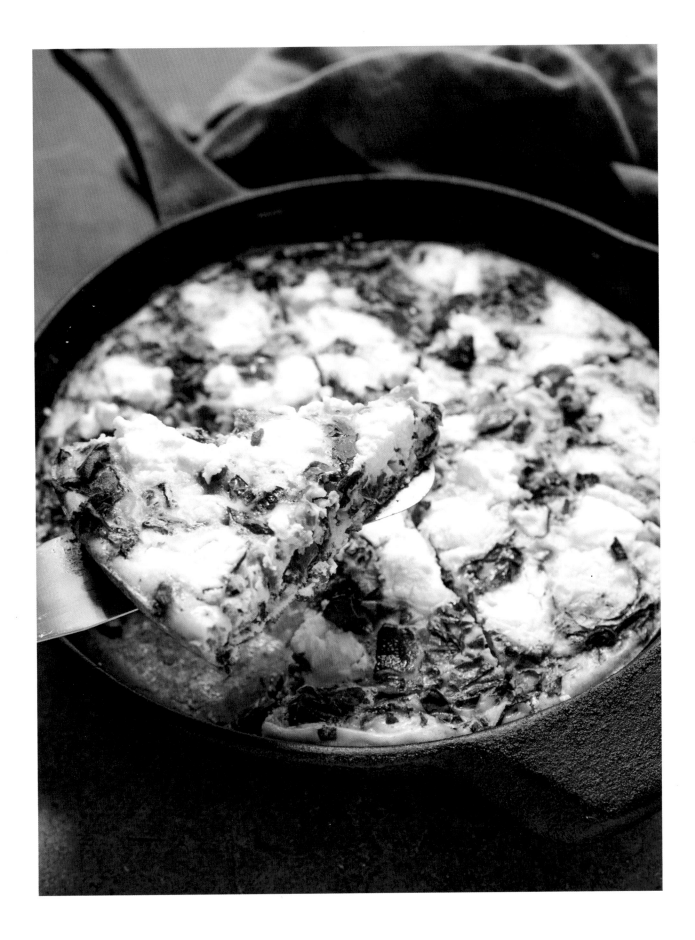

Italian Sausage, Peppers & Spinach Frittata

PREP TIME: 15 minutes | COOK TIME: **40 minutes** | YIELD: **4 servings**

Meat and veggies give this frittata tons of flavor and protein! Mix it up with different greens or any color bell peppers you like. Pair a slice or two of this frittata with a fresh, leafy salad for a well-rounded breakfast.

1 tablespoon cooking fat of choice

1 medium yellow onion, diced

1 medium red bell pepper, sliced into rounds

1/4 teaspoon sea salt

1/4 teaspoon ground black pepper

1 pound ground pork

2 tablespoons Italian Spice Blend (page 330)

1 cup chopped frozen spinach

8 large eggs

1/4 cup full-fat coconut, nut, or dairy milk

4 ounces grated hard cheese, such as Parmigiano-Reggiano or Pecorino Romano (optional)

Preheat the oven to 375°F.

Place the cooking fat, onion, bell pepper, salt, and pepper in an ovenproof 12-inch skillet over medium heat and cook until the onion is translucent and beginning to brown on the edges, 3 to 4 minutes.

Add the ground pork and spice blend to the skillet and cook for 5 to 8 minutes, until no pink remains, breaking the meat up with a spatula as it cooks. Add the spinach and cook for 3 to 5 minutes to warm through and break apart.

While the pork and spinach are cooking, in a large mixing bowl, whisk together the eggs and coconut milk.

Pour the egg mixture into the skillet, over the pork and spinach. Top with the cheese (if using). Transfer the pan to the oven and bake for 15 to 20 minutes, until the eggs are no longer runny, the frittata puffs up a bit, and the edges are golden brown.

DAIRY-FREE?
Omit the cheese.

CALORIES: **627** | FAT: **47 g** | PROTEIN: **43 g** | CARBS: **7 g** | FIBER: **1 g** | NET CARBS: **6 g**

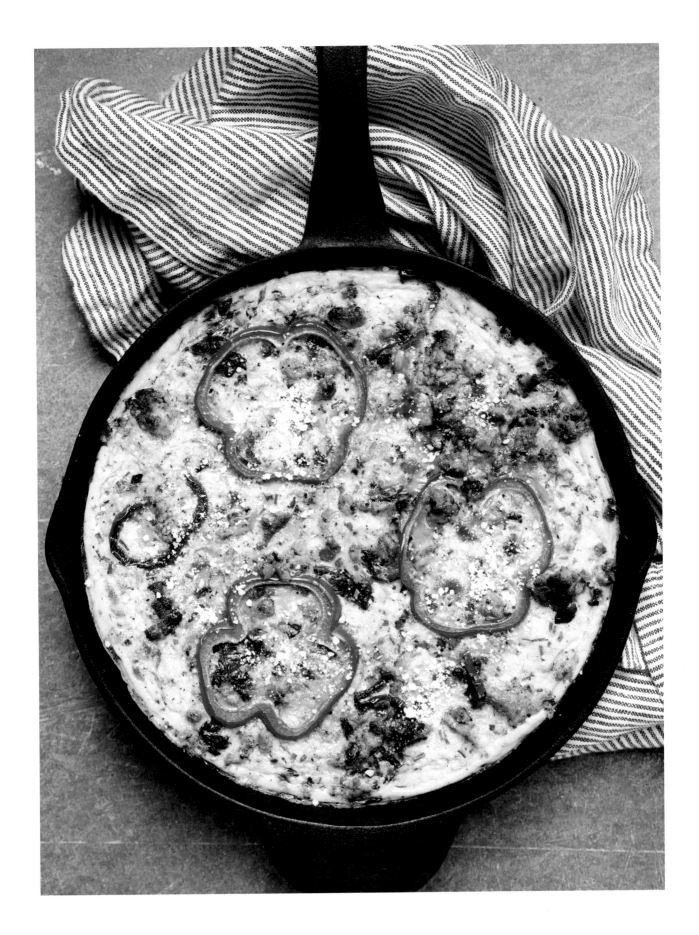

10-Minute Breakfast Hash

PREP TIME: **10 minutes** | COOK TIME: **15 minutes** | YIELD: **4 servings**

Looking for something quick, protein-packed, and egg-free to start your day? This hash is simple and perfect. If Brussels sprouts aren't in season, replace them with some finely sliced Lacinato kale.

1 pound ground pork

1 1/2 tablespoons Italian Spice Blend (page 330)

2 to 3 pinches of ground cinnamon

1 pound Brussels sprouts, trimmed and shredded, or 1 (12-ounce) bag preshredded Brussels sprouts

1/2 teaspoon Trifecta Spice Blend (page 330)

2 ounces goat cheese, crumbled (optional)

Heat a large skillet over medium heat. Place the pork in the hot skillet, season with the Italian Spice Blend and cinnamon, and stir to incorporate. Cook the meat for 5 minutes, breaking it up with a spatula as it cooks.

Add the Brussels sprouts, season with the Trifecta Spice Blend, and continue cooking for another 8 to 10 minutes, until the Brussels sprouts have softened and the meat is cooked through.

Sprinkle the goat cheese on top before serving, if desired.

DAIRY-FREE?
Omit the cheese.

CALORIES: **394** | FAT: **28 g** | PROTEIN: **26 g** | CARBS: **10 g** | FIBER: **4 g** | NET CARBS: **6 g**

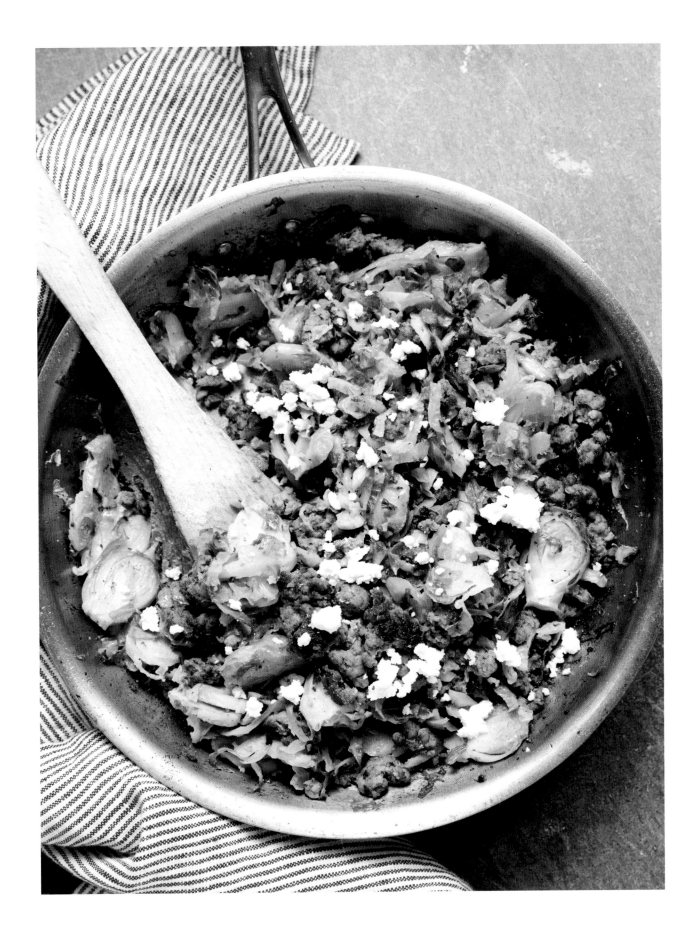

Matcha Chia N'Oatmeal

PREP TIME: 5 minutes, plus time to set | YIELD: **3 servings**

Missing a bowl of soft cereal for breakfast? Try this no-oats oatmeal—what I call n'oatmeal! I enjoy it cold, but you can also warm it up. It's easy to customize to your taste, too. Instead of adding matcha, add some cacao powder and vanilla extract, or try vanilla extract and some frozen blueberries. The base works with lots of options!

1 cup full-fat coconut milk

1 cup water

2 teaspoons matcha powder

2 scoops collagen peptides

5 drops stevia extract

1/4 cup whole chia seeds

1 tablespoon ground chia seeds (optional)

Shredded coconut or coconut flakes, for garnish

Put all the ingredients except the whole and ground chia seeds and the shredded coconut in a blender and blend until smooth. Taste and add more stevia if desired.

Pour the mixture into a large glass mason jar, add the whole chia seeds, cover, and shake well to combine. Refrigerate for 8 hours or overnight to allow the chia seeds to gel.

After it sets, whisk the mixture vigorously to break up the gelled seeds so that they're evenly distributed and the mixture is smooth and thick.

Add the ground chia seeds (if using), cover, and shake to combine. Place in the refrigerator to set for up to 1 hour, until thickened a bit more. If you prefer a thinner consistency, you can omit the ground chia seeds.

Garnish with shredded coconut before serving.

> **FODMAP-FREE?**
> Replace the coconut milk with almond milk or lactose-free whole milk or half and half.

CALORIES: **291** | FAT: **23 g** | PROTEIN: **12 g** | CARBS: **12 g** | FIBER: **9 g** | NET CARBS: **3 g**

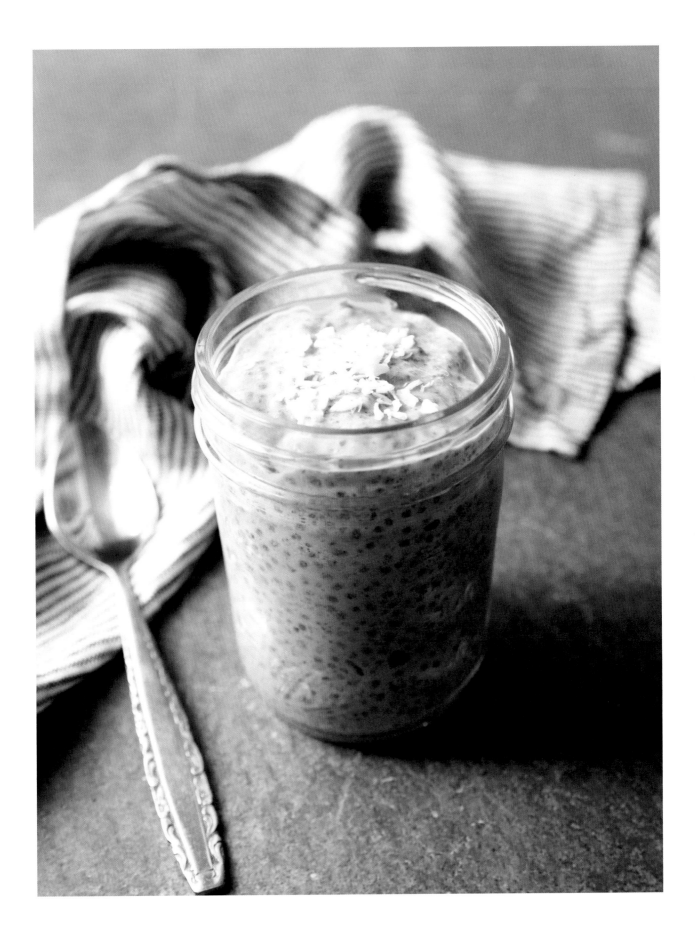

Lemon Blueberry Keto Muffins

PREP TIME: **10 minutes, plus time for the batter to thicken** | COOK TIME: **20 minutes** |
YIELD: **about 8 muffins (1 per serving)**

Unlike typical muffins, these aren't loaded with sugar, and they pack a punch of healthy fats! If you're missing baked goods, try one of these now and then. I recommend freezing them so you aren't tempted to have them more than a couple of times a week—just defrost overnight when you want one.

3 large eggs

1/2 cup full-fat cream cheese or ricotta cheese, room temperature

Grated zest of 3 lemons

Juice of 2 lemons

1 teaspoon pure vanilla extract

1/8 teaspoon green stevia, or 2 or 3 drops stevia extract (optional)

1 1/4 packed cups cashew flour (see Tip)

2 tablespoons coconut flour

1/2 teaspoon baking soda

Pinch of sea salt

1/2 cup fresh blueberries

Preheat the oven to 350°F. Line 8 wells of a standard-size muffin tin with parchment paper liners.

In a food processor or blender, blend together the eggs, cream cheese, lemon zest, lemon juice, vanilla extract, and stevia (if using) until well combined.

In a large mixing bowl, combine the cashew flour, coconut flour, baking soda, and salt. Pour in the wet ingredients and stir to combine. Gently fold in the blueberries. Allow the batter to sit on the countertop for about 10 minutes, until it thickens a bit.

Pour the batter into the prepared wells of the muffin tin, filling all wells evenly. Bake for 20 minutes, or until a toothpick inserted into the center of a muffin comes out clean.

DAIRY-FREE?

You can use dairy-free Kite Hill ricotta; just omit the salt from the recipe.

NOTE

The cashew flour gives these muffins a slightly denser texture than what you may be used to with grain-based muffins, so a smaller portion will be more filling.

TIP

If you can't find cashew flour, you can make your own in a food processor by pulsing raw cashews into a flour-like consistency. (Just don't pulse it so much that it turns into cashew butter!) You can also try making these muffins with almond flour instead.

CALORIES: **313** | FAT: **24 g** | PROTEIN: **10 g** | CARBS: **17 g** | FIBER: **2 g** | NET CARBS: **15 g**

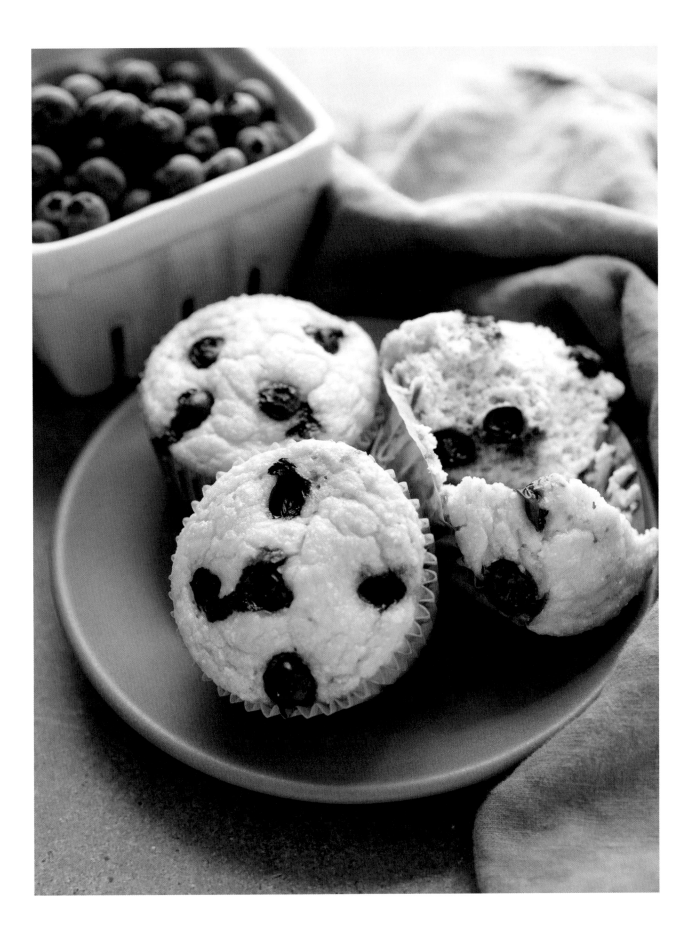

Pumpkin Spice Keto Pancakes

PREP TIME: **15 minutes, plus time for the batter to thicken** | COOK TIME: **35 to 40 minutes** |
YIELD: **12 to 14 pancakes (about 4 per serving)**

These deliciously spiced pancakes are the perfect way to enjoy a weekend morning. To save time in the morning, you can make the batter the night before and refrigerate it overnight to allow it to thicken. Serve these pancakes with some breakfast sausage for a well-balanced meal.

6 large eggs

3/4 cup canned pumpkin (see Note)

1/4 cup plus 2 tablespoons coconut flour

2 teaspoons pumpkin pie spice

1 teaspoon pure vanilla extract

1 teaspoon baking soda

1 teaspoon ground cinnamon, plus extra for garnish

2 pinches of sea salt

10 to 20 drops stevia extract

4 tablespoons ghee (page 336) or butter, divided, plus more for serving

Place all the ingredients except the ghee in a food processor and pulse to combine. Alternatively, place all the ingredients in a medium-sized mixing bowl and whisk vigorously. Allow the batter to sit on the countertop for about 10 minutes, until it thickens a bit.

Melt 1 tablespoon of the ghee in a large skillet over medium-low heat. Pour it into the batter and stir to combine.

Add 1 tablespoon of the ghee to the skillet and return it to the heat. Spoon 3 to 4 tablespoons of batter into the skillet to make 3-inch pancakes. Cook until bubbles begin to appear on the tops of the pancakes, 2 to 3 minutes. Flip the pancakes over and cook for another 2 to 3 minutes, until the bottom is golden brown. Repeat with the remaining batter, adding 1 tablespoon of ghee to the skillet between batches.

Serve with ghee and a sprinkle of cinnamon.

NOTE

When purchasing canned pumpkin for this recipe, make sure it's 100% pumpkin, no other ingredients added. If you use pumpkin from a carton or fresh pumpkin that you cook, your pancake batter will be significantly thinner because those options contain more water. To compensate, you'll likely need to add more coconut flour.

TIP

If you want the taste of maple syrup without a high carb count, blend just 1 teaspoon of maple syrup with 1 tablespoon of nut butter, butter, or ghee to use as a topping.

CALORIES: **417** | FAT: **27 g** | PROTEIN: **19 g** | CARBS: **24 g** | FIBER: **13 g** | NET CARBS: **11 g**

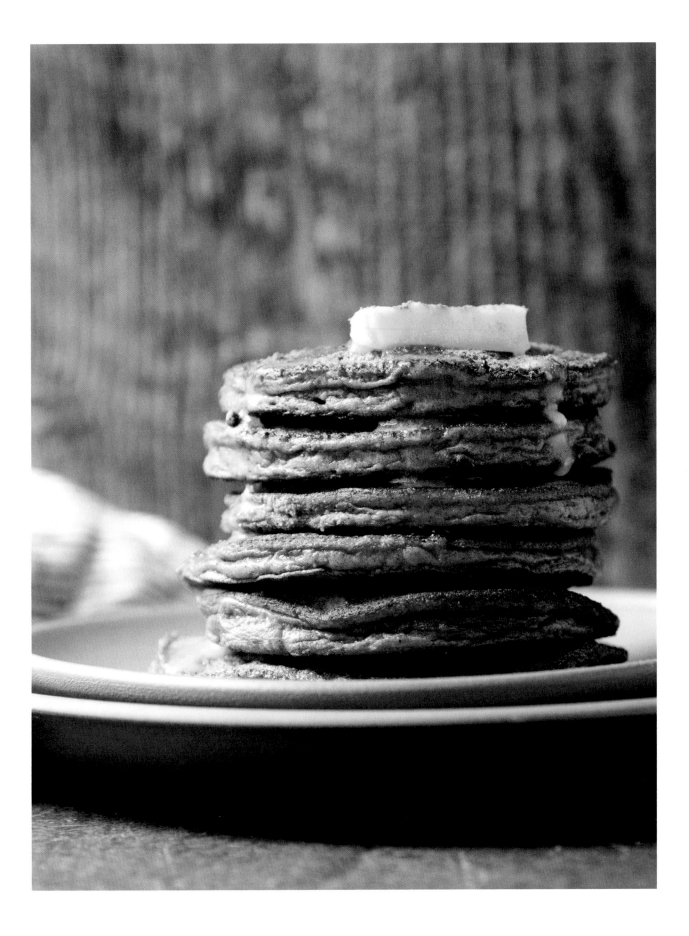

Chocolate Raspberry Smoothie

PREP TIME: **5 minutes** | YIELD: **1 serving**

Berries are a great low-carb fruit to enjoy on your keto diet, especially raspberries! Packed with fiber and flavor, raspberries perfectly balance the creamy chocolate in this smoothie. The collagen adds protein, and you can even add more than I've called for if you like!

3/4 cup water

1/2 packed cup frozen raspberries

4 large ice cubes (approximately 1/2 cup)

1/4 cup full-fat coconut, nut, or dairy milk

1/4 medium avocado, peeled

2 tablespoons cacao powder

2 tablespoons ground chia or flax seeds (see Tip)

2 scoops grass-fed collagen peptides

1/4 teaspoon pure vanilla extract

1/8 teaspoon green stevia, or 2 or 3 drops stevia extract (optional)

Pinch of sea salt

Cacao nibs, for garnish (optional)

Whole fresh raspberries, for garnish (optional)

Place all the ingredients in a blender and blend until smooth. If you prefer a thinner smoothie, add more water or milk to your liking.

Garnish with cacao nibs and fresh raspberries, if desired.

FODMAP-FREE?

Omit the avocado and add one more scoop of grass-fed collagen peptides or 1 tablespoon of nut butter. Replace the coconut milk with almond milk or lactose-free whole milk or half and half.

TIP

I recommend using ground seeds instead of whole seeds because they are more digestible and their nutrients more bioavailable (readily used by the body). Ideally, grind the seeds immediately before using, or grind them in batches each week and keep them in the refrigerator to use in smoothies or to sprinkle on salads.

CALORIES: **444** | FAT: **27 g** | PROTEIN: **28 g** | CARBS: **27 g** | FIBER: **19 g** | NET CARBS: **8 g**

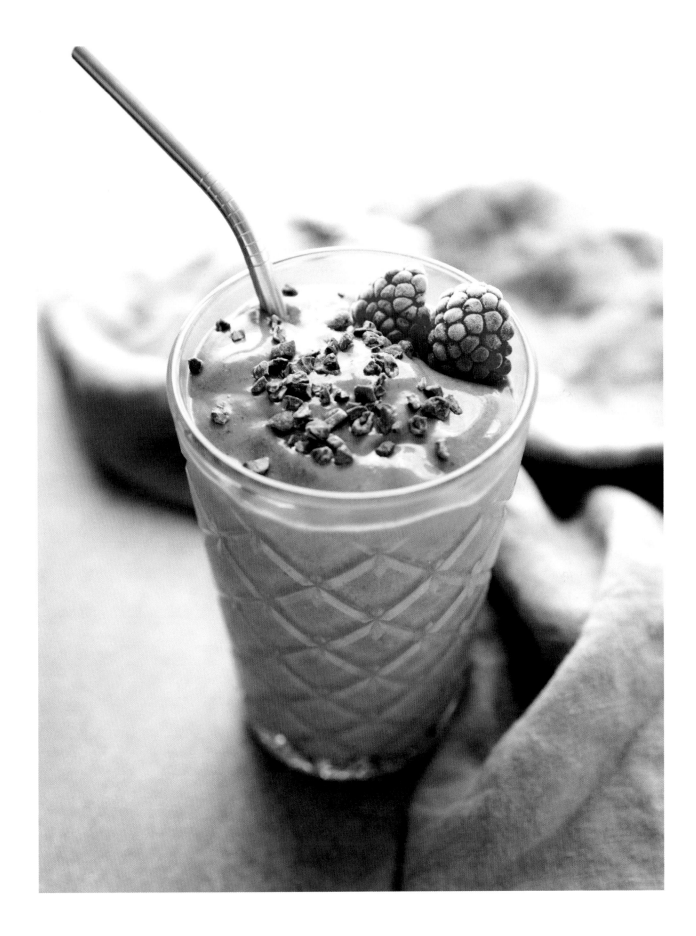

Pumpkin Spice Smoothie

PREP TIME: 5 minutes | YIELD: 2 servings

There's a hidden ingredient in this smoothie that you'd never guess was there unless you were the one blending it: cauliflower! A darling of the keto world, this nutritious veggie easily replaces frozen banana in smoothies to add bulk and vitamins. While it's a hint sweet, this is a veggie-filled breakfast option.

1 cup full-fat coconut, nut, or dairy milk

3/4 cup canned pumpkin (see Note)

1/2 cup frozen riced cauliflower

1 cup water

1 teaspoon ground cinnamon, plus extra for garnish if desired

1 teaspoon pumpkin pie spice

1 teaspoon pure vanilla extract

Small handful of ice (optional)

2 scoops collagen peptides

1/8 teaspoon green stevia, or 2 or 3 drops stevia extract (optional)

1 tablespoon coconut chips, for garnish (optional)

Place all the ingredients except the coconut chips in a blender and blend until smooth. If you prefer a thinner smoothie, add more water or milk to your liking.

Garnish with ground cinnamon and coconut chips before serving, if desired.

NOTE

When purchasing canned pumpkin for this recipe, make sure it's 100% pumpkin, no other ingredients added. If you use pumpkin from a carton or fresh pumpkin that you cook, your smoothie will be significantly thinner because those options contain more water.

CALORIES: **302** | FAT: **24 g** | PROTEIN: **13 g** | CARBS: **12 g** | FIBER: **3 g** | NET CARBS: **9 g**

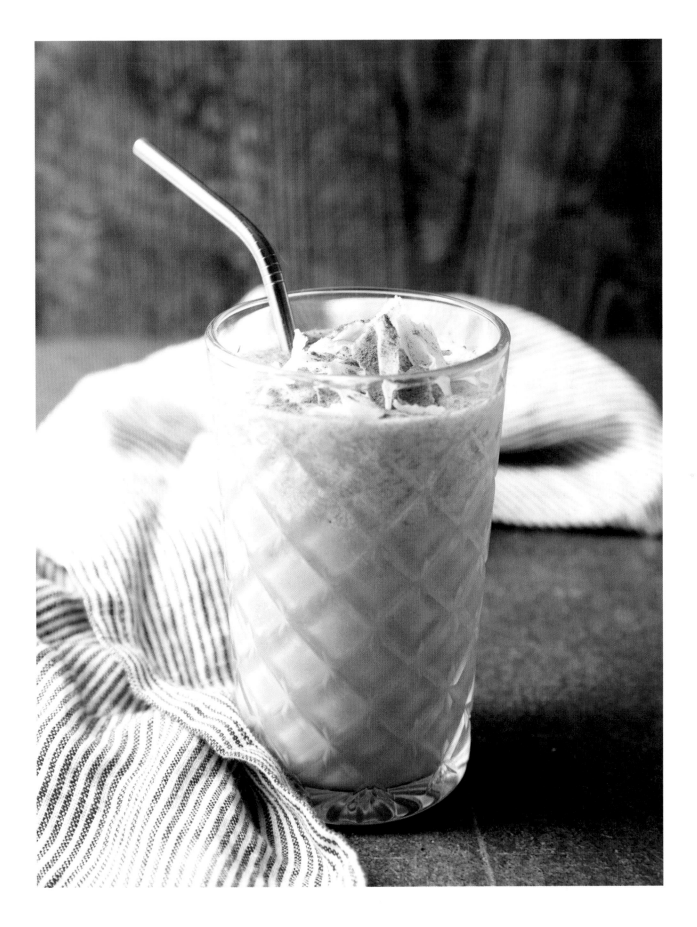

Dreamy Matcha Latte

PREP TIME: 2 minutes | YIELD: **1 serving**

When I first tried matcha, I wasn't totally sure I was a fan, but when I added cacao butter to create this latte, I was completely sold! If you've never tried matcha (a type of green tea powder), this version will hook you. Matcha is loaded with antioxidants—a nutrition bonus to start your day!

1 cup hot water

1/3 cup full-fat coconut, nut, or dairy milk

1 tablespoon cacao butter

1 scoop grass-fed collagen peptides

1/2 to 1 teaspoon matcha powder

2 or 3 drops stevia extract (optional)

Place all the ingredients in a blender and blend until smooth.

FODMAP-FREE?

Replace the coconut milk with almond milk or lactose-free whole milk or half and half.

MAKE IT 21DSD-FRIENDLY

Omit the stevia extract.

NOTES

Cacao butter comes in chunks, so you can estimate the amount. The exact amount isn't critical, and you may find you enjoy a bit more or a bit less.

If you want a stronger matcha flavor, you can go up to 1 teaspoon of matcha; if you want it creamier, you can add more coconut milk.

TIPS

Ceremonial-grade matcha tastes better than culinary-grade matcha, but either will work.

If your latte tastes too "grassy," decrease the amount of matcha powder you use. If it tastes too weak, increase it slightly, about 1/8 teaspoon at a time.

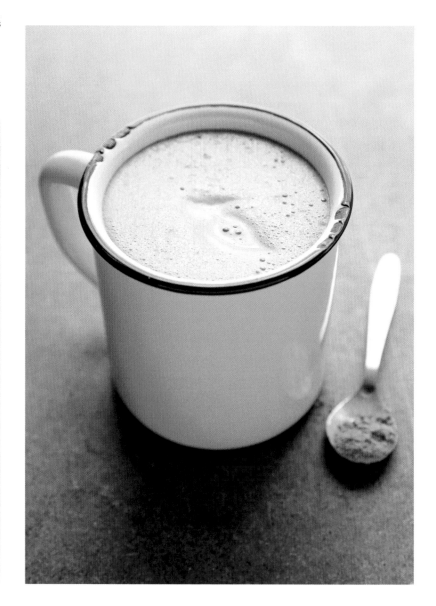

CALORIES: **261** | FAT: **23 g** | PROTEIN: **13 g** | CARBS: **2 g** | FIBER: **0 g** | NET CARBS: **2 g**

Creamy Keto Coffee

PREP TIME: 2 minutes | YIELD: 1 serving

This creamy coffee recipe will quickly become your go-to! Once you try this combination, you'll wonder how you loved coffee any other way. Try it with a pinch of ground cinnamon, some cacao powder, or some vanilla extract to vary the flavor.

1 cup brewed coffee

1/4 to 1/3 cup full-fat coconut, nut, or dairy milk

1 tablespoon cacao butter (see Note)

1 scoop grass-fed collagen peptides

1 scoop MCT powder

2 or 3 drops stevia extract (optional)

Pinch of sea salt

Ground cinnamon, for garnish

Place all the ingredients in a blender and blend until smooth.

Garnish with ground cinnamon.

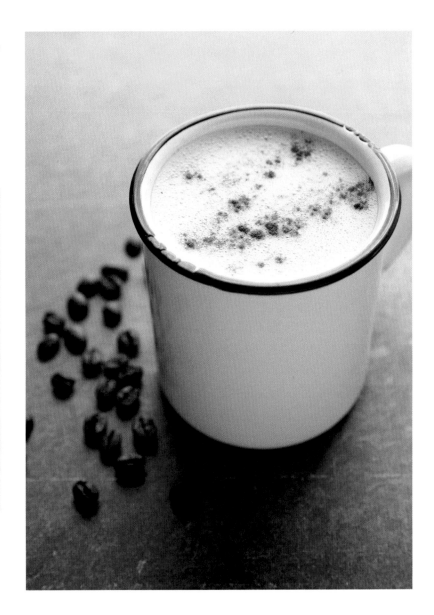

FODMAP-FREE?
Replace the coconut milk with almond milk or lactose-free whole milk or half and half.

MAKE IT 21DSD-FRIENDLY
Omit the stevia extract.

NOTE
Cacao butter comes in chunks, so you can estimate the amount. The exact amount isn't critical, and you may find you enjoy a bit more or a bit less.

TIP
Make it a mocha! Add 1 teaspoon of cacao powder and use only 2 teaspoons of cacao butter.

CALORIES: **320** | FAT: **30 g** | PROTEIN: **11 g** | CARBS: **3 g** | FIBER: **1 g** | NET CARBS: **2 g**

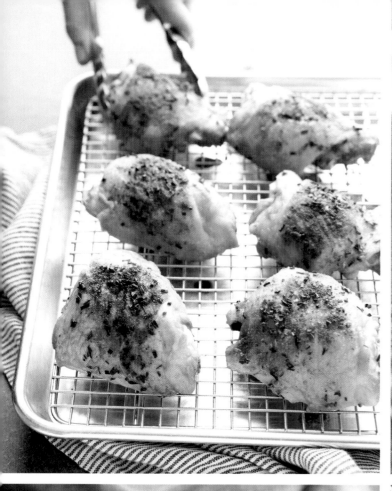

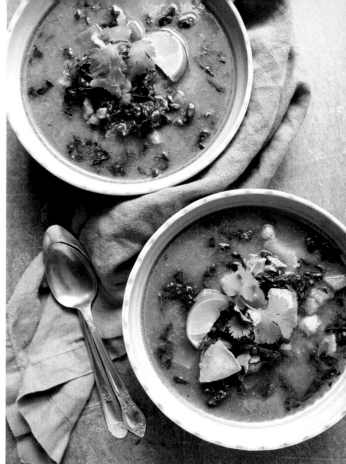

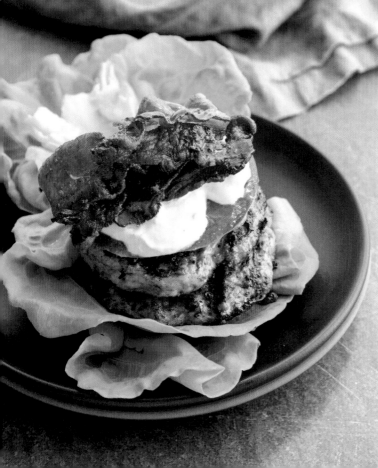

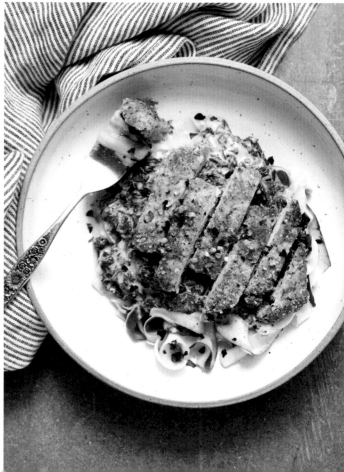

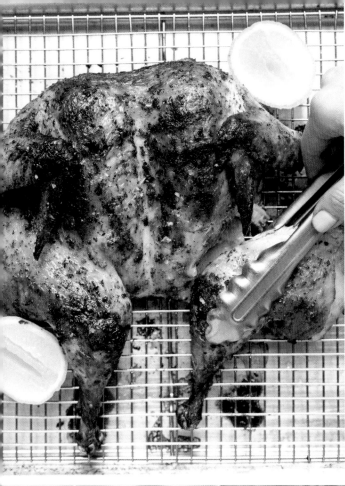

Main Dishes: Chicken

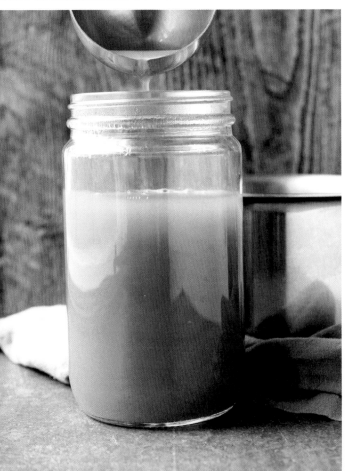

Chicken Salad Collard Wraps

PREP TIME: **20 minutes** | YIELD: **8 wraps (2 per serving)**

When grain-based wraps are out of the picture, collard greens are the perfect way to wrap up chicken (or tuna) salad. But the chicken salad is the real star here—it's delicious freshly made and even better a day or two later!

1 cup finely chopped celery

1/2 cup finely chopped red onions

1/2 cup mayonnaise, homemade (page 335) or store-bought

1 tablespoon Super Garlic Spice Blend (page 330)

2 pounds cooked chicken breast, shredded or finely chopped (see Tips)

Sea salt and ground black pepper

8 to 16 large leaves collard greens

2 cups microgreens, or 1 cup broccoli sprouts, radish sprouts, or other sprouts

In a medium-sized mixing bowl, combine the celery, red onions, mayo, and spice blend. Add the shredded chicken and mix to combine. Taste to check the seasoning and add salt and pepper if desired.

Lay the collard greens flat on a cutting board and remove the stems. Cut away the thick stem most of the way through the leaf, but stop before the top, so the leaf stays connected (you don't want to cut the leaf in half).

After cutting away the stem, there will be a small gap between the sides of the leaf. Overlap these sides so there is no space between them. On each leaf, lay 1/2 cup of the chicken salad mixture and 1/4 cup of the microgreens. If you have smaller leaves or you don't think 1 leaf will be sturdy enough, you can use 2 leaves layered one on top of the other.

Wrap each collard leaf like a burrito, folding the bottom up first, then the sides, then continuing to roll until all the contents are tucked inside. Eat whole or slice in half before serving.

EGG-FREE?

Mash a ripe avocado to use in place of the mayonnaise.

TIPS

To make the easiest chicken ever, butterfly boneless chicken breasts by laying them flat on a cutting board and slicing them in half horizontally, so the pieces are thinner. Place the chicken on a rimmed baking sheet and season lightly on both sides with salt, pepper, and garlic powder. Bake in a preheated 350°F oven for 15 minutes.

To make this recipe even easier, you can use a cooked rotisserie-style chicken from your local grocery store. Look for a chicken without additives or preservatives aside from salt, pepper, and other herbs or seasonings.

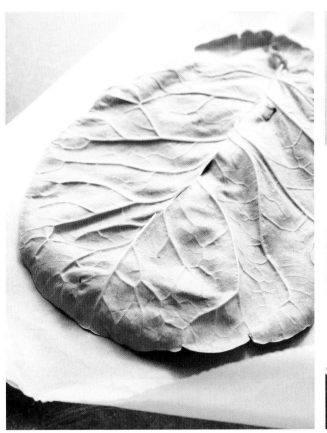 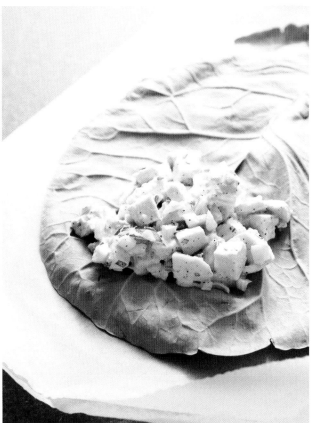

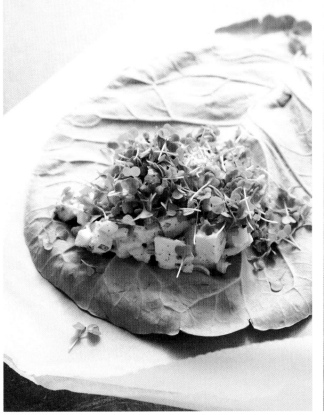 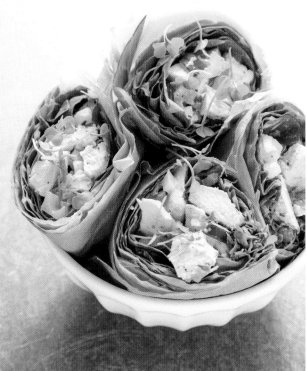

Crispy Chicken Spinach Alfredo

PREP TIME: **25 minutes** | COOK TIME: **35 minutes** | YIELD: **4 servings**

This is a veggie-packed twist on an otherwise not-so-nutritious meal! The greens-loaded cheesy sauce can also be served as a side dish on its own—it's almost like creamed spinach.

4 medium zucchini

1 1/2 pounds boneless, skinless chicken thighs

Sea salt and ground black pepper

1/4 cup cooking fat of choice

FOR THE BREADING

1 cup almond flour or other raw nut or seed meal or flour

2 tablespoons coconut flour

2 tablespoons Super Garlic Spice Blend (page 330)

1 large egg

FOR THE SPINACH ALFREDO SAUCE

5 tightly packed cups finely chopped fresh spinach (about two 5-ounce bags)

1/2 cup full-fat coconut, nut, or dairy milk

1/2 cup grated hard cheese, such as Parmigiano-Reggiano or Pecorino Romano

1 teaspoon granulated garlic

1/4 teaspoon ground black pepper

Sea salt (optional)

FOR GARNISH

Coarse sea salt

Red pepper flakes

Preheat the oven to 375°F. Line a rimmed baking sheet with parchment paper.

Make the zucchini into noodles using a spiral slicer, a handheld julienne peeler, or even a regular vegetable peeler (if using a regular peeler, the noodles will be wide and flat instead of spaghetti shaped). You should get 3 cups of noodles. Set aside.

Prepare the chicken: Tear 2 large sheets of plastic wrap from a roll and place 1 sheet on a large cutting board. Set a chicken thigh on the plastic wrap, then place the second sheet of plastic wrap on top. Using a kitchen mallet, evenly pound the chicken until it's roughly 1/4 inch thick. Repeat this process for all pieces of chicken. Season the chicken on both sides with a few pinches each of salt and pepper.

Place a large, heavy-bottomed sauté pan over medium heat. Melt the cooking fat in the pan and allow it to become hot, about 5 minutes. While the fat is heating, bread the chicken.

Create a breading station for the chicken: In a large shallow bowl or dish, whisk the almond flour, coconut flour, and spice blend until well combined. In a second large shallow bowl or dish, whisk the egg until well beaten. Dip a piece of chicken into the egg to coat it completely, allowing excess egg to drip off. Next, dredge the chicken in the flour mixture to coat it completely, gently shaking off any excess. Repeat this process for all pieces of chicken.

Working in batches, place the chicken in the hot pan and cook for 3 to 4 minutes on each side, until the breading has turned golden brown, adding more oil as needed. Transfer the browned chicken to the prepared baking sheet. Once all of the chicken has been browned, place the baking sheet in the oven and bake for 10 minutes, or until the internal temperature of the chicken reaches 165°F.

Meanwhile, make the alfredo sauce: Combine the spinach, milk, cheese, garlic, and pepper in a large saucepan and heat over medium-low heat, stirring often. Let the sauce reduce slowly for 8 to 10 minutes, until it thickens, then remove the pan from the heat. Taste, add salt if desired, and adjust the seasonings to taste.

Add the zucchini noodles to the alfredo sauce, stir everything together, and return to the heat for 2 to 3 minutes, until the noodles are fork-tender.

Serve the chicken over the zucchini alfredo and garnish with coarse salt and red pepper flakes.

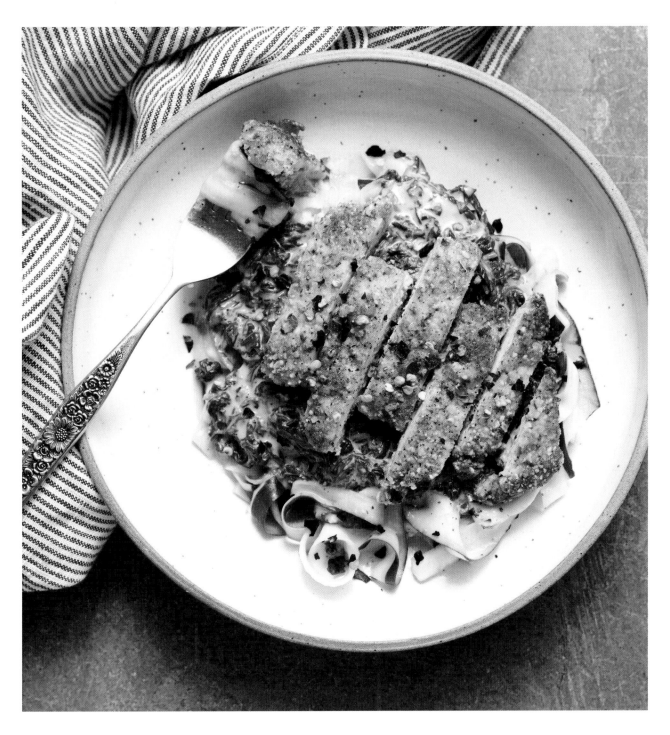

Hidden Veggie Ranch Burgers

PREP TIME: **20 minutes** | COOK TIME: **15 to 30 minutes** | YIELD: **8 burgers (2 per serving)**

Bold herbs and spices pack these burgers with a flavor punch. And they're loaded with low-carb shredded zucchini for extra veggies (read: extra nutrition)! If you like heat, top these with Buffalo sauce by mixing hot sauce with ghee and lemon juice.

FOR THE PATTIES

2 medium zucchini, grated (about 1 cup)

2 pounds ground chicken thigh or turkey (see Note)

1/4 cup chopped fresh chives

3 tablespoons Ranch Spice Blend (page 331)

2 tablespoons chopped fresh parsley

Grated zest of 2 lemons

1/2 teaspoon sea salt

FOR SERVING

1 head iceberg lettuce or butter lettuce, leaves separated

Ranch Dressing (page 347)

Cooked bacon (optional)

Sliced tomato (optional)

Place the grated zucchini in a paper towel or cheesecloth and squeeze out the excess water.

In a large mixing bowl, combine all the ingredients for the patties and mix thoroughly with your hands. Form the meat mixture into 8 equal-sized patties.

Preheat a grill or grill pan to medium-high heat. Grill the burgers for 5 to 6 minutes per side, until the chicken has cooked through and no pink remains. You may need to work in batches, depending on the size of your grill or pan.

Assemble the burgers: Place a burger on a double layer of lettuce leaves, add the ranch dressing, bacon, and tomato (if using), and top with another double layer of lettuce leaves.

NIGHTSHADE-FREE?

Omit the tomato.

NOTE

These burgers taste best when made with ground chicken thigh instead of turkey! If you are unable to find ground chicken thigh, you can make your own: Working in batches, place boneless, skinless chicken thighs in a food processor and pulse until the chicken is the texture of ground meat.

TIP

These patties can be wrapped in plastic wrap or foil and stored in the freezer for up to 6 months. I suggest defrosting them in the refrigerator for 24 hours before using.

CALORIES: **496** | FAT: **34 g** | PROTEIN: **40 g** | CARBS: **6 g** | FIBER: **3 g** | NET CARBS: **3 g**

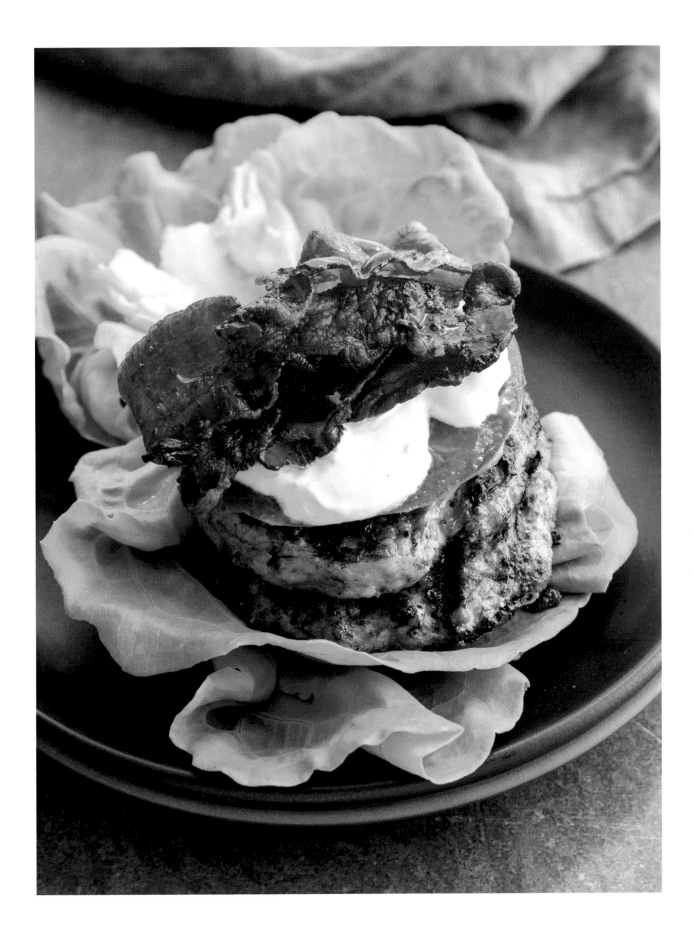

Baby Kale Caesar Salad with Grilled Chicken

PREP TIME: **10 minutes** | YIELD: **4 servings**

Baby kale is relatively new on the salad scene. It's a fantastic way to get lots of vitamins and minerals into your diet without the carbs, and it's perfect in this salad. Chicharrones add just the right crispy crunch to replace bread-based croutons. You'll love this rich, flavorful salad.

8 cups baby kale (see Notes)

2 pounds bone-in, skin-on chicken thighs, grilled or baked (see page 212), then sliced (see Notes)

1/2 cup Caesar Dressing (page 346)

1/4 cup grated hard cheese, such as Parmigiano-Reggiano or Pecorino Romano

FOR SERVING (OPTIONAL)

Chicharrones (pork rinds) (see Notes)

Grated lemon zest

Divide the kale and chicken slices among 4 plates, then drizzle 2 tablespoons of the dressing on each plate. Top with the grated cheese. Add the chicharrones and lemon zest, if desired, before serving.

DAIRY-FREE?
Use the dairy-free version of the Caesar dressing and omit the cheese.

NOTES
If you can't find baby kale, you can use arugula or Lacinato kale. To use Lacinato kale, remove the stems and finely chop the leaves, then squeeze it gently to break down some of its rigidity, so it begins to soften before you mix it with the dressing.

If you're baking or grilling chicken thighs just for this recipe, depending on your protein needs, you may or may not need to use it all. Keep any extra on hand for snacks or easy meals.

The chicharrones provide crunch and replace croutons! They're a delicious addition to this salad, but they're not required. A few brands include 4505 (my favorite), EPIC, and Pork Clouds.

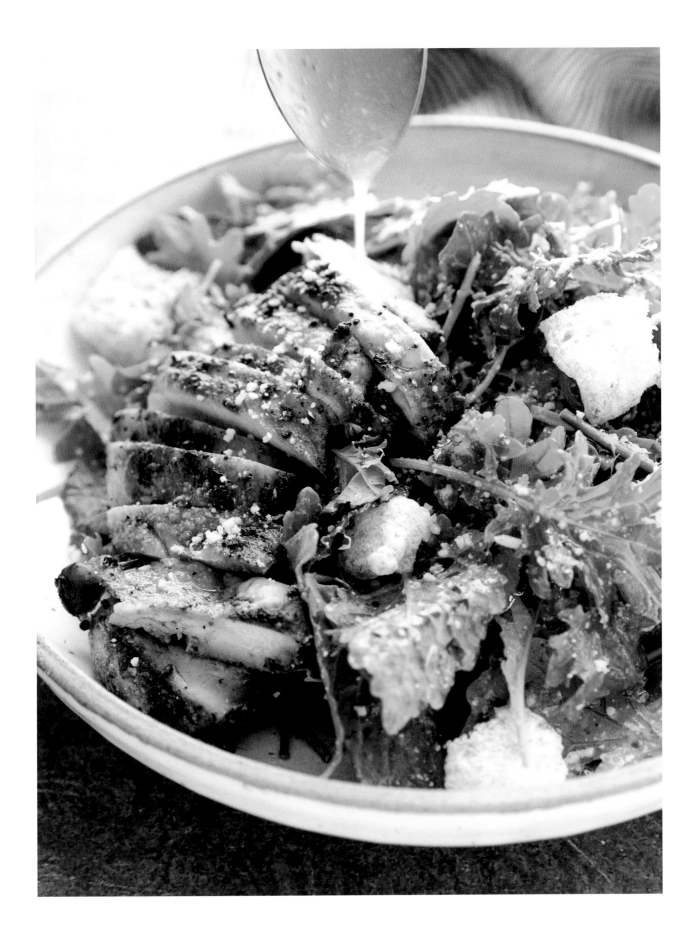

The Best-Tasting Chicken

PREP TIME: 15 minutes, plus time to marinate the chicken | COOK TIME: **1 hour 10 minutes** | YIELD: **6 servings**

For years I tried to re-create the flavor of rotisserie chickens at home, and every time I failed—until now. Two simple steps make this chicken next-level amazing: the overnight marinade and the quick trip to the grill. You'll never want chicken another way again!

3 tablespoons Greek Spice Blend (page 330)

2 tablespoons extra-virgin olive oil, plus more for brushing

Juice of 1 lemon

1 whole chicken (3 1/2 to 4 pounds)

2 or 3 generous pinches of sea salt

2 tablespoons cooking fat of choice

TIPS

Save the bones from your chicken (including the backbone!) to make broth (page 220). I recommend freezing both raw and cooked bones until you fill a gallon-sized bag, then using them for your broth.

If you don't want to grill the chicken first, you can skip that step and simply roast the chicken for 10 minutes more, but the grilling step is what truly makes it "The Best-Tasting Chicken"!

In a small bowl, combine the spice blend, olive oil, and lemon juice. Set aside.

Spatchcock (split) the chicken: Remove any organs (sometimes found in a paper or plastic wrapping) from the inside of the chicken. Place the whole chicken breast side down on a large cutting board. Using kitchen shears or a large, sharp knife, cut along one side of the backbone, then turn the chicken around and cut down the other side. Remove the backbone, then flip the chicken over and firmly press down on the breastbone to flatten.

Place the chicken in a large roasting pan and season generously on both sides with the sea salt. Next, coat both sides of the chicken evenly with the oil mixture. Cover and marinate for at least 1 hour or overnight in the refrigerator (overnight is recommended).

Preheat the oven to 375°F. Preheat a grill or grill pan to high heat.

Brush the hot grill or grill pan with the cooking fat, then sear the chicken skin side down for 8 to 10 minutes, until the skin is charred.

Transfer the chicken to a clean roasting pan, skin side up, and put in the oven for 1 hour, or until the internal temperature of the chicken reaches 165°F. (Test the temperature by inserting the thermometer into a meaty part of the leg, avoiding the bone.)

Remove the chicken from the oven and transfer it to a cutting board. Brush it liberally with olive oil and let rest for at least 10 minutes before serving.

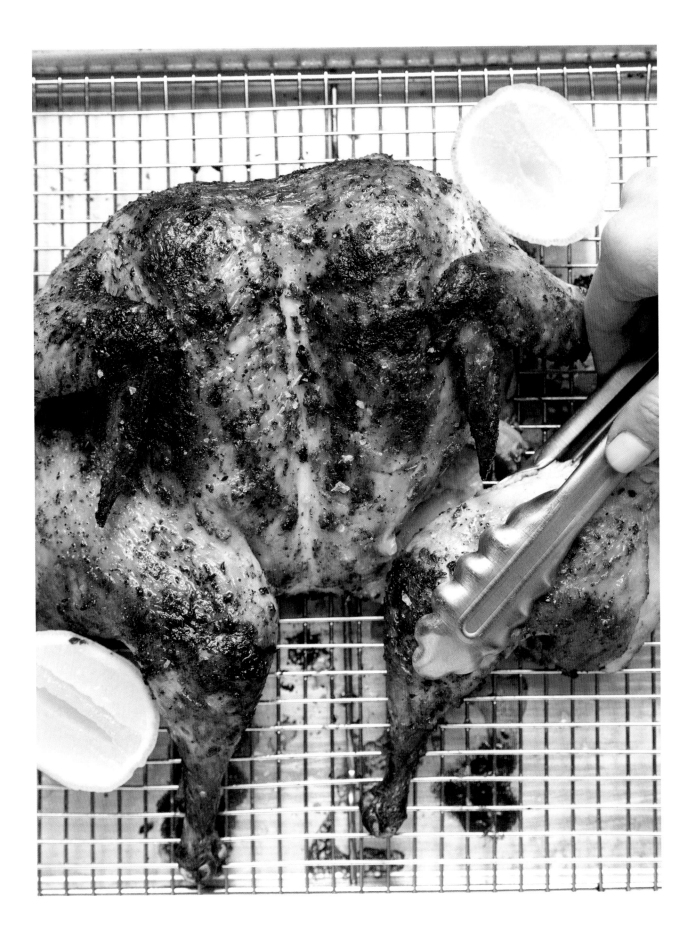

Keto Chicken Tenders

PREP TIME: **15 minutes** | COOK TIME: **40 minutes** | YIELD: **24 tenders (4 per serving)**

Traditional breading is loaded with carbs, and fried foods at restaurants are cooked in inflammatory oils—not ideal. This easy at-home recipe comes to the rescue! I recommend making a double batch; you'll find yourself enjoying leftovers for days. Reheat them in the oven or a toaster oven for the best texture.

1/4 cup cooking fat of choice

1 1/2 cups unsweetened shredded coconut

2 tablespoons coconut flour

1 tablespoon Trifecta Spice Blend (page 330)

2 teaspoons paprika

2 large eggs

2 pounds chicken tenders (see Note)

Prepared yellow mustard, for serving

Preheat the oven to 375°F. Line a rimmed baking sheet with foil, then place a wire baking rack on top of it and set aside.

Place a large, heavy-bottomed sauté pan over medium-high heat. Using just enough fat to coat the bottom of the pan, melt the cooking fat and allow it to become hot (but not smoking), about 5 minutes. While the fat is heating up, bread the chicken.

Create a breading station for the chicken: In a large shallow bowl or dish, whisk the coconut, coconut flour, and spices until well combined. In a second large shallow bowl or dish, whisk the eggs until well beaten.

Dip a piece of chicken into the egg to coat it completely, allowing the excess egg to drip off. Next, dredge the chicken in the flour mixture to coat it completely, gently shaking off any excess. Repeat this process for all the tenders.

Working in batches, place the chicken tenders in the hot pan and cook for 3 to 4 minutes on each side, until the breading has turned golden brown, adding more cooking fat to the pan as needed. Transfer the browned tenders to the wire rack on the baking sheet and space them out evenly.

Once all of the chicken has been browned, place the baking sheet in the oven and bake for 15 minutes, or until the internal temperature of the chicken reaches 165°F. Serve with mustard on the side.

NIGHTSHADE-FREE?
Omit the paprika.

NOTE
If you can't find precut chicken tenders, you can use boneless, skinless chicken breast sliced into roughly 1 by 4-inch strips.

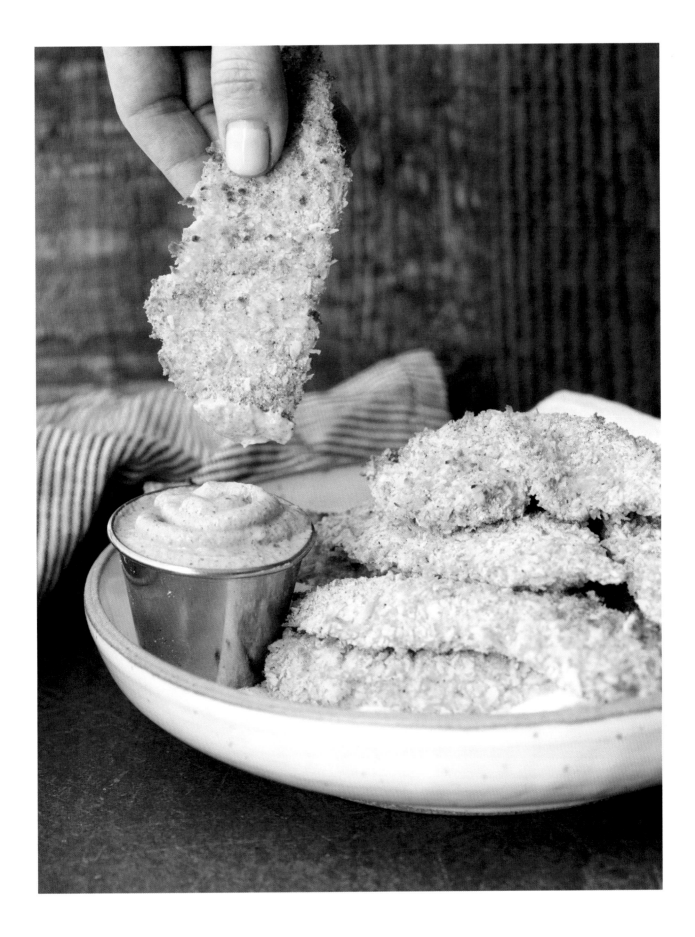

Cacio e Pepe Spaghetti Squash with Grilled Chicken Thighs

PREP TIME: **5 minutes** | COOK TIME: **50 minutes** | YIELD: **6 servings**

Even though I grew up with an Italian father, somehow I was never introduced to cacio e pepe (literally "cheese and pepper") until I took a trip to Italy, where I enjoyed it more than a few times. It's so simple to make this classic with spaghetti squash instead of pasta, and it's delicious as a main course with chicken or as a side dish with other proteins.

1 medium spaghetti squash (about 3 pounds)

1/4 cup (1/2 stick) butter (see Note)

1 cup finely grated hard cheese, such as Parmigiano-Reggiano or Pecorino Romano, plus extra for garnish

1/2 teaspoon ground black pepper

Sea salt

2 pounds bone-in, skin-on chicken thighs, grilled or baked (see page 212), then sliced

Preheat the oven to 375°F.

Make the spaghetti squash noodles: Slice the spaghetti squash in half crosswise. Scoop out the seeds, then sprinkle the cut sides with salt and pepper. Place both halves face down on a rimmed baking sheet and roast for 35 to 45 minutes, until the flesh of the squash is translucent and the skin begins to soften and easily separates from the "noodles" inside.

Allow the squash to cool enough that you can handle it (or carefully use tongs to hold it while still hot), then scoop out the "noodles" into a large serving bowl. Set aside.

Melt the butter in a large skillet and add the spaghetti squash noodles, cheese, and pepper, tossing everything together until the cheese begins to melt and coats the noodles.

Garnish with a pinch or two of sea salt and more black pepper and grated cheese, and serve with the chicken thighs.

> **NOTE**
> If you don't want to use butter, use 2 tablespoons of ghee (page 336) combined with 1/4 cup of full-fat coconut milk.

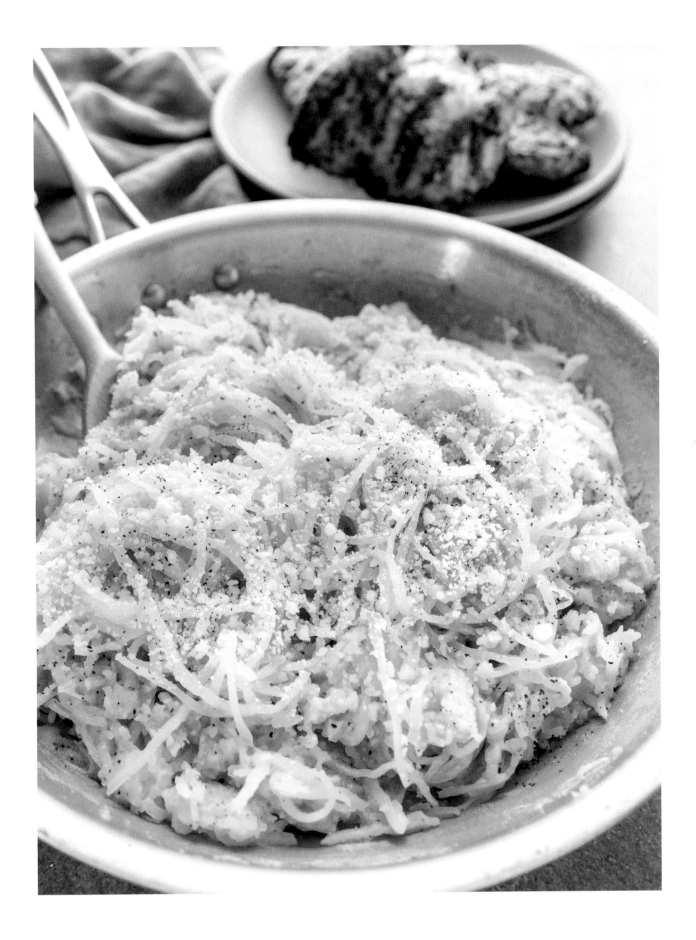

Skillet Chicken Cacciatore

PREP TIME: **15 minutes** | COOK TIME: **1 hour** | YIELD: **6 servings**

With just a few fresh ingredients, this classic chicken dish comes together easily on the stovetop while finishing in the oven, no extra attention required. The pop of pesto takes it over the top, and you'll have enough sauce in the pan to serve this over zoodles or spaghetti squash noodles.

2 tablespoons cooking fat of choice

2 medium yellow onions, sliced

1 medium bell pepper, any color, sliced

Sea salt and ground black pepper

8 large cloves garlic, grated or minced

4 bone-in, skin-on chicken legs (about 2 pounds)

1 1/2 teaspoons dried oregano leaves, divided

1 tablespoon extra-virgin olive oil

1 (26.46-ounce) box chopped tomatoes (see Note)

2 tablespoons balsamic vinegar

FOR GARNISH

Juice of 1/2 lemon

Dried oregano leaves

Grated hard cheese, such as Parmigiano-Reggiano or Pecorino Romano (optional)

2 tablespoons Pesto (page 343) or chopped fresh basil

FOR SERVING (OPTIONAL)

Lemon wedges

Preheat the oven to 375°F.

Melt the cooking fat in 12-inch oven-safe skillet over medium heat. Add the onions and bell pepper, season with a few pinches each of salt and pepper, and cook for 7 to 9 minutes, until the onions become translucent and begin to brown. Stir every few minutes so the onions and peppers don't burn.

Add the garlic and cook for 1 to 2 more minutes, until the garlic starts to turn golden brown.

Season both sides of the chicken with a few pinches each of salt and pepper and 1 teaspoon of the oregano. Reduce the heat to medium-low if it seems the veggies are becoming overly browned or are at risk of burning.

Push the onions, pepper, and garlic to one side of the pan and add two of the chicken legs, skin side down, on the bare part of the pan. Move the onions, pepper, and garlic on top of the chicken, then add the two remaining chicken legs to the other side of the pan, skin side down. Spread the onions, pepper, and garlic back over all the chicken legs, so the chicken is fully covered.

Brown the chicken for 5 to 6 minutes, until the skin starts to crisp up. Flip the chicken, drizzle it with the olive oil, and add the tomatoes and vinegar, filling in the space around the chicken legs. Add a few generous pinches each of salt and pepper and the remaining 1/2 teaspoon of oregano.

Transfer the skillet to the oven and bake for 30 to 40 minutes, until the chicken reaches an internal temperature of 165°F. If you want to crisp up the skin, turn the oven to broil and place the skillet under the broiler for about 5 minutes.

Garnish with fresh lemon juice, dried oregano, grated cheese (if desired), and peso. Serve with lemon wedges if desired.

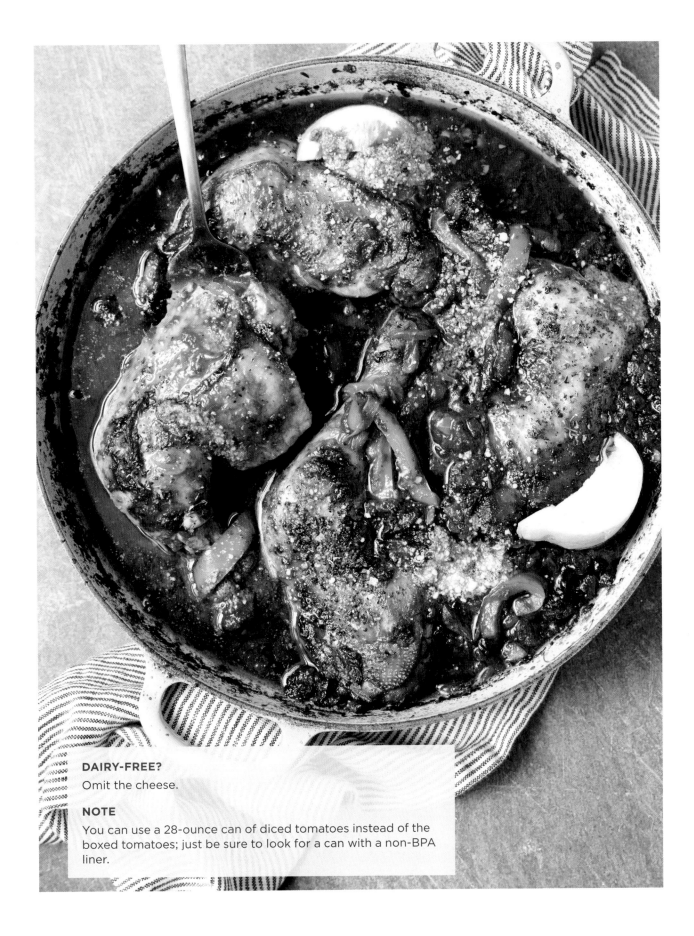

DAIRY-FREE?

Omit the cheese.

NOTE

You can use a 28-ounce can of diced tomatoes instead of the boxed tomatoes; just be sure to look for a can with a non-BPA liner.

Weeknight Roasted Chicken

PREP TIME: **5 minutes** | COOK TIME: **45 minutes** | YIELD: **6 servings**

This method for preparing chicken thighs is a go-to for any low-carb household—it couldn't be easier! Choose any spices you love (clearly garlic is a favorite of mine) and roast away! You can even season half the pan one way and half another to enjoy a different flavor for leftovers during the week.

3 pounds bone-in, skin-on chicken thighs

1/4 cup spice blend of choice (pages 330 to 331) (see Note)

Preheat the oven to 375°F. Set a wire baking rack on a rimmed baking sheet.

Season both sides of the chicken thighs with the spice blend. Place them skin side up on the wire rack and bake for about 45 minutes, until the internal temperature of the chicken reaches 165°F. Check the chicken after 15 minutes to make sure the spices aren't burning—if they look overly browned, brush some olive oil or other cooking fat on top of the thighs to moisten and cover with foil for the remainder of the baking time.

Remove the chicken from the oven and let it cool.

Store the chicken in an airtight container in the refrigerator for up to 5 days.

NOTE

If you're avoiding nightshades and/or FODMAPs, make sure that you use a spice blend without these.

TIP

To reheat the thighs and re-crisp the skin, carefully cut around the bone to remove it, then flatten out the thigh and place it skin side down in a skillet over medium-high heat for a few minutes to crisp, then flip and cook for another 2 minutes, or until warmed through.

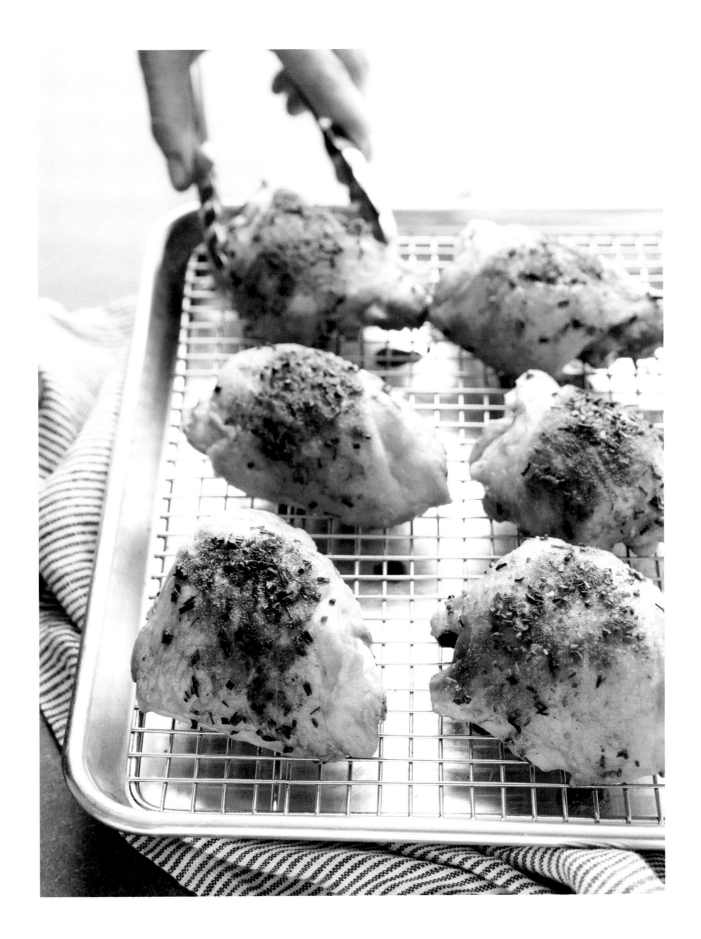

White Chicken Chili

PREP TIME: 25 minutes | COOK TIME: **30 minutes (Instant Pot), 50 minutes (stovetop), or 4 hours (slow cooker)** | YIELD: **6 servings**

If you're looking for a hearty dish that's more filling than a typical soup, this recipe is for you. This broth-based chili is perfect for the whole family. You can make it spicier by adding more jalapeños or milder by leaving them out.

4 slices bacon, chopped into 1/2-inch pieces

1 jalapeño pepper, finely diced

1 medium yellow onion, diced

4 cloves garlic, smashed or roughly chopped

Sea salt and ground black pepper

10 ounces button mushrooms, stemmed and quartered

1 medium carrot, finely diced

2 teaspoons dried oregano leaves

2 teaspoons ground coriander

2 teaspoons ground cumin

2 to 3 cups chicken broth, homemade (page 220) or store-bought, divided

2 teaspoons arrowroot or tapioca starch (optional; see Tip)

1 1/2 pounds boneless, skinless chicken thighs

2 cups chopped zucchini (1/3-inch cubes, 2 to 3 medium zucchini)

FOR GARNISH

1/4 cup chopped fresh cilantro leaves

1/4 cup sliced green onions

1 medium avocado, sliced

FOR SERVING

1 lime, cut into wedges

TO MAKE THIS ON THE STOVETOP:

Place the bacon in a large enameled cast-iron Dutch oven or other heavy-bottomed pot over medium heat. Cook, stirring occasionally, until the fat has rendered, 6 to 8 minutes.

Add the jalapeño and onion and cook until the onion is translucent, 3 to 4 minutes. Add the garlic, season generously with salt and pepper, and cook for 1 to 2 minutes, stirring to combine the ingredients.

Add the mushrooms and cook for 5 to 6 minutes, until softened, then add the carrot, oregano, coriander, and cumin to the pot. Cook until the vegetables begin to brown a bit, about 5 minutes.

Add 2 cups of the broth and the arrowroot (if using) and stir to combine. Add the chicken thighs on top of the vegetables, pressing them down so they're covered by the broth. Add 1/2 to 1 cup more broth if necessary to cover the chicken. Cover and cook for 15 minutes, or until the chicken is cooked through. Add more salt and pepper to taste if necessary.

Remove the chicken thighs from the pot and place on a cutting board or plate, then shred them using 2 forks. Return the shredded chicken to the pot and stir to combine. Add more salt and pepper to taste if necessary.

Continue to cook, uncovered, for 10 minutes, or until the liquid has reduced to your desired consistency. Add the zucchini and cook for about 2 minutes to warm through.

Garnish with cilantro, green onions, and sliced avocado before serving. Serve with lime wedges.

TO MAKE THIS IN A SLOW COOKER:

Cook the bacon in a skillet over medium heat, stirring occasionally, until the fat has rendered, 6 to 8 minutes.

CALORIES: **395** | FAT: **27 g** | PROTEIN: **26 g** | CARBS: **11 g** | FIBER: **2 g** | NET CARBS: **9 g**

Add the jalapeño, onion, and garlic, season generously with salt and pepper, and cook for 1 to 2 minutes.

Transfer the bacon and vegetables, along with the rendered fat, to a slow cooker and add all of the remaining ingredients except for the garnishes and zucchini. Cook on low for 3 to 4 hours. Add the zucchini and remove the chicken. Shred the chicken with 2 forks, then mix it back into the chili. Garnish with cilantro, green onions, and sliced avocado before serving. Serve with lime wedges.

TO MAKE THIS IN AN INSTANT POT OR OTHER MULTICOOKER:

Set the Instant Pot to the sauté function (normal). Once the pot is hot, place the bacon in the pot and cook, stirring occasionally, until the fat has rendered, 6 to 8 minutes. Add the jalapeño, onion, and garlic, season generously with salt and pepper, and cook for 1 to 2 minutes.

Add just 1 cup of chicken broth. Add the remaining ingredients except the zucchini to the pot, reset the cooker to manual, and cook on high pressure for 20 minutes. When cooking is finished, allow the cooker to depressurize on its own; don't flip the valve to release it.

Add the zucchini and remove the chicken. Shred the chicken with 2 forks, then mix it back into the chili. Garnish with cilantro, green onions, and sliced avocado before serving. Serve with lime wedges.

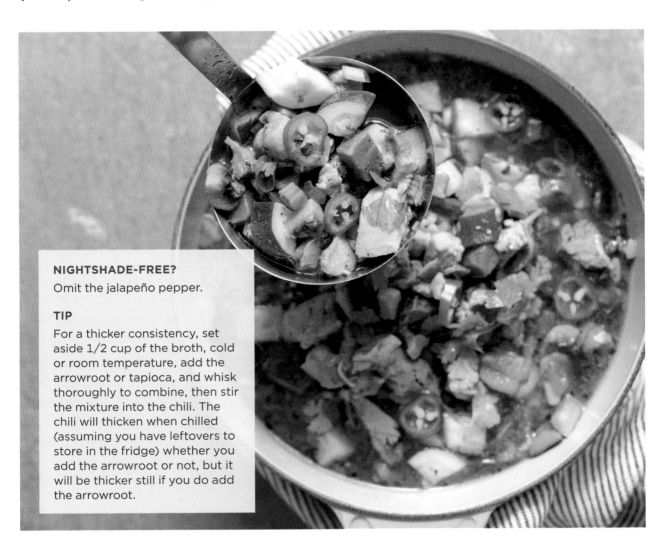

NIGHTSHADE-FREE?
Omit the jalapeño pepper.

TIP
For a thicker consistency, set aside 1/2 cup of the broth, cold or room temperature, add the arrowroot or tapioca, and whisk thoroughly to combine, then stir the mixture into the chili. The chili will thicken when chilled (assuming you have leftovers to store in the fridge) whether you add the arrowroot or not, but it will be thicker still if you do add the arrowroot.

Thai Red Curry Soup

PREP TIME: **20 to 25 minutes** | COOK TIME: **15 minutes (Instant Pot), 25 minutes (stovetop), or 3 to 4 hours (slow cooker)** | YIELD: **6 servings**

This soup is a meal in a bowl! Packed with protein from the chicken and tons of leafy greens, it's satisfying and super simple to make. Keep red curry paste on hand as a pantry staple (I love Thai Kitchen brand) and use it for this dish as well as the Thai Meatballs on page 244.

2 tablespoons cooking fat of choice, divided

2 medium carrots, roughly chopped

1 large yellow onion, diced

1 (1-inch) piece of fresh ginger, peeled and minced or grated

Sea salt

4 cloves garlic, smashed

2 pounds boneless, skinless chicken thighs, cut into 1 1/2-inch pieces

4 cups chicken broth, homemade (page 220) or store-bought

1 (13.5-ounce) can full-fat coconut milk

3 tablespoons red curry paste

2 or 3 dashes of fish sauce

3 cups chopped kale

Chopped fresh cilantro leaves, for garnish

1 lime, cut into wedges, for serving

SERVING SUGGESTION
Serve with a side of Cilantro Cauli-Rice (page 282).

TO MAKE THIS ON THE STOVETOP:

Melt 1 tablespoon of the cooking fat in a large stockpot over medium heat. Add the carrots, onion, and ginger, lightly season with salt, and cook for 4 to 5 minutes, until tender. Add the garlic and cook for 1 minute more.

Make a hole in the veggie mixture and add the remaining tablespoon of cooking fat. Add the chicken, season with salt, and cook for 4 to 5 minutes, until the chicken begins to brown.

Add the broth, coconut milk, red curry paste, and fish sauce and stir to combine. Bring to a boil, then turn the heat down to low and simmer for 10 minutes. Stir in the kale and cook for 5 minutes more.

Garnish with cilantro and serve with lime wedges.

TO MAKE THIS IN A SLOW COOKER:

Put all of the ingredients except the kale in a slow cooker. Cook on low for 3 to 4 hours. Stir in the kale and heat for 5 minutes. Garnish with cilantro and serve with lime wedges.

TO MAKE THIS IN AN INSTANT POT OR OTHER MULTICOOKER:

Set the Instant Pot to the sauté function (normal). Place the carrots, onion, garlic, ginger, and a few pinches of sea salt in the pot and cook for 4 to 5 minutes, until tender.

Add the remaining ingredients except the kale to the pot, season lightly with salt, and cook on the soup setting for 5 minutes. When cooking is finished, allow the cooker to depressurize on its own; don't flip the valve to release it. Stir in the kale and heat for 5 minutes.

Garnish with cilantro and serve with lime wedges.

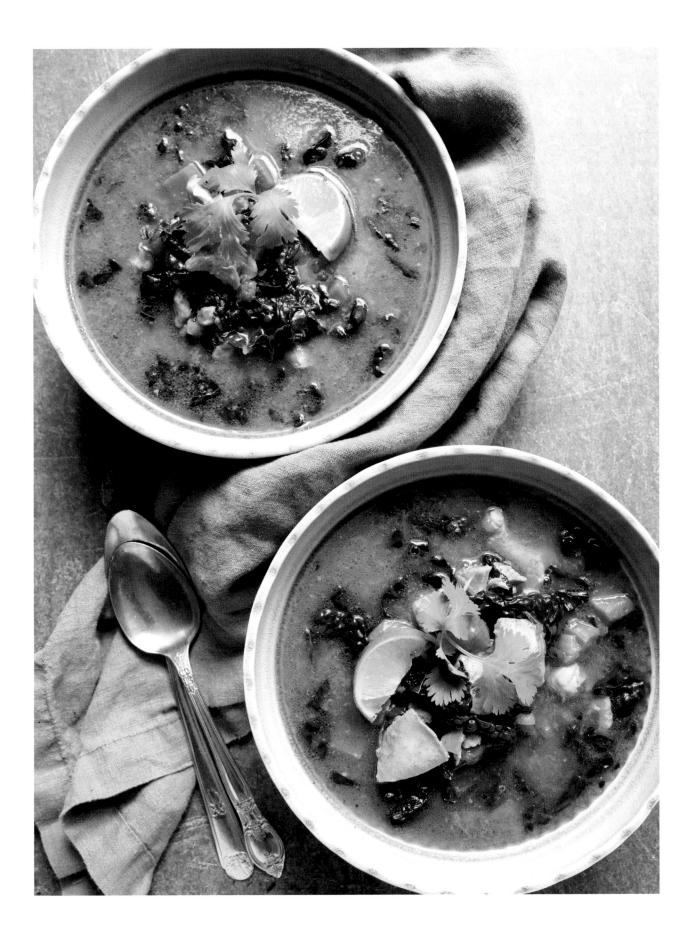

Simple Shredded Chicken

PREP TIME: **5 minutes** | COOK TIME: **6 to 8 hours (slow cooker), 12 minutes (Instant Pot)** | YIELD: **8 servings**

When you want to be sure you've got protein on hand for a variety of recipes, this is a perfect go-to recipe. Mix this chicken with some mayonnaise and seasonings or chopped veggies for a quick chicken salad, or use it to make some quick tacos any night of the week.

4 pounds boneless, skinless chicken thighs

Sea salt

2 cups chicken broth, homemade (page 220) or store-bought

10 cloves garlic, peeled

TO MAKE THIS IN A SLOW COOKER:

Season the chicken with the salt on both sides. Place the meat, broth, and garlic in a slow cooker and cook on low for 6 to 8 hours.

Remove the chicken from the slow cooker, reserving any liquid. Allow it to cool slightly, then shred it with 2 forks. Taste the shredded meat and spoon some of the reserved liquid over it if needed for additional flavor.

TO MAKE THIS IN AN INSTANT POT:

Season the chicken with the salt on both sides. Place it in the multicooker and add the broth and garlic. Cook on high pressure for 12 minutes. When cooking is finished, allow the cooker to depressurize on its own; don't flip the valve to release it.

Store in an airtight container in the refrigerator for up to 5 days.

FODMAP-FREE?
Omit the garlic.

TIP
Preparing this chicken ahead of time is a great way to make weeknight meals easy. When you're ready to eat, sear it in a skillet with some cooking fat and season as desired for the meal you're preparing.

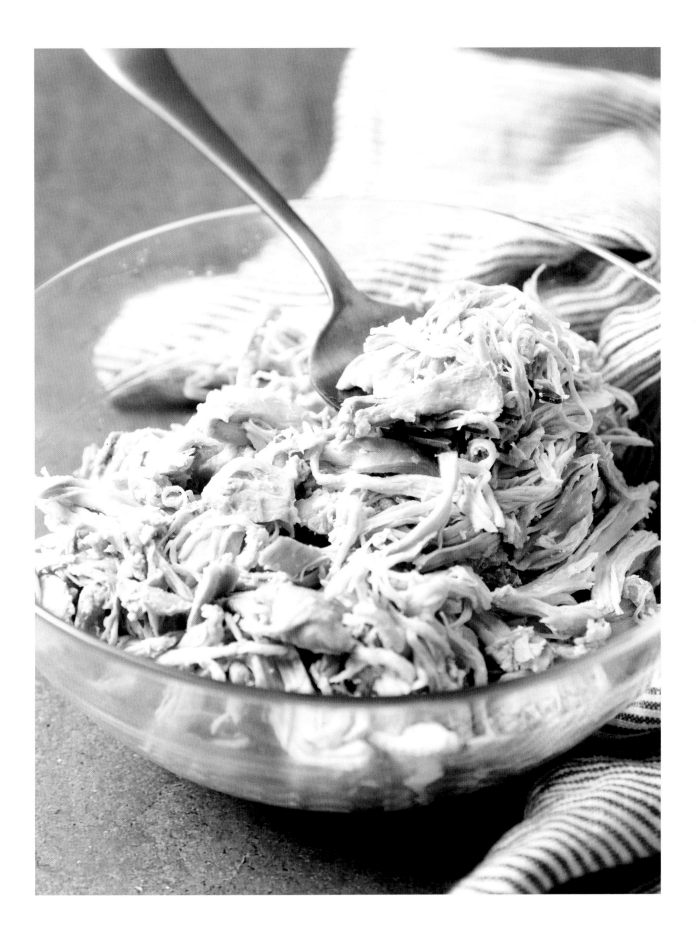

Chicken Broth

PREP TIME: 5 minutes | COOK TIME: **8 to 24 hours (slow cooker), 2 hours (Instant Pot)** |
YIELD: **2 to 3 quarts if slow cooked, 4 quarts if cooked in an Instant Pot (1 cup per serving)**

The best way to make use of the carcass from a whole chicken and other chicken bones is to save them in a gallon-sized zip-top bag in the freezer and use them to make broth. This is a great way to both save money and get extra minerals and electrolytes into your diet.

4 quarts filtered water

1 1/2 to 2 pounds chicken bones with cartilage (see Note)

Cloves from 1 head of garlic, peeled and smashed with the side of a knife

2 tablespoons apple cider vinegar

2 teaspoons sea salt (optional)

TO MAKE THIS IN A SLOW COOKER:

Place all of the ingredients in a slow cooker. Set the heat to high and bring to a boil, then turn the heat down to low. Cook for at least 8 hours and up to 24 hours—the longer it cooks, the better.

Turn off the slow cooker and allow the broth to cool.

TO MAKE THIS IN AN INSTANT POT:

Place all of the ingredients in the multicooker. Cook on high pressure for 2 hours. When cooking is finished, allow the cooker to depressurize on its own; don't flip the valve to release it.

Strain the broth through a fine-mesh strainer or cheesecloth. Pour the cooled broth into glass jars and store in the refrigerator for up to a few days. You can also store it in plastic containers in the freezer until you're ready to use it. Make sure the broth has cooled completely before freezing.

Before using the broth, chip away at the top and discard any fat that has solidified.

FODMAP-FREE?
Omit the garlic.

NOTE
Chicken feet work extremely well to create a gelatinous broth, but if you don't have chicken feet, a carcass from a whole chicken works, as do bones saved from previous meals. Chicken wing bones and necks also work great for making broth.

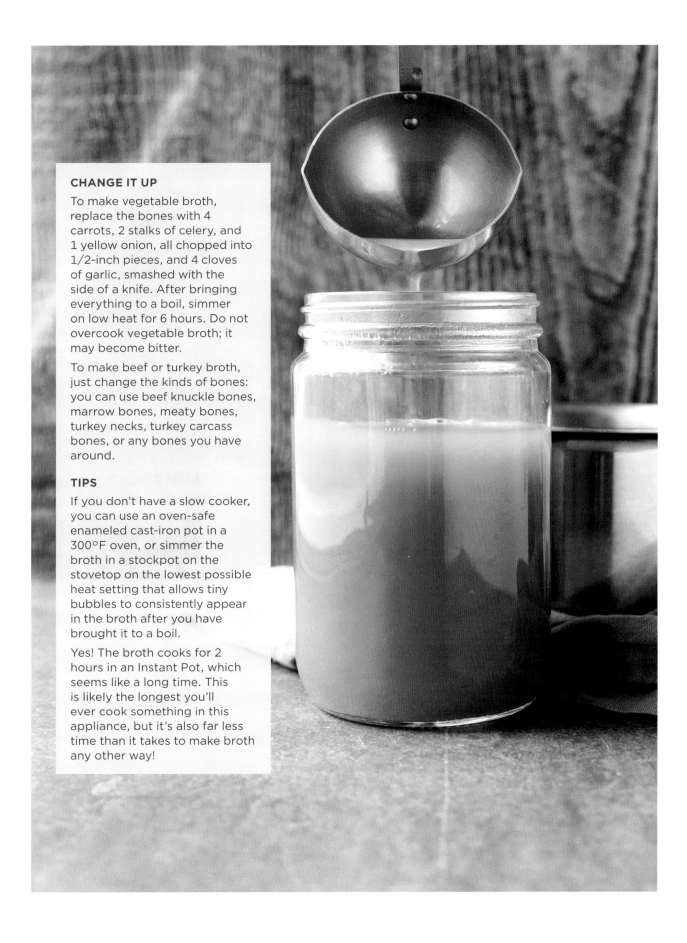

CHANGE IT UP

To make vegetable broth, replace the bones with 4 carrots, 2 stalks of celery, and 1 yellow onion, all chopped into 1/2-inch pieces, and 4 cloves of garlic, smashed with the side of a knife. After bringing everything to a boil, simmer on low heat for 6 hours. Do not overcook vegetable broth; it may become bitter.

To make beef or turkey broth, just change the kinds of bones: you can use beef knuckle bones, marrow bones, meaty bones, turkey necks, turkey carcass bones, or any bones you have around.

TIPS

If you don't have a slow cooker, you can use an oven-safe enameled cast-iron pot in a 300°F oven, or simmer the broth in a stockpot on the stovetop on the lowest possible heat setting that allows tiny bubbles to consistently appear in the broth after you have brought it to a boil.

Yes! The broth cooks for 2 hours in an Instant Pot, which seems like a long time. This is likely the longest you'll ever cook something in this appliance, but it's also far less time than it takes to make broth any other way!

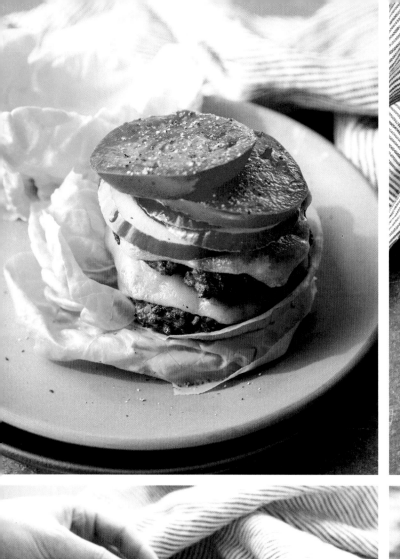

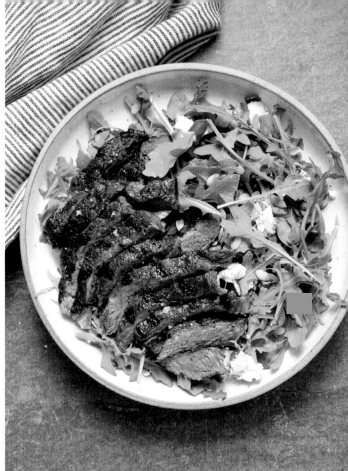

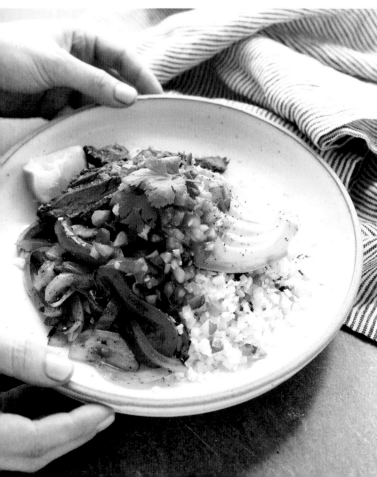

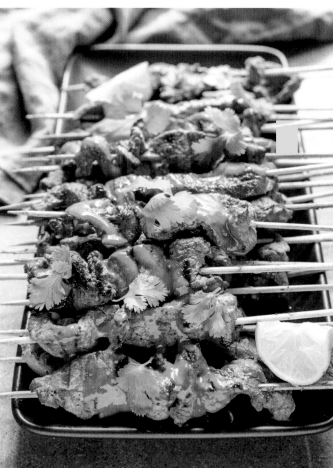

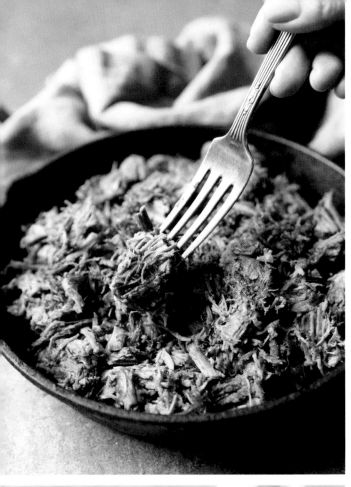

Main Dishes: Beef

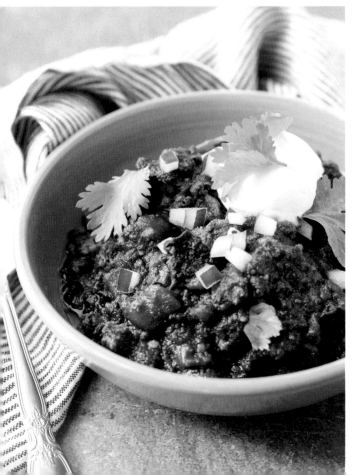

Umami Steak & Arugula Salad

PREP TIME: **15 minutes, plus time to marinate the steak** | COOK TIME: **10 minutes** | YIELD: **4 servings**

This is hands-down the easiest and best marinade you'll ever make for steak! This flavor combination works with nearly any protein, and the flavor infuses quickly, in an hour if that's all you have. Don't skip this simple recipe—it'll quickly become your go-to way to prepare steak.

2 pounds rib eye, hanger steak, or skirt steak

2 to 3 tablespoons coconut aminos

1 tablespoon Trifecta Spice Blend (page 330)

6 cups fresh arugula

1/4 cup pumpkin seeds, pine nuts, or sunflower seeds

4 ounces blue cheese, goat cheese, or feta (optional)

1/2 cup Balsamic Vinaigrette (page 344)

Coarse sea salt, for garnish

Marinate the steak: In a large baking dish, coat the steak evenly in the coconut aminos and the spice blend. Cover and place in the refrigerator to marinate for at least 20 minutes or up to 4 hours.

When you're ready to grill the steak, preheat a grill or grill pan to high heat. Cook the steak for 3 to 5 minutes per side, depending on the thickness and desired level of doneness. Set the cooked steak aside to rest for 10 minutes, then slice it against the grain into thin strips.

While the steak is resting, assemble the rest of the ingredients in large bowls for the salad.

Add the sliced steak on top of the salad and serve while the steak is still warm. Garnish with coarse sea salt.

DAIRY-FREE?
Omit the cheese.

TIP
To pack in even more nutrition without more carbs, add microgreens to this salad! I recommend about 1/4 cup per person.

CALORIES: **695** | FAT: **49 g** | PROTEIN: **54 g** | CARBS: **7 g** | FIBER: **1 g** | NET CARBS: **6 g**

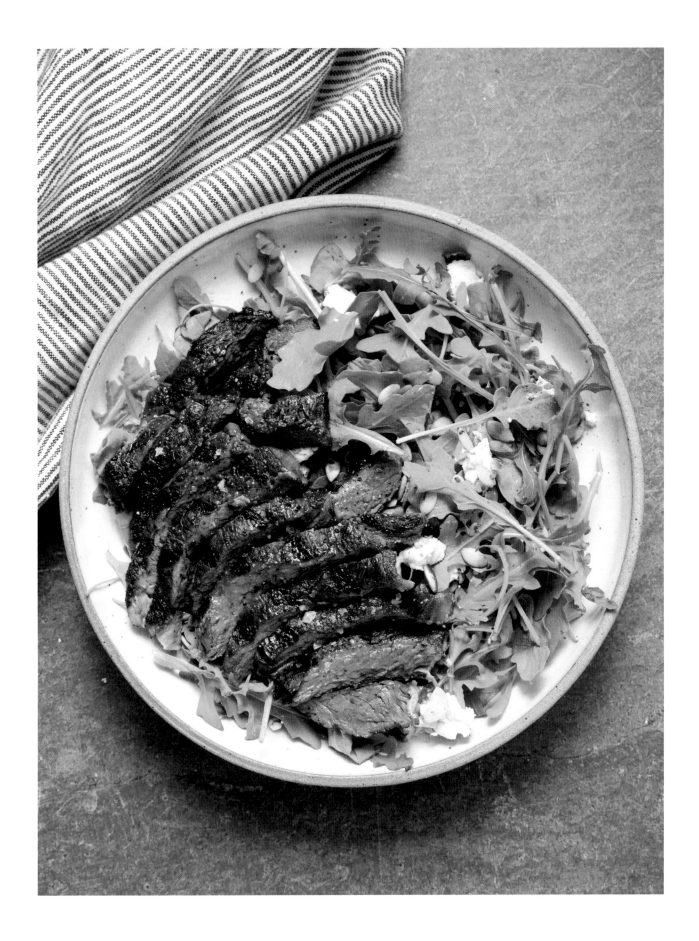

Beef Fajita Bowl

PREP TIME: 15 minutes, plus time to marinate the steak | COOK TIME: **15 minutes** | YIELD: **4 servings**

The fresh garlic, spices, and citrus in the marinade for this fajita steak take the flavor in this bowl over the top. Paired with sliced avocado and salsa you make yourself using the recipe on page (or a store-bought version) and served over cauliflower rice, this bowl is hearty and satisfying!

FOR THE MARINADE

2 tablespoons extra-virgin olive oil

Juice of 4 limes

1/2 teaspoon sea salt

1/2 teaspoon ground black pepper

1 tablespoon Taco & Fajita Spice Blend (page 331)

2 cloves garlic, minced or grated

2 pounds skirt or flank steak

2 medium red bell peppers, sliced

1 large yellow onion, sliced

FOR SERVING

1 batch Cilantro Cauli-Rice (page 282)

Sliced avocado

Pico de gallo or Quick Salsa (page 306)

Chopped fresh cilantro leaves

Lime wedges

MAKE THE MARINADE:

In a large glass baking dish, whisk together the olive oil, lime juice, salt, pepper, spice blend, and garlic.

MARINATE THE STEAK:

Place the steak in the baking dish with the marinade and massage the marinade into it. Cover and place in the refrigerator to marinate for at least 20 minutes or up to overnight.

When you're ready to grill the steak, preheat a grill or grill pan to high heat. Cook the steak for 3 to 5 minutes per side, depending on the thickness and desired level of doneness. Set the cooked steak aside to rest for 10 minutes.

While the steak is resting, grill the bell peppers and onion until they are soft and have grill marks, about 5 minutes, turning as needed to prevent burning. (Alternatively, you can cook the peppers and onions in a skillet with a bit of olive oil, salt, and pepper while you grill the steak.)

To serve, slice the steak against the grain into thin strips and divide the cauli-rice among 4 bowls. Place the steak strips on the cauli-rice and add the grilled peppers and onion. Top with sliced avocado, pico de gallo, and fresh cilantro, and squeeze the lime wedges over the top.

CALORIES: **454** | FAT: **23 g** | PROTEIN: **49 g** | CARBS: **12 g** | FIBER: **2 g** | NET CARBS: **10 g**

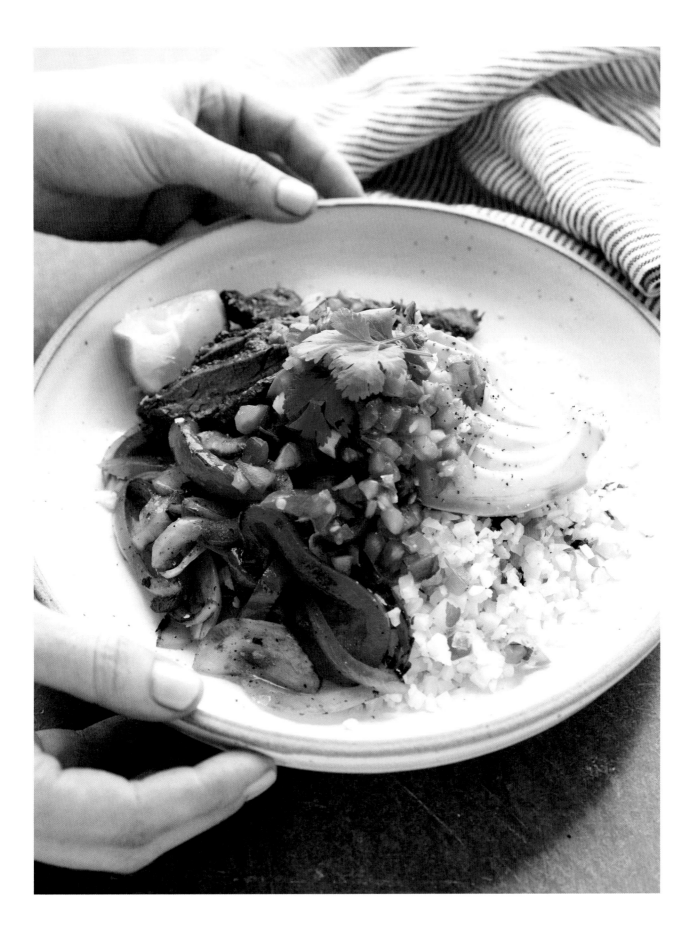

Power Bacon Cheeseburgers

PREP TIME: 15 minutes | COOK TIME: **10 minutes** | YIELD: **8 patties (1 per serving)**

Liver is a fantastic superfood, packed with B vitamins, choline, and iron, but it's often hard to incorporate into everyday meals. These burgers are the perfect way to get the benefits of liver while enjoying a tasty burger. Your family will love these and won't notice the secret ingredient!

1/2 pound bacon (about 8 slices)

1/4 pound chicken livers

1 1/4 pounds ground beef, 85% lean

4 cloves garlic, grated or minced

2 tablespoons ketchup, homemade (page 340) or store-bought

1 teaspoon granulated garlic

1 teaspoon granulated onion

1 teaspoon ground cumin

1 teaspoon paprika

1/2 teaspoon ground black pepper

1/2 to 1 teaspoon sea salt (see Tip)

8 slices cheddar cheese (optional)

1 head Boston/butter or iceberg lettuce, leaves separated, for serving

TOPPINGS (OPTIONAL)

Bacon-y Caramelized Onions (page 294)

Sliced red onion

Sliced tomato

Place the bacon and liver in a food processor and blend until the meat is finely ground.

In a large mixing bowl, mix together the bacon-and-liver mixture, beef, garlic, ketchup, spices, and salt. Divide the mixture into 8 portions and shape into 1/4-inch-thick patties.

Grill the burgers over medium-high heat for about 5 minutes per side, until cooked to 145°F in the center. Top the patties with the cheddar cheese (if using) and allow it to melt.

To serve, place one or two cooked burgers on layered lettuce leaves, then add the toppings and more lettuce if you like.

DAIRY-FREE?

Omit the cheese.

TIP

If you know that the bacon you're using is on the saltier side, start with just 1/2 teaspoon salt. If the burgers seem to need more salt the first time you make these, just add more when you make them again!

CALORIES: **404** | FAT: **32 g** | PROTEIN: **27 g** | CARBS: **3 g** | FIBER: **1 g** | NET CARBS: **2 g**

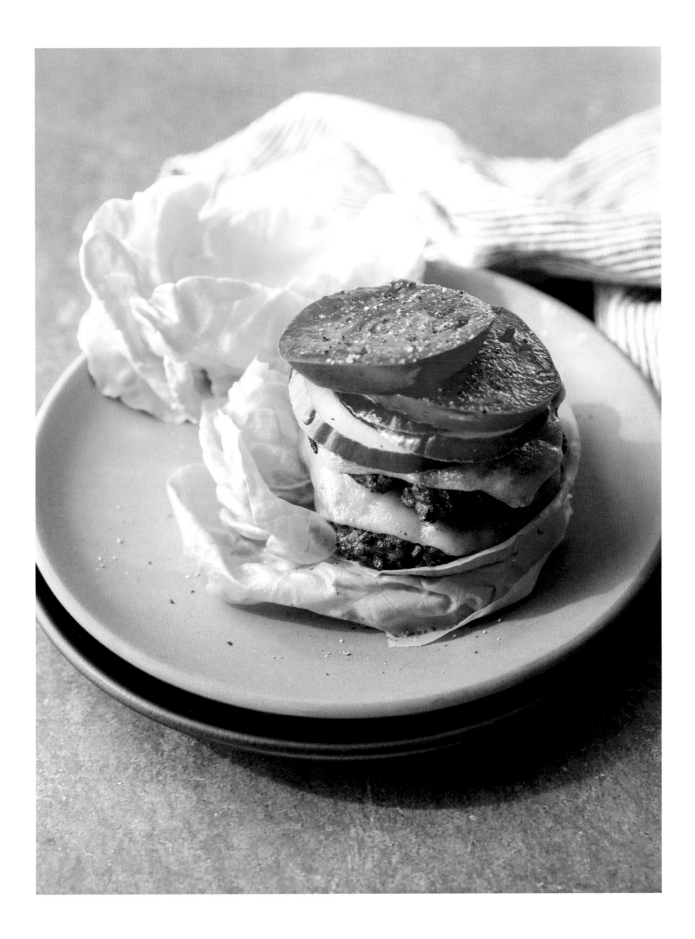

Sloppy Joe Chili

PREP TIME: 20 minutes | COOK TIME: 40 minutes (stovetop), 30 minutes (Instant Pot), or 3 to 4 hours (slow cooker) | YIELD: 6 servings

Growing up, we ate a lot of a popular canned sloppy joe brand that was loaded with junky ingredients—yikes! I wanted to re-create the same amazing flavors in a healthy dish that's more like a chili than a sandwich, and this recipe is it! It's super easy to make and major comfort food!

FOR THE SPICE BLEND

1 tablespoon smoked paprika

1 teaspoon granulated garlic

1 teaspoon granulated onion

1/2 teaspoon sea salt

1/2 teaspoon ground black pepper

FOR THE SLOPPY JOE MIXTURE

2 slices thick-cut bacon, chopped

1 large yellow onion, finely diced

1 medium green bell pepper, finely diced

1 medium red bell pepper, finely diced

Sea salt and ground black pepper

Pinch of ground cinnamon

1 clove garlic, minced or grated

4 portobello mushrooms, cut into 1/2-inch pieces

2 pounds ground beef, 85% lean

1 (28-ounce) can diced tomatoes

3 tablespoons coconut aminos

2 tablespoons ketchup, homemade (page 340) or store-bought

1 tablespoon apple cider vinegar

2 teaspoons Dijon mustard

FOR GARNISH

1 small red onion, diced

1/3 cup full-fat sour cream (optional)

TO MAKE THIS ON THE STOVETOP:

In a small bowl, mix together all the ingredients for the spice blend. Set aside.

Place the bacon in a large stockpot over medium-high heat. Cook, stirring occasionally, until the fat has rendered, about 4 minutes.

Add the onion and bell peppers, lightly season with salt and pepper, add the cinnamon, and sauté until the onions are translucent and beginning to brown, about 5 minutes. Add the garlic and cook for 1 minute more, until fragrant.

Turn the heat down to medium, add the mushrooms, and lightly season with salt and pepper. Cook for 5 minutes, then stir in the spice blend and add the beef. Let the meat cook for a few minutes to begin to brown, then add the diced tomatoes, coconut aminos, ketchup, vinegar, mustard, and cinnamon. Stir to combine, then turn the heat down to medium-low and simmer for 15 to 20 minutes, until the meat is cooked through.

To serve, spoon the sloppy joe mixture onto serving plates and garnish with the red onion and sour cream, if desired.

TO MAKE THIS IN A SLOW COOKER:

In a small bowl, mix together all the ingredients for the spice blend. Set aside.

Place the bacon in a skillet or sauté pan over medium-high heat and cook, stirring occasionally, until the fat has rendered, about 4 minutes.

Transfer the bacon and the rendered fat to a slow cooker with all of the remaining ingredients and the spice blend. Cook on low for 3 to 4 hours.

CALORIES: **421** | FAT: **24 g** | PROTEIN: **34 g** | CARBS: **20 g** | FIBER: **5 g** | NET CARBS: **15 g**

TO MAKE THIS IN AN INSTANT POT OR OTHER MULTICOOKER:

Use 1 (6-ounce) can tomato paste instead of 1 (28-ounce) can diced tomatoes.

In a small bowl, mix together all the ingredients for the spice blend. Set aside.

Set the Instant Pot to the sauté function (normal). Once hot, place the bacon in the pot and cook, stirring occasionally, until rendered, 3 to 4 minutes. Add the onion, bell peppers, and garlic, lightly season with salt and pepper, and sauté until translucent and beginning to brown, about 5 minutes.

Add the remaining ingredients and the spice blend to the pot, reset the cooker to manual, and cook on high pressure for 20 minutes. When cooking is finished, allow the cooker to depressurize on its own; don't flip the valve to release it.

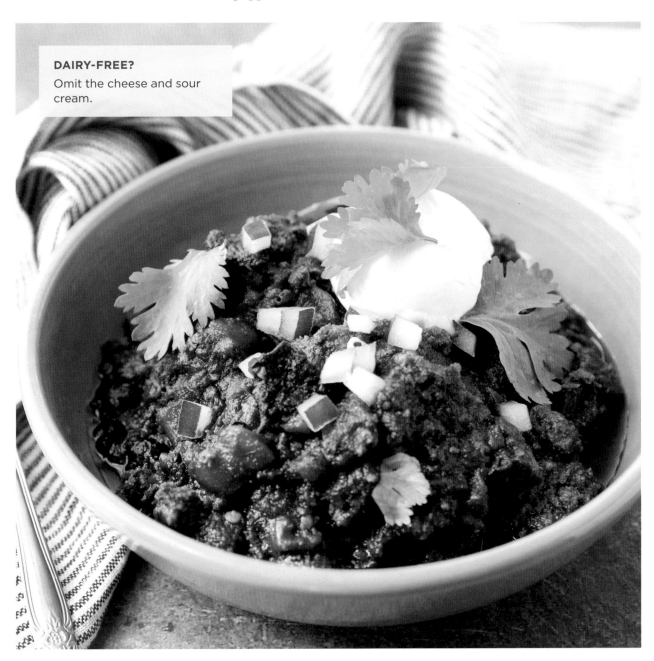

DAIRY-FREE?
Omit the cheese and sour cream.

Mediterranean Meatloaf

PREP TIME: 15 minutes | COOK TIME: **1 hour 15 minutes** | YIELD: **8 servings**

Meatloaf is a classic filling and satisfying meal for the whole family, but this one has a twist: tons of amazing Mediterranean flavor! The blend of herbs and spices in this meatloaf will excite your palate, and it tastes great both freshly made and as reheated leftovers.

8 ounces mushrooms, any kind

1 tablespoon cooking fat of choice

1 small yellow onion, diced

1 medium carrot, peeled and diced

1 stalk celery, diced

Sea salt and ground black pepper

1/2 cup fresh cilantro, leaves and stems, finely chopped

1/4 cup fresh mint, leaves only, finely chopped (about 1/2 ounce)

2 tablespoons coconut flour

2 teaspoons paprika

2 teaspoons Trifecta Spice Blend (page 330)

1 teaspoon ground cinnamon

1 teaspoon ground cumin

1/2 teaspoon sea salt

1/2 teaspoon ground black pepper

2 pounds ground beef or turkey

2 large eggs, beaten

FOR TOPPING

8 slices bacon (about 12 ounces), cut in half

Fresh cilantro leaves

2 tablespoons ketchup, homemade (page 340) or store-bought

Preheat the oven to 375°F.

Wipe any dirt off the mushrooms and place them (including the stems) in a food processor. Pulse until they're in very small pieces—not quite as small as grains of rice, but almost! Set aside.

Melt the cooking fat in a medium-sized skillet over medium heat. Add the onion, carrot, and celery, season with a few pinches each of salt and pepper, and cook, stirring every few minutes, for 7 to 9 minutes, until the onion and celery become translucent and begin to brown and the carrot softens. Add the mushrooms to the skillet and cook for about 5 minutes, until they brown and release most of their water.

While the mushrooms are cooking, in a small mixing bowl, combine the fresh herbs, coconut flour, spices, and salt and pepper.

Place the ground meat in a large mixing bowl and then pour the eggs over it. Sprinkle half of the herb-and-spice mixture evenly over the meat and combine the ingredients with your hands. Add the cooked vegetables and mushrooms, then add the remaining herb-and-spice mixture. Mix with your hands to incorporate all the ingredients.

TO COOK IN A LOAF PAN:
Place the meat mixture in a 8 by 4-inch loaf pan and place the bacon slices on the top. Set the loaf pan on a rimmed baking sheet.

TO COOK ON A WIRE BAKING RACK:
Set a wire baking rack on a rimmed baking sheet. Form the meat mixture into the shape of a loaf and place on the rack. Place the bacon on top of the meat.

CALORIES: **473** | FAT: **37 g** | PROTEIN: **30 g** | CARBS: **6 g** | FIBER: **2 g** | NET CARBS: **4 g**

Cover the loaf with foil and bake until its internal temperature reaches 160°F, about 1 hour, removing the foil halfway through to allow the bacon to crisp up.

At the end of baking, if the bacon needs more time to brown, switch the oven to broil for 2 to 3 minutes. (If you're cooking the meatloaf in a loaf pan, you may need to drain the pan about three-quarters of the way through baking, as the meatloaf may release a fair amount of liquid.)

Garnish with cilantro and drizzle with ketchup before serving.

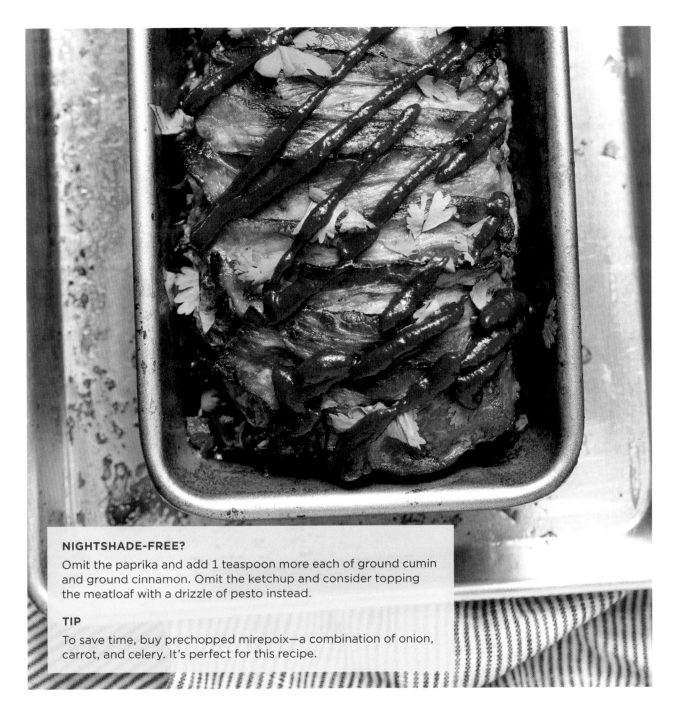

NIGHTSHADE-FREE?

Omit the paprika and add 1 teaspoon more each of ground cumin and ground cinnamon. Omit the ketchup and consider topping the meatloaf with a drizzle of pesto instead.

TIP

To save time, buy prechopped mirepoix—a combination of onion, carrot, and celery. It's perfect for this recipe.

Beef Satay Skewers

PREP TIME: **30 minutes, plus time to marinate the steak** | COOK TIME: **15 minutes** | YIELD: **6 servings**

Delicious Thai flavors combine to make these skewers a great option not only for dinner but also for parties or events. Make extra satay sauce and use it for the Shrimp Pad Thai on page 264 to simplify that recipe even further.

FOR THE MARINADE

1/2 cup full-fat coconut milk

3 tablespoons coconut aminos

2 to 3 dashes of fish sauce

1/2 small yellow onion, finely chopped

2 cloves garlic, grated or minced

1 teaspoon ground cumin

1/4 teaspoon ground ginger

Pinch of red pepper flakes

Pinch of sea salt

Pinch of ground black pepper

2 pounds sirloin steak, sliced

1 medium red onion, cut into 1 1/2-inch chunks

FOR THE SATAY SAUCE

1/2 cup coconut aminos

1/2 cup unsweetened peanut, almond, or sunflower seed butter

1/4 cup rice vinegar

2 to 3 dashes of fish sauce

1/2 teaspoon toasted sesame seeds

1/4 teaspoon ground black pepper

1/4 teaspoon sea salt

1/4 teaspoon red pepper flakes

FOR GARNISH

1/4 cup chopped fresh cilantro leaves

1 lime, cut into wedges

MAKE THE MARINADE:

Whisk together all the ingredients for the marinade in a large mixing bowl.

MARINATE THE STEAK:

Place the steak in the bowl with the marinade and massage the marinade into it. Cover and place in the refrigerator to marinate overnight.

When you're ready to grill the steak, soak 12 to 16 (depending on how many slices of meat you have) bamboo or wooden skewers for 10 minutes and preheat a grill or grill pan to medium-high heat. Thread the marinated steak pieces on the skewers, alternating them with the onion pieces.

Grill the skewers for 4 to 6 minutes on each side, or to your desired level of doneness, so the steak is seared but not burned. Remove from the heat, cover with foil, and let rest for 5 minutes.

While the skewers are resting, make the satay sauce: Whisk together all the ingredients for the sauce in a small mixing bowl.

Garnish the skewers with cilantro, squeeze lime juice over the meat, and serve with the satay sauce on the side.

NIGHTSHADE-FREE?
Omit the red pepper flakes from the sauce and marinade.

TIP
Save time: ask your butcher to preslice the meat for you into "stir-fry or fajita strips."

CALORIES: **605** | FAT: **30 g** | PROTEIN: **57 g** | CARBS: **19 g** | FIBER: **3 g** | NET CARBS: **16 g**

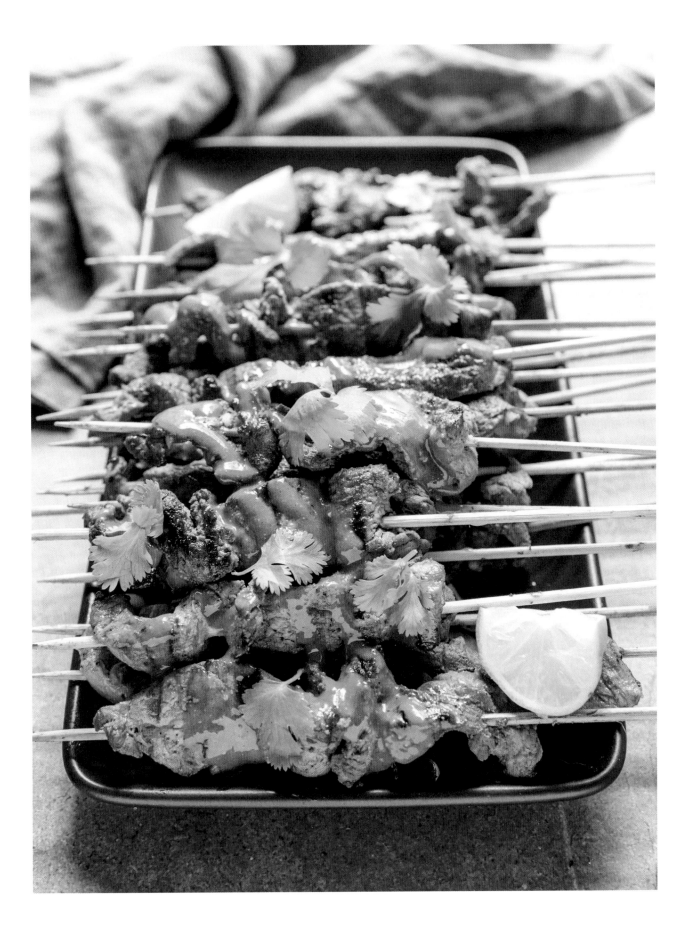

Meat & Greens Bowl

PREP TIME: 10 minutes | COOK TIME: 30 minutes | YIELD: 6 servings

This twist on a traditional meat sauce is a quick and easy way to pack in the dark leafy greens! Prep a double batch to reheat for easy meals all week. Try it over cauliflower rice, roasted broccoli, or any other veggies you like.

2 pounds ground beef, pork, or turkey, or a combination

1 tablespoon Italian Spice Blend (page 330)

1 bunch Italian kale, removed from stem and finely chopped

1 (24-ounce) jar sugar-free pasta sauce

Sea salt and ground black pepper

4 large zucchini

Fresh basil leaves, for garnish (optional)

Grated hard cheese, such as Parmigiano-Reggiano or Pecorino Romano, for garnish (optional)

Place the ground meat in a large skillet over medium-high heat. Add the spice blend, stir to combine, and cook until the meat is browned through, 5 to 8 minutes.

Add the kale and cook until softened, about 3 minutes. Turn the heat down to medium, add the pasta sauce, and simmer until the sauce is heated through, 5 to 10 minutes, stirring occasionally. Add salt and pepper to taste, then remove the pan from the heat.

While the sauce is cooking, make the zucchini into noodles using a spiral slicer, a handheld julienne peeler, or even a regular vegetable peeler (if using a regular peeler, the noodles will be wide and flat instead of spaghetti-shaped). You should get about 4 cups of noodles.

Fill a large pot with 1 inch of water and place a steamer basket in the pot. Cover and bring to a boil over high heat. Add the noodles to the basket and steam for 3 minutes. Transfer the noodles to a colander to drain and allow to cool slightly.

Place the noodles in a large bowl and top with the meat-and-greens sauce. Garnish with the basil and grated cheese, if desired.

DAIRY-FREE?
Omit the cheese.

CALORIES: **405** | FAT: **22 g** | PROTEIN: **35 g** | CARBS: **21 g** | FIBER: **3 g** | NET CARBS: **18 g**

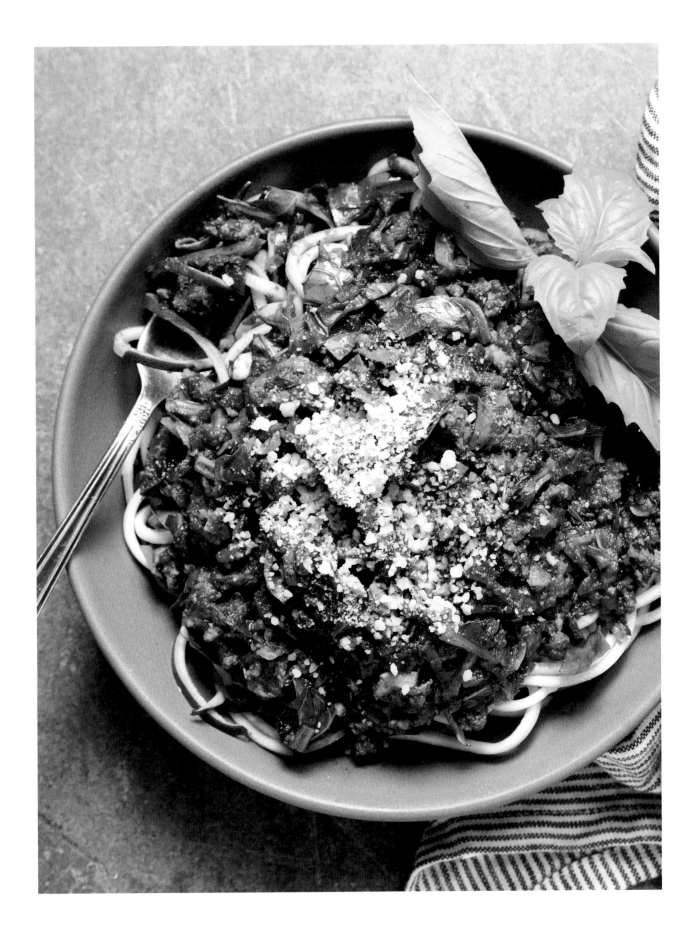

Spiced Stuffed Eggplant

PREP TIME: 5 minutes | COOK TIME: 40 minutes | YIELD: 4 servings

Eggplant is a super-versatile low-carb vegetable, perfect for stuffing! If you've been looking for an easy recipe for lamb, this is it, but you can also make this with other ground meats if you prefer. The feta adds a pop of bright, briny flavor, but if you're dairy-free, try some chopped olives on top.

1 large eggplant (about 1 1/4 pounds)

2 tablespoons extra-virgin olive oil

Sea salt

FOR THE STUFFING

2 teaspoons cooking fat of choice

1 small yellow onion, diced

Sea salt and ground black pepper

4 cloves garlic, minced or grated

1 pound ground lamb, beef, or turkey

1 tablespoon dried oregano leaves

2 teaspoons paprika

1 teaspoon ground cumin

1/2 teaspoon ground cinnamon

1 small tomato, chopped

FOR SERVING

2 ounces feta cheese (optional)

2 tablespoons chopped fresh cilantro leaves

1 lemon, halved

Preheat the oven to 375°F.

Slice the eggplant in half lengthwise, then score both halves in one direction and then the other by cutting about 1/2 inch deep. Rub the olive oil on both halves and season lightly with sea salt. Place the eggplant in a roasting pan or oven-safe skillet flesh side down and roast for 25 to 30 minutes, until the flesh is soft but not mushy/overcooked.

While the eggplant roasts, prepare the stuffing: Melt the cooking fat in a skillet over medium heat. Add the onion, season with a few pinches each of salt and pepper, and cook, stirring every few minutes, for 7 to 9 minutes, until the onion becomes translucent and begins to brown. Add the garlic and cook for 1 to 2 minutes more, until the garlic starts to turn golden brown.

Add the ground meat and seasonings to the pan and cook for 8 to 10 minutes, until browned through, breaking it up with a wooden spoon as it cooks and ensuring that the spices are evenly incorporated into the meat. Remove the pan from the heat and set aside.

When the eggplant is done roasting, remove it from the oven, carefully scoop out the flesh (do not discard the skins), and add the flesh to the skillet with the browned meat. Stir to combine, then spoon the meat-and-eggplant mixture back into the eggplant skins.

Place the chopped tomato on top of the stuffed eggplant. Return the eggplant to the oven and roast for 10 minutes to warm through.

Garnish with feta cheese (if desired), cilantro, and a squeeze of fresh lemon.

CALORIES: **448** | FAT: **36 g** | PROTEIN: **21 g** | CARBS: **14 g** | FIBER: **7 g** | NET CARBS: **7 g**

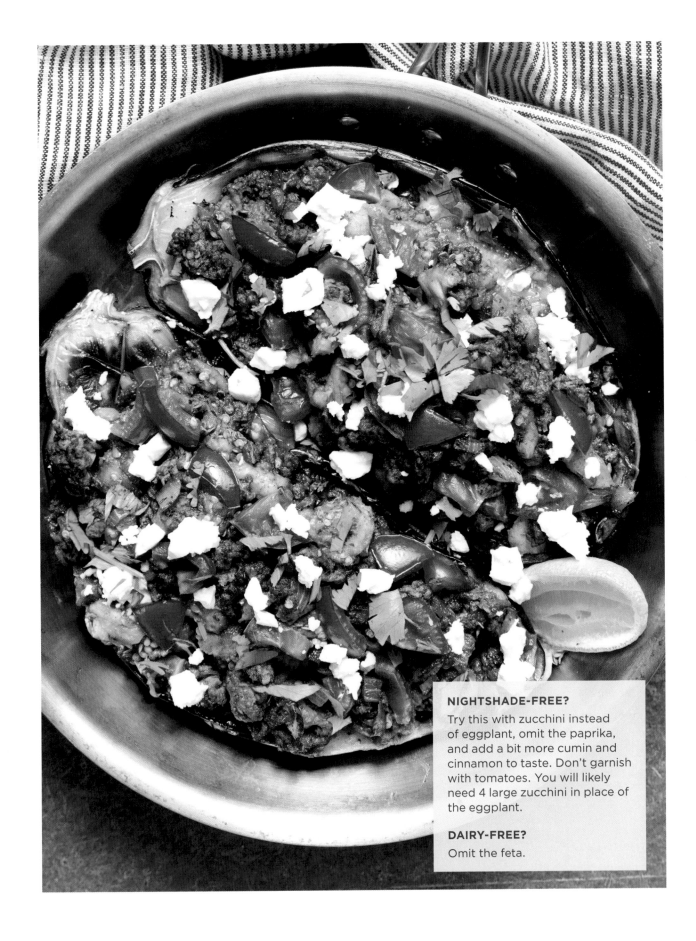

NIGHTSHADE-FREE?
Try this with zucchini instead
of eggplant, omit the paprika,
and add a bit more cumin and
cinnamon to taste. Don't garnish
with tomatoes. You will likely
need 4 large zucchini in place of
the eggplant.

DAIRY-FREE?
Omit the feta.

Simple Shredded Beef

PREP TIME: 5 minutes | COOK TIME: 6 to 8 hours (slow cooker), 30 minutes (Instant Pot) | YIELD: 12 servings

When you want to be sure you've got protein ready-made and on hand for a variety of recipes, this is a perfect go-to recipe. Once it's shredded, sear this beef in a hot cast-iron skillet just before eating, or use it to make some quick tacos by adding Taco & Fajita Spice Blend (page 331).

4 pounds beef pot roast, brisket, or stew meat

Sea salt

2 cups chicken broth, homemade (page 220) or store-bought, or beef broth

10 cloves garlic, peeled

TO MAKE THIS IN A SLOW COOKER:

Season the beef with the salt on all sides. Place the meat, broth, and garlic in a slow cooker and cook on low for 6 to 8 hours.

Remove the beef from the slow cooker, reserving any liquid. Allow it to cool slightly, then shred it with 2 forks. Taste the shredded meat and spoon some of the reserved liquid over it if needed for additional flavor.

TO MAKE THIS IN AN INSTANT POT:

Season the beef with the salt on both sides and cut it into 2- to 3-inch pieces. Place it in the multicooker and add the broth and garlic. Cook on high pressure for 30 minutes. When cooking is finished, allow the cooker to depressurize on its own; don't flip the valve to release it.

Store in an airtight container in the refrigerator for up to 5 days.

FODMAP-FREE?
Omit the garlic.

TIP
Preparing this beef ahead of time is a great way to make weeknight meals easy. When you're ready to eat, sear it in a skillet with some cooking fat and season as desired for the meal you're preparing.

CALORIES: **450** | FAT: **29 g** | PROTEIN: **44 g** | CARBS: **1 g** | FIBER: **0 g** | NET CARBS: **1 g**

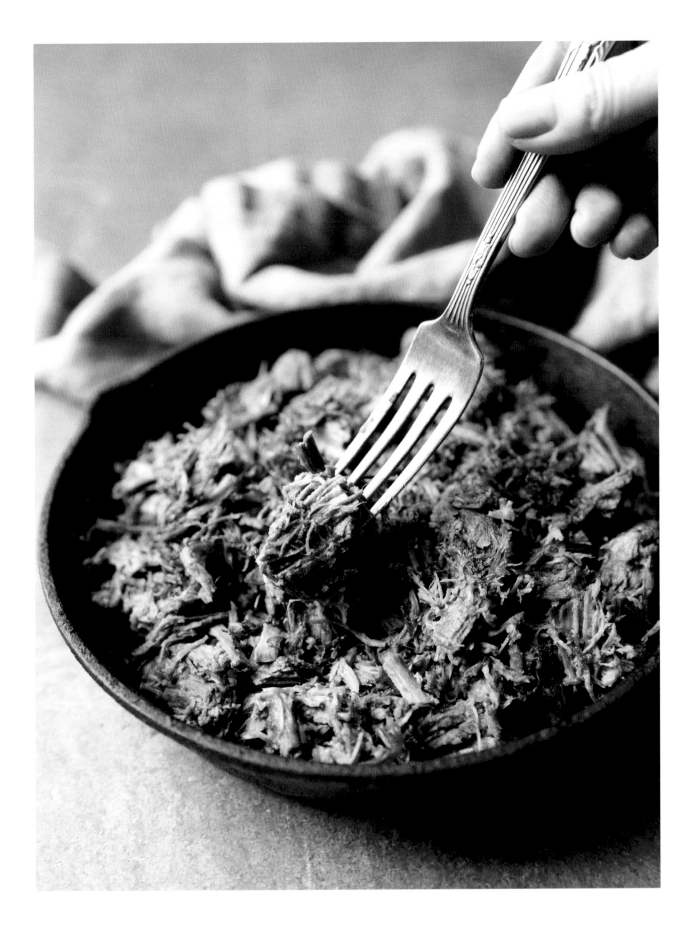

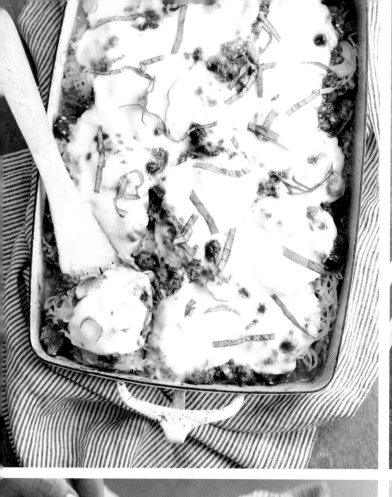
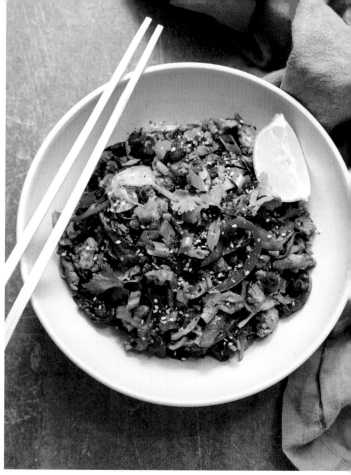
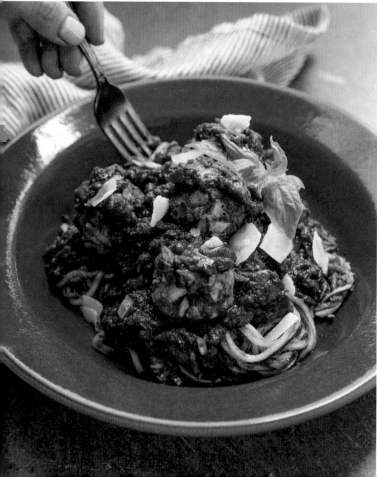
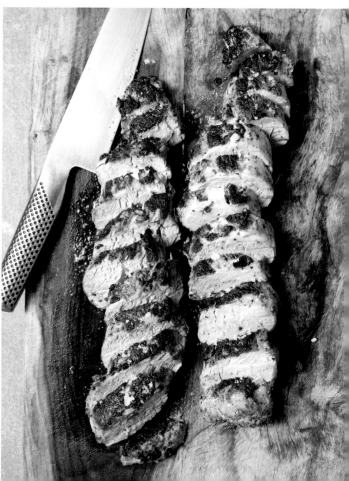

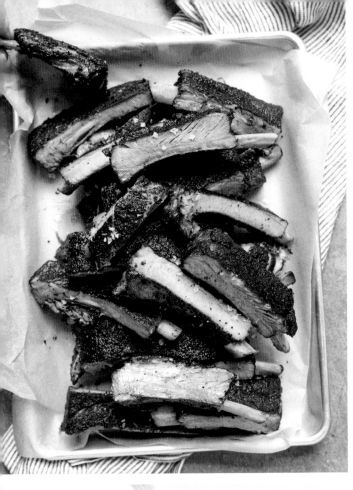

Main Dishes: Pork

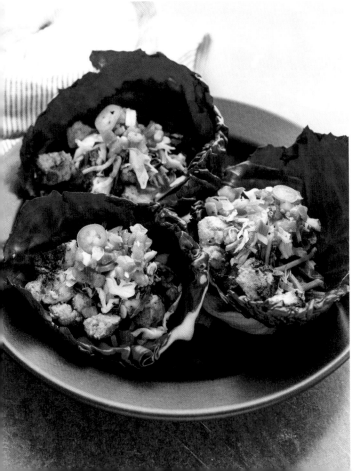

Thai Meatballs

PREP TIME: **15 minutes** | COOK TIME: **20 minutes** | YIELD: **2 dozen meatballs (4 per serving)**

Basic ground meat takes on new life in this bold meatball recipe. Enjoy these with any simple vegetable side, or enjoy them as a quick protein-and-fat snack anytime. I think they're especially delicious when made with all pork, but use any protein combination you like!

2 tablespoons coconut aminos (see Tips)

1 tablespoon red curry paste

2 to 3 dashes of fish sauce

Grated zest of 1 lime

1/4 cup finely chopped fresh cilantro leaves

1/4 cup minced green onions (about 1 green onion)

1 teaspoon grated or minced garlic (about 2 cloves)

1 teaspoon sea salt

1/4 teaspoon ginger powder

1 pound ground pork (see Tips)

1 pound ground chicken or turkey, preferably dark meat for the best flavor (see Tips)

FOR GARNISH (OPTIONAL)
Chopped fresh cilantro leaves
Sesame seeds
Sliced green onions

FOR SERVING
Cilantro Cauli-Rice (page 282)

Preheat the oven to 375°F.

In a small mixing bowl, combine the coconut aminos, red curry paste, fish sauce, lime zest, cilantro, green onions, garlic, salt, and ginger powder. Stir to mix well.

In a large mixing bowl, combine the chicken and pork and mix well with your hands. Add the marinade and use your hands to mix it with the meat until well combined. Form the meat mixture into twenty-four meatballs (about 1 1/3 ounces each) and place on a rimmed baking sheet.

Bake for 20 minutes, or until cooked through.

Remove the meatballs from the oven and garnish with cilantro, sesame seeds, and green onions, if desired. Serve with cauliflower rice.

TIPS

If you use Big Tree brand coconut aminos, use less salt.

You can also use 2 pounds of one type of ground meat if you prefer. In that case, I recommend using ground pork for the best flavor.

CALORIES: **323** | FAT: **22 g** | PROTEIN: **27 g** | CARBS: **2 g** | FIBER: **1 g** | NET CARBS: **1 g**

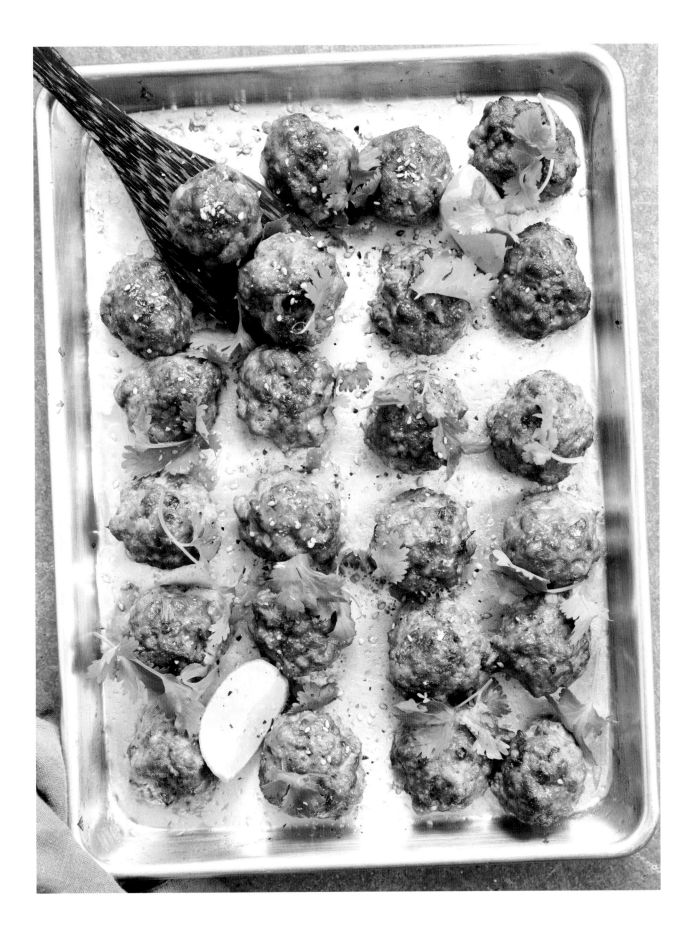

Tacos al Pastor

PREP TIME: 15 minutes, plus time to marinate the pork | COOK TIME: 15 minutes | YIELD: 4 servings

You know how tacos at a restaurant are so, so delicious, but you can't quite figure out how they get so much flavor into them? Here's how: a good marinade and a bit of time! With a bit of forethought, you can enjoy that amazing flavor at home with these tacos.

FOR THE MARINADE

4 cloves garlic, peeled

2 chipotle peppers in adobo sauce (see Tip)

1 small yellow onion, roughly chopped

1/2 cup fresh lime juice (about 4 limes)

1/4 cup apple cider vinegar

1 tablespoon extra-virgin olive oil

1 teaspoon dried oregano leaves

1 teaspoon ground cumin

1/2 teaspoon sea salt

2 pounds boneless pork leg roast or pork butt, cut into 1/2-inch pieces

1 head purple cabbage, leaves separated, for serving

FOR TOPPING (OPTIONAL)

Spicy Citrus Slaw (page 280)

Pico de gallo or Quick Salsa (page 306)

Chopped red onion

Chopped fresh cilantro leaves

Sliced jalapeño pepper

MAKE THE MARINADE:

Place the marinade ingredients in a food processor or high-speed blender and blend until smooth.

Place the pork in a large bowl and pour the marinade over it. Massage the marinade into the pork, cover, and place in the refrigerator to marinate for at least 1 hour or up to overnight.

When you're ready to cook the pork, preheat the oven to 375°F. Line a rimmed baking sheet with foil, then place a wire baking rack on top of it.

Remove the pork from the marinade and pat it dry with a paper towel. Evenly space the meat on the baking rack, then place it in the oven and roast for 10 minutes.

Place an oven rack just under the broiler and set the oven to broil. Transfer the baking sheet to just under the broiler and broil on high for 2 to 5 minutes, until the meat has crisped up and browned a bit.

Spoon the pork onto the cabbage leaves and top with slaw, pico de gallo, red onion, cilantro, and jalapeño, if desired.

TIP
Freeze the remainder of the peppers in adobo for later use. If you can't find these peppers (sold in a can), you can use 1 tablespoon of ground chipotle chili pepper instead.

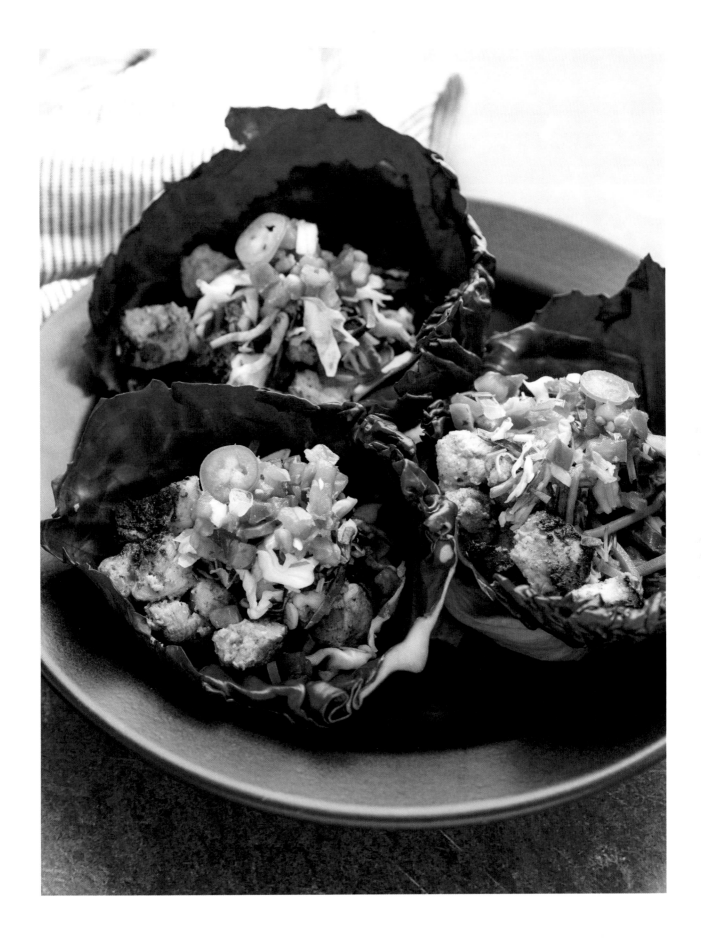

Super Garlic Stir-Fry Bowl

PREP TIME: 20 minutes | **COOK TIME: 35 minutes** | **YIELD: 6 servings**

This is one of my go-to easy weeknight meals, and I think it'll become one for you and your family, too! With just a handful of fresh ingredients and lots of pantry items, you can pull together some bold Asian flavors that will satisfy your takeout craving without all the carbs.

2 pounds ground pork

1/4 cup Super Garlic Blend (page 330)

1/2 teaspoon ginger powder

1 medium red bell pepper, thinly sliced

1 small red onion, thinly sliced

4 cloves garlic, minced or grated

4 cups shredded cabbage (about 1 head; see Tip)

1/4 cup coconut aminos

2 to 3 dashes of fish sauce

FOR GARNISH

Chopped fresh cilantro leaves

Sesame seeds

Sliced green onions

FOR SERVING

Lime wedges

In a large bowl, combine the ground pork, spice blend, and ginger powder and mix well with your hands.

Place the ground pork in a 12-inch skillet and cook over medium-high heat for about 10 minutes, until the meat has cooked through, breaking it up with a wooden spoon as it cooks. Remove the meat from the pan and set aside.

Add the bell pepper and onion to the skillet. Cook for about 5 minutes, until the onion starts to turn translucent and the pepper softens. Add the garlic and cook for 1 to 2 minutes more, until the garlic starts to turn golden brown.

Return the meat to the skillet, then add the shredded cabbage, coconut aminos, and fish sauce and stir to combine. Cook for about 5 minutes, until the cabbage softens slightly.

Garnish with chopped cilantro, sesame seeds, and sliced green onions. Serve lime wedges on the side.

NIGHTSHADE-FREE?
Omit the red bell pepper.

TIP
To save time and effort, buy pre-shredded cabbage. Some of these mixtures come with both green and purple cabbage and sometimes even some carrot (as shown in the picture), and they're perfect for this dish.

CALORIES: **481** | FAT: **32 g** | PROTEIN: **29 g** | CARBS: **19 g** | FIBER: **6 g** | NET CARBS: **13 g**

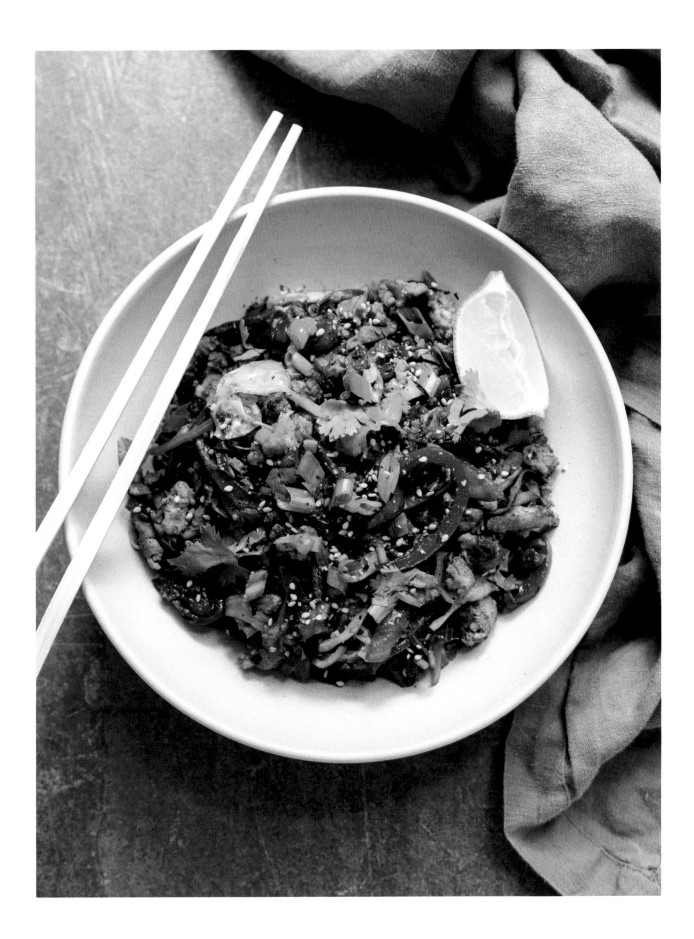

Spaghetti Bolognese Bake

PREP TIME: 25 minutes | COOK TIME: **50 minutes** | YIELD: **8 servings**

What could be better than a hearty Bolognese? A Bolognese casserole! This baked dish is super satisfying and perfect for feeding a family or a crowd—or one person with lots of leftovers. This dish freezes and reheats beautifully, so make a big batch to enjoy comfort food anytime.

1 medium spaghetti squash (about 3 pounds)

Sea salt and ground black pepper

4 slices bacon, chopped

1 medium carrot, finely diced

1 medium yellow onion, finely diced

1 stalk celery, finely diced

4 cloves garlic, minced or grated

1 pound ground pork

1 pound ground veal or beef

2 tablespoons Greek Spice Blend (page 330)

1/2 cup full-fat coconut milk

1/4 cup dry white wine (optional)

6 ounces tomato paste

16 ounces fresh mozzarella, sliced into 1/4-inch rounds (see Note)

Thinly sliced fresh basil, for garnish (optional)

NIGHTSHADE-FREE?
Use 6 ounces canned pumpkin instead of tomato paste.

DAIRY-FREE?
Omit the cheese.

MAKE IT 21DSD-FRIENDLY
Omit the white wine.

CHANGE IT UP
Make this using zucchini noodles (see page 198) instead of spaghetti squash.

Preheat the oven to 375°F.

Slice the spaghetti squash in half lengthwise. Scoop out the seeds, then sprinkle the cut sides with salt and pepper. Place both halves face down on a rimmed baking sheet and roast for 35 to 45 minutes, until the flesh of the squash is translucent and the skin begins to soften and easily separates from the "noodles" inside. Allow the squash to cool enough that you can handle it, then scoop out the "noodles" into a large roasting pan. Set aside.

While the squash is roasting, make the sauce: In a large skillet over medium-high heat, cook the bacon until the fat has rendered and the bits are crispy, about 8 minutes. Add the carrot, onion, and celery and sauté for about 8 minutes, until the onion and celery are translucent. Add the garlic and cook for 1 minute more, or until fragrant.

Add the pork, veal, and spice blend and cook until the meat is browned and cooked through, about 10 minutes. Add the coconut milk, white wine (if using), and tomato paste. Turn the heat down to medium-low and simmer, stirring occasionally, for 20 minutes, or until the sauce has thickened and any alcohol has evaporated. Add salt and pepper to taste. Remove from the heat.

Add the sauce to the roasting pan with the spaghetti squash noodles and mix well to combine. Lay the slices of cheese on top.

Place an oven rack just under the broiler and set the oven to broil. Place the roasting pan in the oven just under the broiler for 2 to 5 minutes, until the cheese is melted and lightly browned.

Garnish with thinly sliced fresh basil, if desired.

Store leftovers in an airtight container in the refrigerator for up to 5 days or in the freezer for up to 6 weeks. To defrost, place in the refrigerator overnight, then reheat before serving.

CALORIES: **539** | FAT: **38 g** | PROTEIN: **36 g** | CARBS: **12 g** | FIBER: **2 g** | NET CARBS: **10 g**

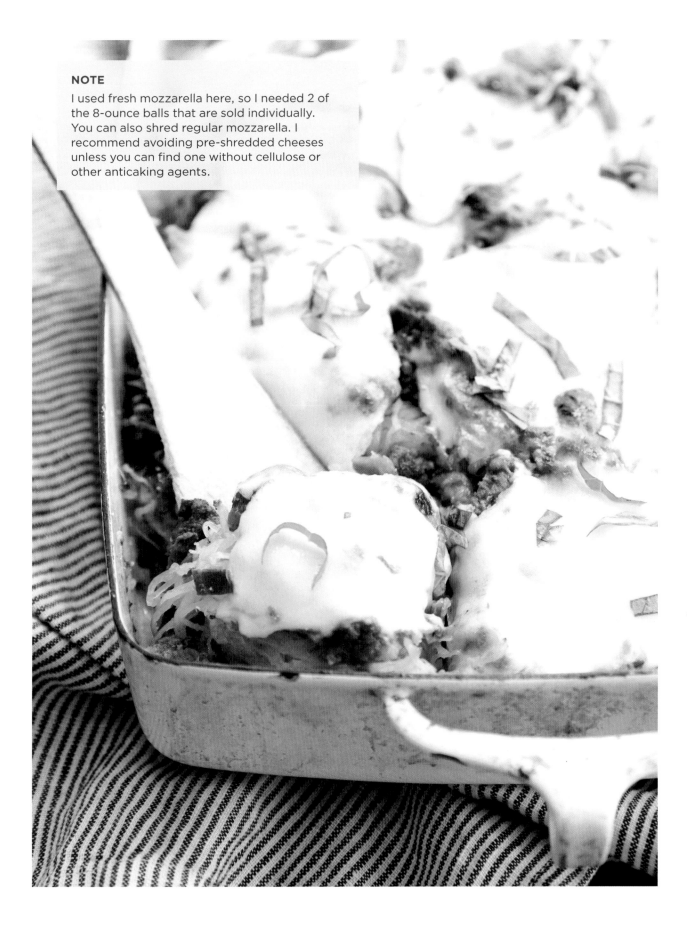

NOTE

I used fresh mozzarella here, so I needed 2 of the 8-ounce balls that are sold individually. You can also shred regular mozzarella. I recommend avoiding pre-shredded cheeses unless you can find one without cellulose or other anticaking agents.

Meatballs Marinara

PREP TIME: **20 minutes** | COOK TIME: **25 minutes** | YIELD: **2 dozen meatballs (4 per serving)**

Meatballs made at restaurants often include breadcrumbs, which aren't keto-friendly. This is a simple way to make meatballs at home with some zucchini noodles and sauce—easy-peasy. Make extra to keep this quick protein source on hand for weeknight meals or snacks anytime.

2 pounds ground pork

3 tablespoons Italian Spice Blend (page 330)

4 cloves garlic, grated or minced

1 small yellow onion, finely diced

Grated zest of 1 lemon

4 large zucchini

3 cups marinara, homemade (page 338) or store-bought (use a no-sugar–added variety), warmed

FOR GARNISH (OPTIONAL)

1/2 cup grated hard cheese, such as Parmigiano-Reggiano or Pecorino Romano

1/4 cup chopped fresh basil

DAIRY-FREE?

Omit the cheese.

CHANGE IT UP

Swap out the pork for ground beef or a combination of ground pork and ground chicken.

TIP

Double or triple this recipe to have extras for leftovers. Store in an airtight container in the fridge for up to 5 days or in the freezer for later use.

Preheat the oven to 375°F.

Make the meatballs: In a medium-sized mixing bowl, combine the ground pork, spice blend, garlic, and onion. Mix well with your hands until the spice mixture is evenly dispersed.

Form the meat into twenty-four 1 1/3-ounce meatballs, about the size of golf balls, and place them in a 9 by 13-inch baking dish or on a rimmed baking sheet. Bake for 20 minutes, or until cooked through.

While the meatballs are baking, make the zucchini into noodles using a spiral slicer, a handheld julienne peeler, or even a regular vegetable peeler (if using a regular peeler, the noodles will be wide and flat instead of spaghetti-shaped). You should get 4 cups of noodles.

Fill a large pot with 1 inch of water and place a steamer basket in the pot. Cover and bring to a boil over high heat. Add the noodles to the basket and steam for 3 minutes. Transfer the noodles to a colander to drain off the excess liquid as they cool slightly.

Place the noodles in a large bowl and toss them with the marinara sauce. Top with the meatballs and garnish with the grated cheese and basil, if desired.

CALORIES: **551** | FAT: **36 g** | PROTEIN: **31 g** | CARBS: **27 g** | FIBER: **6 g** | NET CARBS: **21 g**

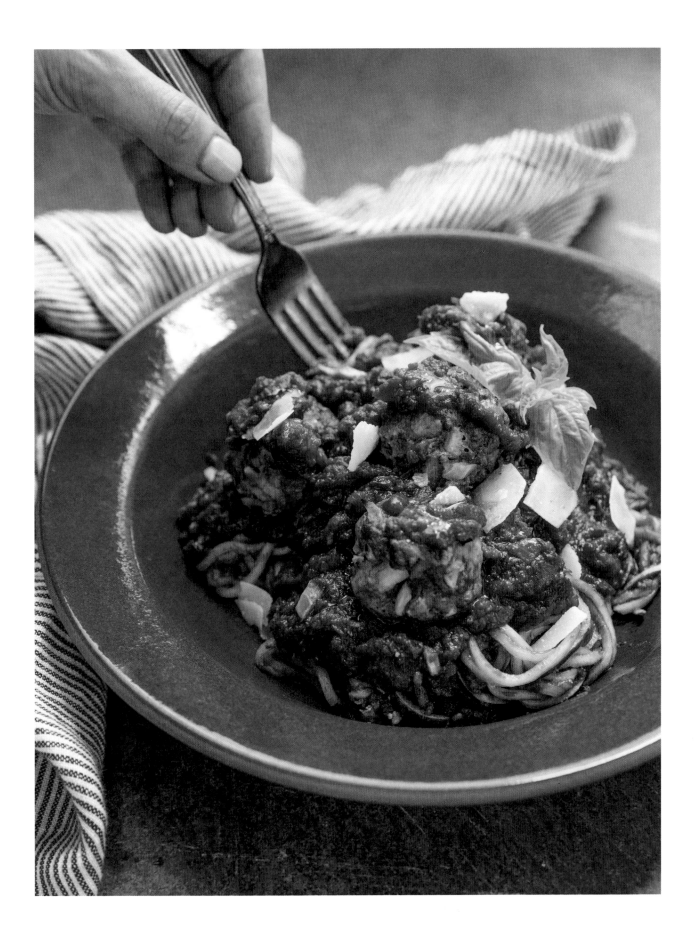

Cocoa BBQ Ribs

PREP TIME: **10 minutes, plus time to marinate the ribs** | COOK TIME: **3 hours** | YIELD: **8 servings**

Making a giant rack of ribs (or two) can seem really intimidating, but trust me, this recipe is the easiest and best way to make ribs in a regular oven! This is a great way to feed a crowd or keep to eating keto for a game day or party. Brush on some BBQ Sauce (page 341) for an extra flavor boost!

2 racks St. Louis–style pork ribs (5 to 6 pounds total) (see Note)

1/2 cup Cocoa BBQ Spice Blend (page 331)

Coat both sides of each rack of ribs heavily with the spice blend, wrap tightly with foil, and let sit in the refrigerator for at least 3 hours, preferably overnight.

Preheat the oven to 275°F.

Remove the ribs from the refrigerator and, keeping them foil-wrapped, place them in the oven on a rimmed baking sheet, foil seam up. Cook for 2 to 3 hours, until the rib meat easily separates from the bone. Remove the ribs from the oven and unwrap them from the foil, then return them to the rimmed baking sheet.

Place an oven rack directly under the broiler and turn the broiler to high. Place the rack of ribs directly under the broiler and broil for 5 minutes, or until the outsides of the ribs are crispy.

Alternatively, instead of broiling, you can crisp the ribs in a grill pan: Heat the grill pan over high heat. Once the pan is hot, add the ribs and cook for 5 minutes, or until the outsides of the ribs are crispy.

NOTE
You can make these using baby back ribs if you prefer. Simply adjust the cooking time to 2 hours, then add more time as needed until the ribs are tender.

CALORIES: **582** | FAT: **36 g** | PROTEIN: **60 g** | CARBS: **0 g** | FIBER: **0 g** | NET CARBS: **0 g**

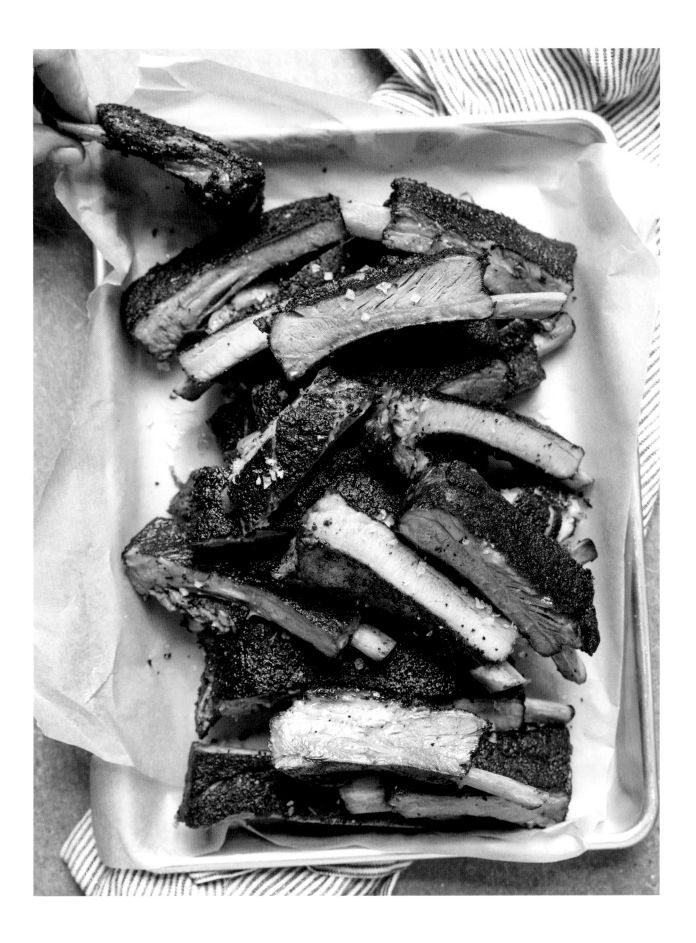

NUTS | EGGS | **NIGHTSHADES** | **FODMAPS** | DAIRY | **21DSD-FRIENDLY**

Cajun Pork Tenderloin

PREP TIME: **5 minutes** | COOK TIME: **20 to 25 minutes** | YIELD: **4 servings**

The addition of Cajun spice transforms the classic flavor combination of pork and mustard! This is a perfect weeknight meal prepared with pantry ingredients that make this simple protein taste fantastic. Enjoy this pork with a salad or a side of Spicy Roasted Asparagus with Lemon (page 292) or Creamy Cauliflower Purée (page 284) for a complete meal.

2 tablespoons Cajun Spice Blend (page 331)

2 tablespoons Dijon mustard

2 tablespoons ghee (page 336)

2 pork tenderloins (1 1/2 to 2 pounds total)

Coarse sea salt, for garnish

Preheat the oven to 375°F.

In a small mixing bowl, combine the spice blend, mustard, and ghee. Brush the mixture evenly onto the pork tenderloins.

Place a large cast-iron or other oven-safe skillet on the stovetop over medium-high heat.

When the pan is hot, sear the tenderloins on both sides until lightly browned, about 2 minutes per side.

Transfer the pan to the oven and roast the tenderloins for 15 to 20 minutes, until the internal temperature of the pork reaches at least 145°F. Garnish with coarse sea salt before serving.

NIGHTSHADE-FREE?
Use the Super Garlic (page 330) or Ranch Spice Blend (page 331) instead of the Cajun Spice Blend.

CALORIES: **295** | FAT: **10 g** | PROTEIN: **46 g** | CARBS: **0 g** | FIBER: **0 g** | NET CARBS: **0 g**

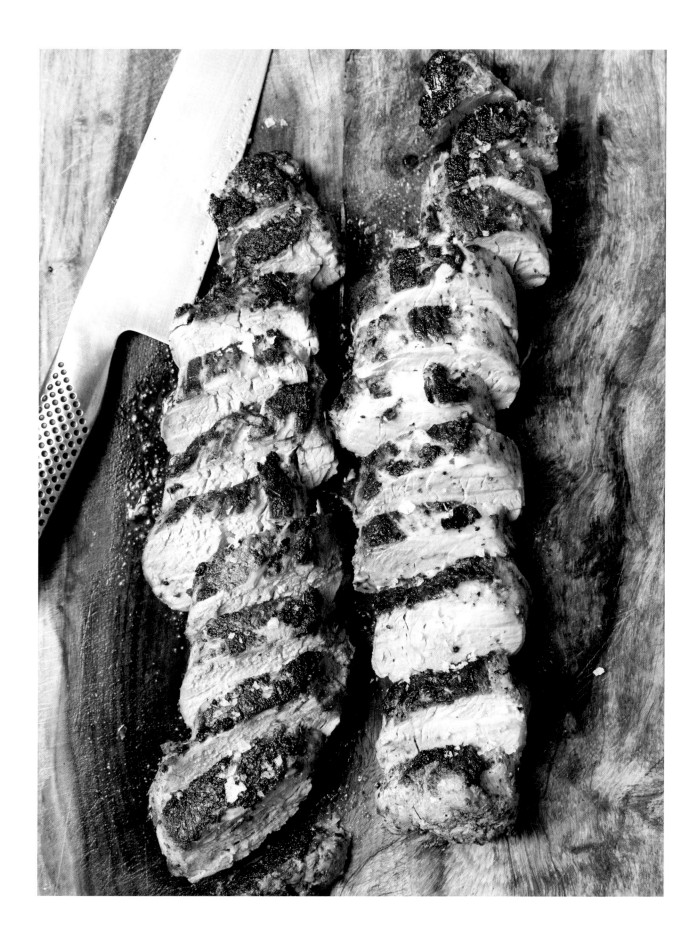

Simple Shredded Pork

PREP TIME: 5 minutes | COOK TIME: **6 to 8 hours (slow cooker), 35 minutes (Instant Pot)** | YIELD: **8 servings**

Like the Shredded Beef recipe on page 240, this is a perfect go-to recipe to ensure that you've got a protein ready-made and on hand for a variety of recipes. Once it's shredded, sear this pork in a hot cast-iron skillet just before eating, or use it to make some quick tacos by adding Taco & Fajita Spice Blend (page 331).

4 pounds pork shoulder roast

Sea salt

2 cups chicken broth, homemade (page 220) or store-bought

10 cloves garlic, peeled

4 bay leaves

TO MAKE THIS IN A SLOW COOKER:

Season the pork shoulder liberally with the salt on all sides. Place the meat, broth, garlic, and bay leaves in a slow cooker and cook on low for 6 to 8 hours.

Remove the pork from the slow cooker, reserving any liquid. Allow the meat to cool slightly, then shred it with two forks. Taste the shredded meat and spoon some of the reserved liquid over it if needed for additional flavor.

TO MAKE THIS IN AN INSTANT POT OR OTHER MULTICOOKER:

Season the pork shoulder liberally with the salt on all sides and cut it into 2- to 3-inch pieces. Place it in the multicooker and add the broth, garlic, and bay leaves. Cook on high pressure for 35 minutes. When cooking is finished, allow the cooker to depressurize on its own; don't flip the valve to release it.

FODMAP-FREE?
Omit the garlic.

TIP
Preparing this pork ahead of time is a great way to make weeknight meals easy. When you're ready to eat, sear it in a skillet with some cooking fat to brown and crisp it up. Season as desired for the meal you're preparing.

CALORIES: **628** | FAT: **39 g** | PROTEIN: **63 g** | CARBS: **2 g** | FIBER: **0 g** | NET CARBS: **2 g**

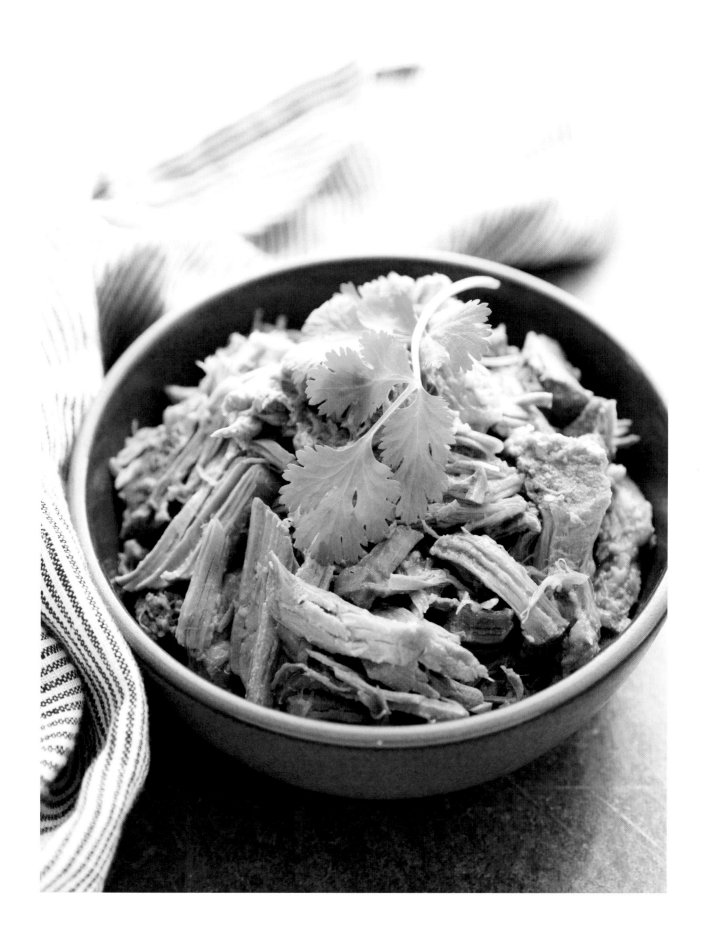

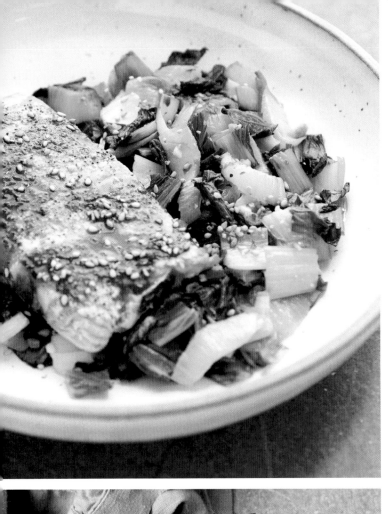
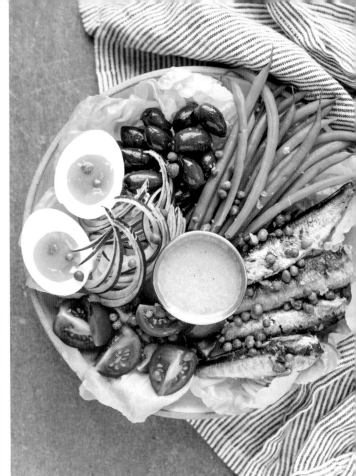
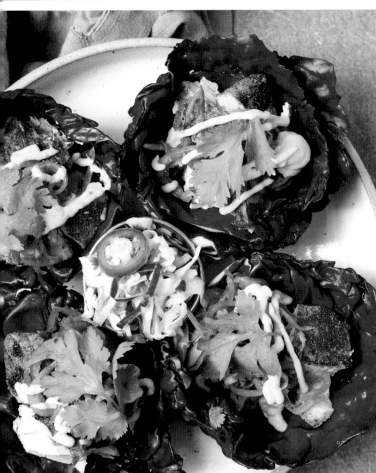
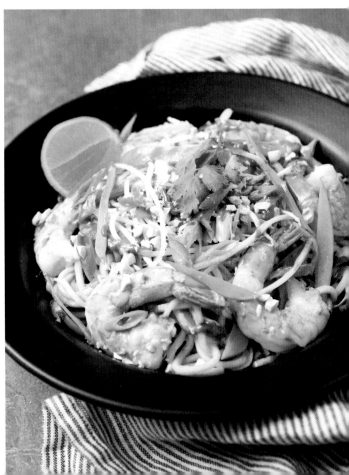

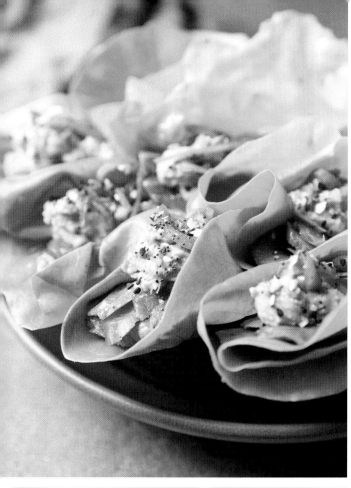

Main Dishes: Seafood

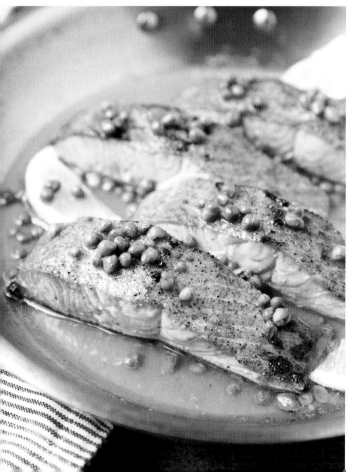

NUTS | EGGS | **NIGHTSHADES** | **FODMAPS** | DAIRY | **21DSD-FRIENDLY**

Blackened Fish Tacos

PREP TIME: 10 minutes | COOK TIME: **10 minutes** | YIELD: **8 tacos (2 per serving)**

Tacos are a perfect keto-friendly food when you swap out the high-carb shells for cabbage or lettuce. I love the extra crunch from fresh cabbage, but use any "wrapper" you like. Fish cooks really quickly, so this dish is a perfect option for a weeknight when you're pressed for time.

4 (6-ounce) boneless salmon (skin-on) or halibut fillets

Sea salt

2 teaspoons Taco & Fajita Spice Blend (page 331)

1 head red cabbage, leaves separated

1/2 cup Marinated Onions (page 290)

1/4 cup roughly chopped fresh cilantro leaves

FOR SERVING

Spicy Citrus Slaw (page 280)

Sliced avocado or Avocado Crema (page 342)

4 lime wedges

Set an oven rack directly below the broiler and turn the oven to the low broil setting. Heat a large oven-safe skillet (preferably cast iron) over medium-high heat.

Lightly season the skin side of the salmon with salt and season the other side with the spice blend. Place the salmon skin side down in the dry, hot pan and sear for 3 minutes.

Transfer the pan to the oven, directly below the broiler. Broil for 4 to 5 minutes, until the fish is opaque. Remove the pan from the oven and flake the fish with a fork. Set the skin aside to eat separately.

Assemble the tacos: Using 1 or 2 large cabbage leaves per taco, layer on the fish, marinated onions, and cilantro. Serve with the citrus slaw, avocado, and lime wedges.

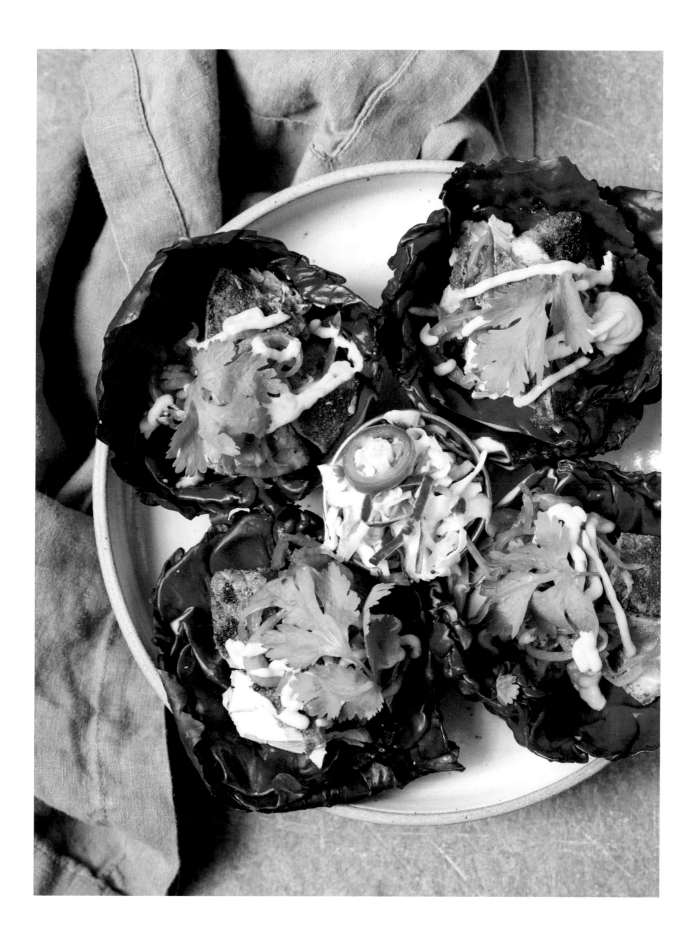

NUTS | EGGS | NIGHTSHADES | FODMAPS | DAIRY | 21DSD-FRIENDLY

Shrimp Pad Thai

PREP TIME: 15 minutes | COOK TIME: 10 minutes | YIELD: 4 servings

Thai food is delicious, but a traditional pad Thai is very high in carbs—not keto-friendly! This is an easy low-carb version to make at home. Make the sauce ahead of time to have a quick-fix meal on hand for later in the week. Bonus: This sauce works perfectly as a satay sauce for the Beef Satay Skewers on page 234!

4 large zucchini or yellow squash

1 cup snow peas, sliced lengthwise into thin strips

4 dozen extra-large shrimp, peeled and deveined (see Note)

FOR THE SAUCE

3/4 cup coconut aminos

1/2 cup unsweetened peanut butter, almond butter, sunflower butter, or tahini

4 drops fish sauce

1/2 teaspoon minced or grated garlic

1/4 teaspoon minced fresh ginger

Juice of 1 lime

Sea salt and ground black pepper

FOR GARNISH

1 tablespoon chopped peanuts

1/4 cup chopped fresh cilantro

1/2 cup bean sprouts (optional)

Make the zucchini into noodles using a spiral slicer, a handheld julienne peeler, or even a regular vegetable peeler (if using a regular peeler, the noodles will be wide and flat instead of spaghetti-shaped). You should get 4 cups of noodles.

Fill a large pot with 1 inch of water and place a steamer basket in the pot. Cover and bring to a boil over high heat. Add the noodles to the basket and steam for 3 minutes. Using tongs, transfer the noodles to a colander (leave the boiling water in the pot) to drain off the excess liquid as they cool slightly. Place the snow peas on top of the noodles in the colander.

Place the shrimp in the steamer basket over the still-boiling water and cook for 4 to 5 minutes, until pink all the way through. The exact cooking time will vary depending on the size of the shrimp. Remove from the heat and set aside.

In a small mixing bowl, whisk together the sauce ingredients until well combined. Add salt and pepper to taste.

Place the noodles, snow peas, sauce, and shrimp in a large skillet over medium-high heat and toss gently to combine. Cook for 2 to 3 minutes, until heated through.

To serve, garnish with chopped peanuts, cilantro, and bean sprouts, if desired.

TIP

When whisking the sauce together, it will take a bit of time to get all of the ingredients to incorporate into a smooth mixture. Just keep whisking! It will look a bit clumpy for a while, then magically it'll become smooth.

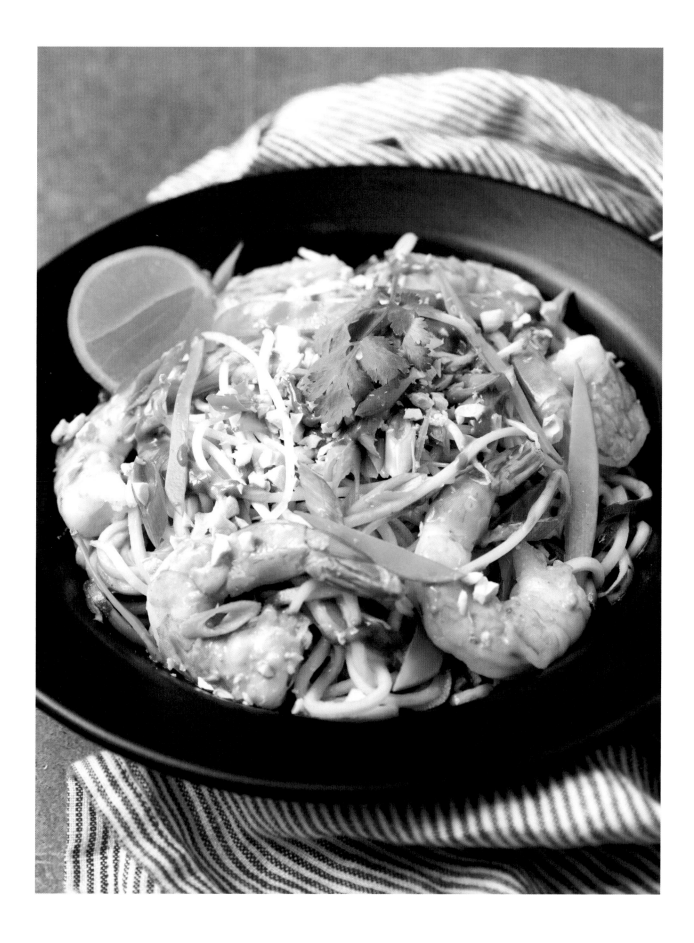

Lemon Caper Salmon

PREP TIME: **5 minutes** | COOK TIME: **10 minutes** | YIELD: **4 servings**

This classic flavor combination highlights the delicate taste of salmon in an easy one-pan recipe. Serve this alongside Creamy Cauliflower Purée (page 284) and a green salad. Or swap this salmon for the grilled chicken on Baby Kale Caesar Salad (page 202) or for the sardines in Niçoise Salad (page 274).

4 (6-ounce) wild salmon fillets

Sea salt and ground black pepper

2 teaspoons Trifecta Spice Blend (page 330)

4 tablespoons butter or ghee (page 336), divided

Juice of 2 lemons

1 teaspoon Dijon mustard

1/3 cup capers (about one 2-ounce jar)

Freshly cracked black pepper, for garnish

Lemon slices, for serving

Set an oven rack directly below the broiler and turn on the oven to the broil setting.

Use a paper towel to pat the salmon dry on both sides. Lightly season the skin side of the salmon with salt and pepper and season the other side with the spice blend.

Melt 1 tablespoon of the butter in a large oven-safe skillet, preferably stainless-steel, over high heat. Place the salmon skin side down and sear for 2 minutes. Transfer the pan to the oven, directly under the broiler. Broil for 4 minutes, until the salmon is opaque in the center or cooked to your liking.

While the salmon broils, place the remaining butter in a small microwave-safe bowl and melt it by microwaving it on high in 30-second increments. Whisk in the lemon juice and mustard.

Remove the pan from the oven and add the lemon mustard sauce, spooning it over the fish. Add the capers and garnish with pepper. Serve with lemon slices.

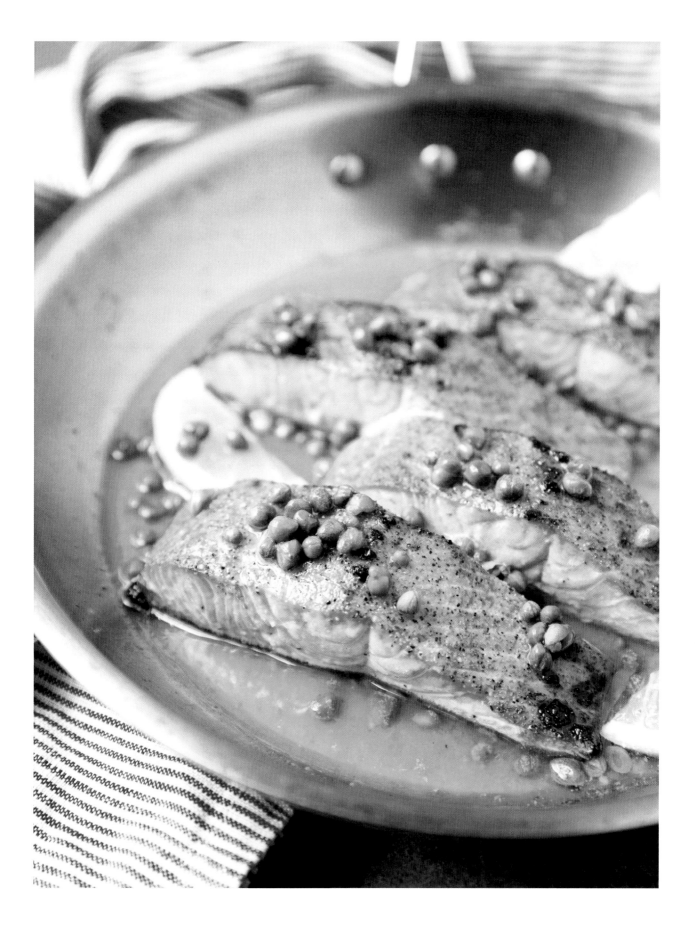

NUTS | EGGS | **NIGHTSHADES** | **FODMAPS** | DAIRY | **21DSD-FRIENDLY**

Sole Italiano

PREP TIME: **10 minutes** | COOK TIME: **20 minutes** | YIELD: **4 servings**

This simple weeknight meal takes ho-hum fish and turns it into a beautiful family meal. I love this served over zucchini noodles or Creamy Cauliflower Purée (page 284). For a spicy version, use an arrabbiata tomato sauce or add some red pepper flakes to the pan when you're cooking the onions and garlic.

2 tablespoons ghee (page 336) or butter

2 medium yellow onions, sliced

4 large cloves garlic, grated or minced

2 pounds lemon sole or other whitefish fillets

1/2 teaspoon Trifecta Spice Blend (page 330)

1 (24-ounce) jar sugar-free pasta sauce

2 tablespoons capers

Lemon wedges, for serving (optional)

Place an oven rack directly under the broiler and turn on the oven to the broil setting.

Melt the ghee in a large oven-safe skillet over medium heat. Add the onions and cook for 5 to 7 minutes, until they become translucent and begin to brown. Add the garlic and cook for 1 to 2 minutes, until the garlic starts to turn golden brown. Remove the onions from the pan and set aside.

Season each side of the sole with the spice blend. Add the sole to the pan and cook for 1 to 2 minutes, until it starts to brown. Flip the sole and return the onions to the pan, placing them around and on top of the fish. Add the pasta sauce and capers to the skillet around the fish.

Transfer the pan to the oven and broil for 5 minutes, until the fish is white all the way through and flaky, or cooked to your liking. If desired, add a squeeze of fresh lemon juice before serving.

268   **MAIN DISHES: SEAFOOD**   CALORIES: **429** | FAT: **13 g** | PROTEIN: **47 g** | CARBS: **29 g** | FIBER: **6 g** | NET CARBS: **23 g**

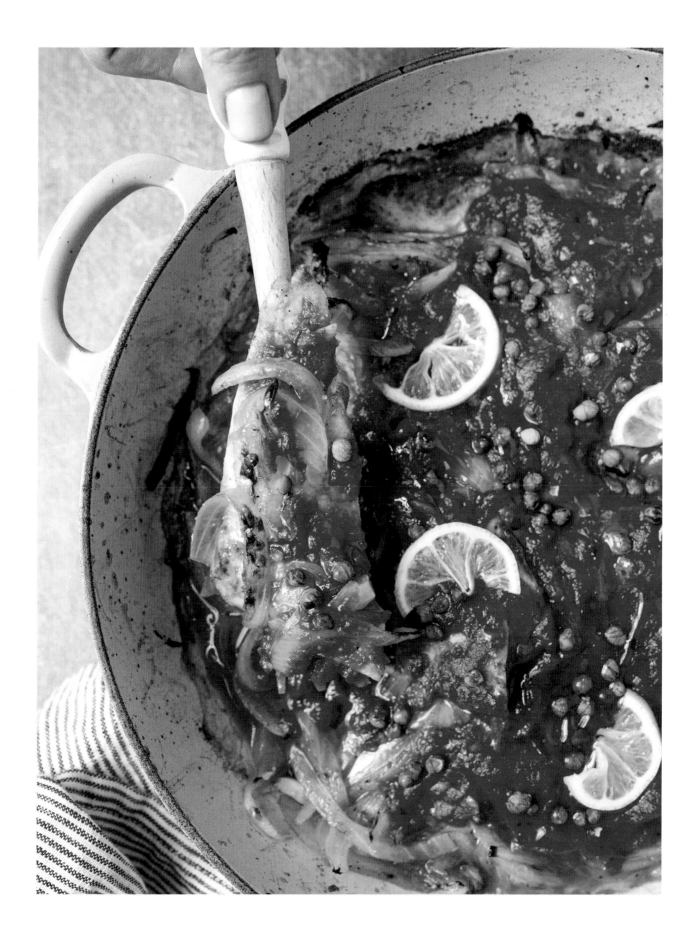

Glazed Salmon with Seared Bok Choy

PREP TIME: 10 minutes | COOK TIME: 16 minutes | YIELD: 4 servings

This easy salmon recipe is perfect for a weeknight when you're stopping at the grocery store and bringing home just a few items to cook up. Swap cod for the salmon if you prefer, and any hearty greens will work if bok choy isn't available—like green cabbage, Lacinato kale, or Swiss chard.

2 pounds wild salmon fillets

1 teaspoon Trifecta Spice Blend (page 330)

1 tablespoon coconut oil

1 pound baby bok choy, chopped (see Note)

2 teaspoons coconut aminos

Sea salt

1 tablespoon water

FOR THE DEGLAZING LIQUID

1/4 cup coconut aminos

1/4 cup fresh lemon juice

1 tablespoon coconut oil

1 teaspoon fish sauce

2 cloves garlic, grated or minced

1/4 teaspoon ginger powder

FOR GARNISH (OPTIONAL)

2 teaspoons sesame seeds

Place an oven rack directly under the broiler and turn on the oven to the broil setting. Heat a large oven-safe skillet (preferably cast-iron) over high heat.

Use a paper towel to pat the salmon dry on both sides. Sprinkle both sides lightly with the spice blend.

Place the salmon skin side down in the preheated dry skillet and sear for 2 minutes. Transfer the pan to the oven and broil for 4 minutes, until the salmon is opaque in the center or cooked to your liking. Remove the salmon from the pan once it's cooked so that you can deglaze the pan.

In a small bowl, mix together all the deglazing liquid ingredients. Return the pan to the stovetop over high heat and pour in the deglazing liquid. Use a whisk to remove the seared bits from the bottom of the pan to flavor the sauce. Let the sauce reduce for 4 to 5 minutes, until it becomes thick and sticky, stirring occasionally.

Heat a separate large skillet over medium-high heat. Add the coconut oil, then the bok choy and coconut aminos. Season lightly with salt and add the water. Cover and cook for 4 to 5 minutes, until the bok choy is fork-tender, tossing halfway through.

To serve, divide the bok choy and salmon among 4 plates and drizzle the sauce over the top. Garnish with sesame seeds, if desired.

HOW TO DEGLAZE A PAN

Pour a liquid such as broth into a very hot pan that has flavor-filled bits of food seared on the bottom. Whisk the liquid to remove the bits from the bottom of the pan and help flavor the sauce. Allow the liquid to simmer rapidly over high heat for a few minutes, then strain the sauce before serving.

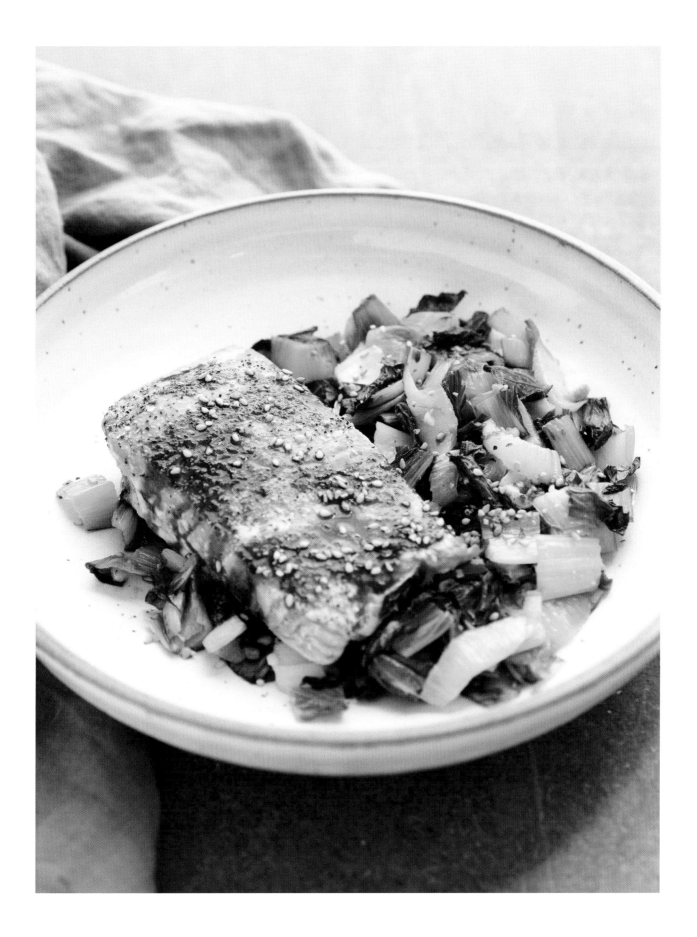

Deli Tuna Salad

PREP TIME: 15 minutes | YIELD: 4 servings

Perhaps this comes as no surprise, but growing up in New Jersey meant I ate a ton of bagel sandwiches. While the high-carb bagels are out on keto, my favorite parts, the tuna salad and spices, are in! The flavors of this recipe take me back to enjoying a heaping helping of tuna salad and "everything" spices from my local deli.

1 medium carrot, peeled

1/2 small red onion

3 (5-ounce) cans tuna (reserve the liquid)

1/4 cup mayonnaise, homemade (page 335) or store-bought (see Note)

1/2 teaspoon Trifecta Spice Blend (page 330)

1 stalk celery, finely chopped

1 head butter lettuce, for serving

FOR SERVING

Red onion slices

Tomato slices

FOR GARNISH

Bagel Spice Blend (page 330)

TO MAKE WITH A FOOD PROCESSOR:

Fit your food processor with the shredding disc and shred the carrot and red onion. Remove the shredding blade and fit the processor with the chopping blade. Add the tuna, 1 tablespoon of the liquid from the cans, the mayonnaise, and the Trifecta Spice Blend. If you prefer creamier tuna salad, use more of the liquid from the cans of tuna. Pulse 6 to 10 times, until well combined. Add the celery and stir to combine.

TO MAKE BY HAND:

Shred the carrot and red onion with a box grater or finely mince them by hand. Place the carrot and onion in a large mixing bowl and add the tuna, 1 tablespoon of the liquid from the cans, the mayonnaise, the Trifecta Spice Blend, and the celery. If you prefer creamier tuna salad, use more of the liquid from the cans of tuna. Stir to combine.

Taste and add additional seasoning if desired. Spoon the tuna onto 4 lettuce leaves (you can layer 2 leaves if you like) and serve with slices of red onion and tomato. Garnish with the Bagel Spice Blend.

> **NOTE**
> If you're not making your own mayonnaise (see page 335), I recommend buying 100% avocado oil mayonnaise. Two brands I like are Sir Kensington's and Primal Kitchen.

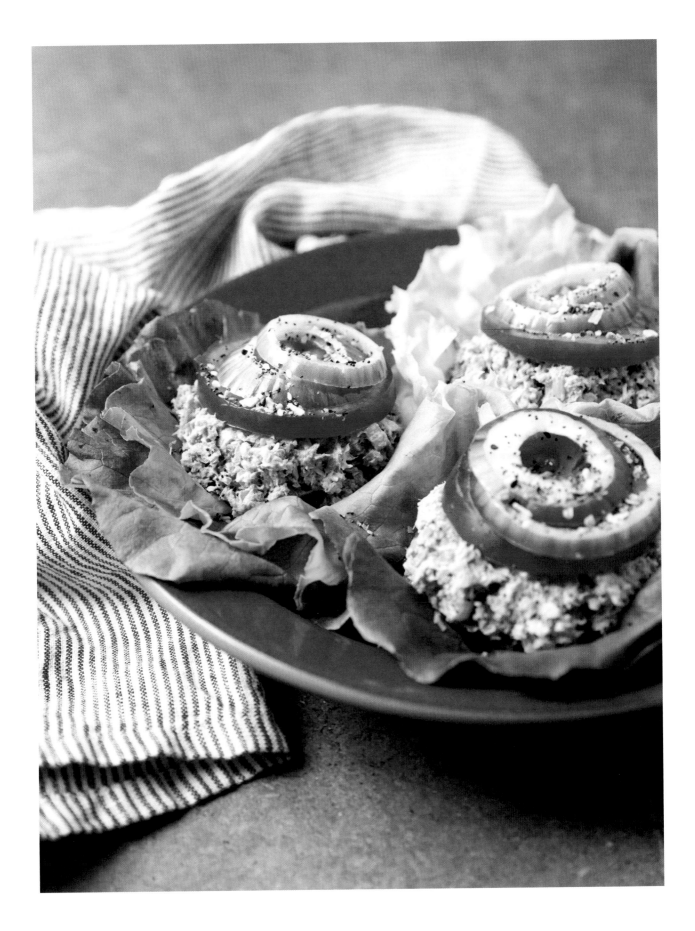

Niçoise Salad

PREP TIME: **5 minutes** | COOK TIME: **20 minutes** | YIELD: **4 servings**

If you enjoy a chunky salad with more toppings than lettuce, this is a great option for you! You can swap canned tuna or cooked fish or chicken for the sardines if you prefer, but sardines are a power-packed superfood rich in healthy omega-3s, and they're easy to keep on hand so you can have this salad anytime.

4 large eggs

3 cups water

8 ounces green beans, trimmed

Sea salt

1 head butter lettuce, cut into bite-sized pieces

1 cup cherry tomatoes, halved

1/2 cup pitted Kalamata olives

1/2 medium red onion, thinly sliced

4 (4-ounce) cans sardines packed in olive oil, drained

FOR THE DRESSING

3 tablespoons lemon juice (about 2 lemons)

1/4 cup extra-virgin olive oil

1/2 teaspoon Dijon mustard

Sea salt and ground black pepper

HARD-BOIL THE EGGS:

Fill a medium-sized saucepan two-thirds full with water, cover, and bring to a boil over high heat. When the water comes to a boil, gently place the eggs in the pot using a slotted spoon. Boil for 8 minutes for slightly runny centers or 10 minutes for hard-boiled. While the eggs boil, fill a large bowl with water and ice. Place the eggs in the ice bath immediately after cooking to halt the cooking process. Set aside.

COOK THE GREEN BEANS:

Fill a large bowl with ice water and set aside. In a large saucepan, bring the 3 cups of water to a boil. Add the green beans and a pinch of salt. Cook until the green beans are slightly cooked but still firm, about 3 minutes. Transfer the beans to the ice water to stop the cooking process and let sit for about 2 minutes to cool. Drain.

Place the lettuce on a large serving platter. Arrange the cherry tomatoes, olives, onion slices, eggs, and sardines in small piles on top of the lettuce.

Whisk together all the dressing ingredients in a small bowl. Add salt and pepper to taste. Pour the dressing over the salad and enjoy.

CALORIES: **490** | FAT: **32g** | PROTEIN: **35g** | CARBS: **20g** | FIBER: **10g** | NET CARBS: **10g**

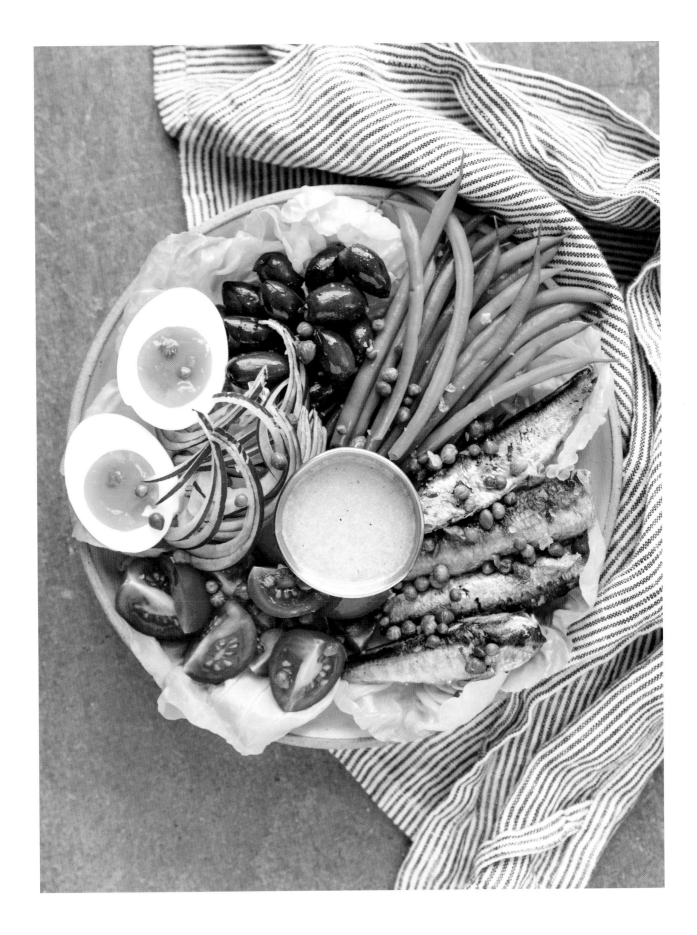

Salmon Avocado Roll-Ups

PREP TIME: 5 minutes | YIELD: **about 8 roll-ups (4 per serving)**

Smoked salmon is a perfect easy protein source to have on hand at all times. You can pair it with scrambled eggs for breakfast or enjoy it in these roll-ups for breakfast or lunch—or even a snack. For even more crunch, add a slice of cucumber to each roll-up!

1 medium avocado, peeled, pitted, and smashed (see Tip)

Juice of 1/2 lemon

Pinch of sea salt

2 tablespoons minced chives

8 ounces smoked salmon

1 head Boston or Bibb lettuce, leaves separated

1/4 cup Marinated Onions (page 290)

Bagel Spice Blend (page 330), for garnish (optional)

In a small bowl, combine the avocado, lemon juice, salt, and chives.

Assemble the roll-ups: Place a few slices of smoked salmon on a lettuce leaf, then top with the avocado mixture and the marinated onions. Sprinkle with the spice blend, if desired. Repeat with the remaining ingredients.

TIP

You can use 1/2 cup of cream cheese in place of the avocado if you prefer!

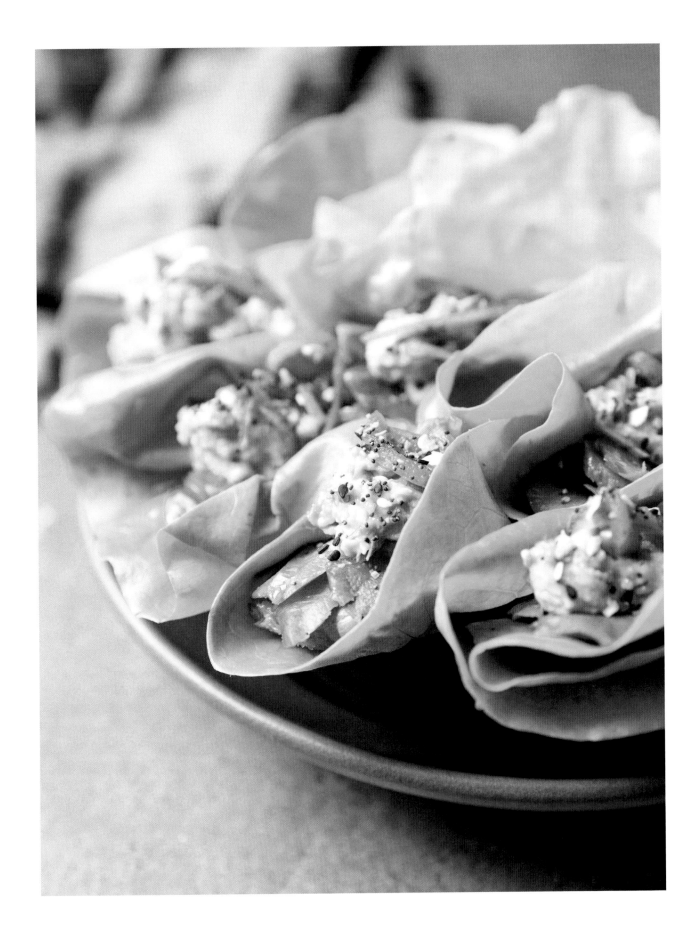

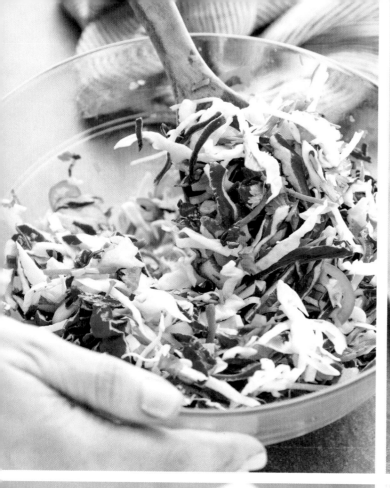
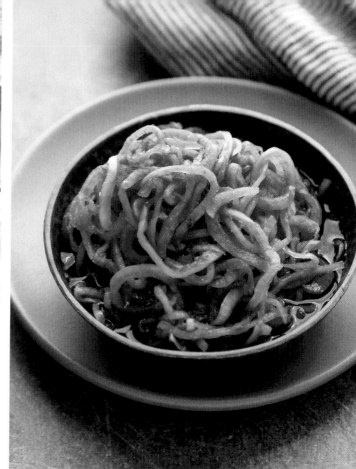
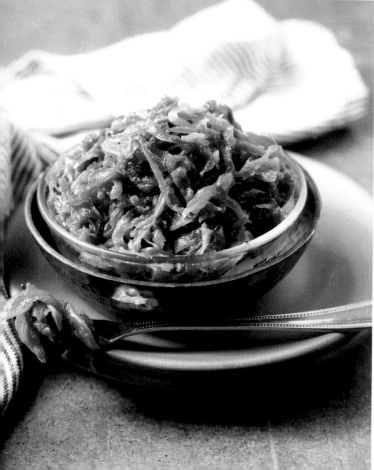
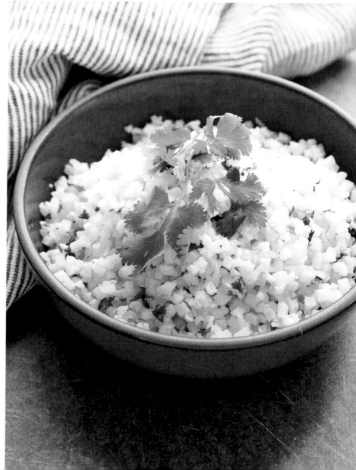

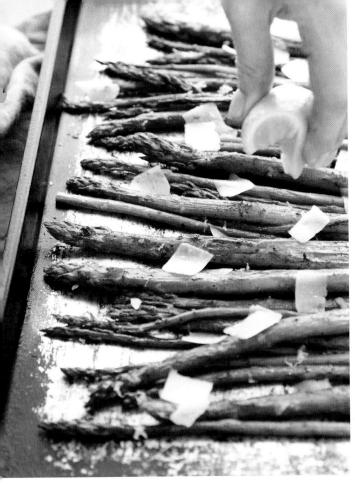

Sides

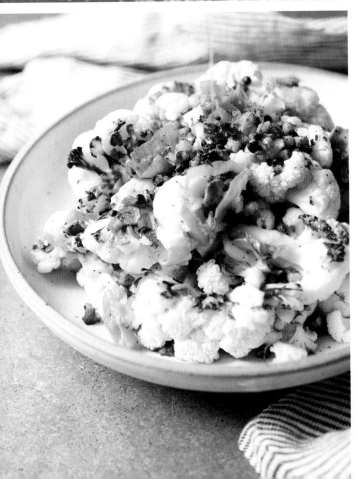

Spicy Citrus Slaw

PREP TIME: **15 minutes** | YIELD: **4 servings**

If you're looking for a simple, fresh side dish that you can pair with not only tacos but almost any easy protein, this one is for you! Top salads with it to add crunch, or pair it with some sausage for a quick and easy meal. Add more jalapeños for more heat or leave them out for a milder flavor.

1 tablespoon extra-virgin olive oil

Grated zest of 1 lemon

Grated zest of 1 lime

1 tablespoon lemon juice

1 tablespoon lime juice

A few pinches of sea salt

1 (16-ounce) bag coleslaw mix
(or about 1/2 head of cabbage and
1 carrot, shredded)

1 jalapeño pepper, sliced, seeded if
desired for less heat (optional)

In a large mixing bowl, combine the olive oil, lemon and lime zest, lemon and lime juice, and salt, and whisk until well mixed. Add the slaw mix and jalapeño (if using) and toss until the ingredients are evenly distributed.

NIGHTSHADE-FREE?
Omit the jalapeño.

CALORIES: **82** | FAT: **4 g** | PROTEIN: **2 g** | CARBS: **13 g** | FIBER: **5 g** | NET CARBS: **8 g**

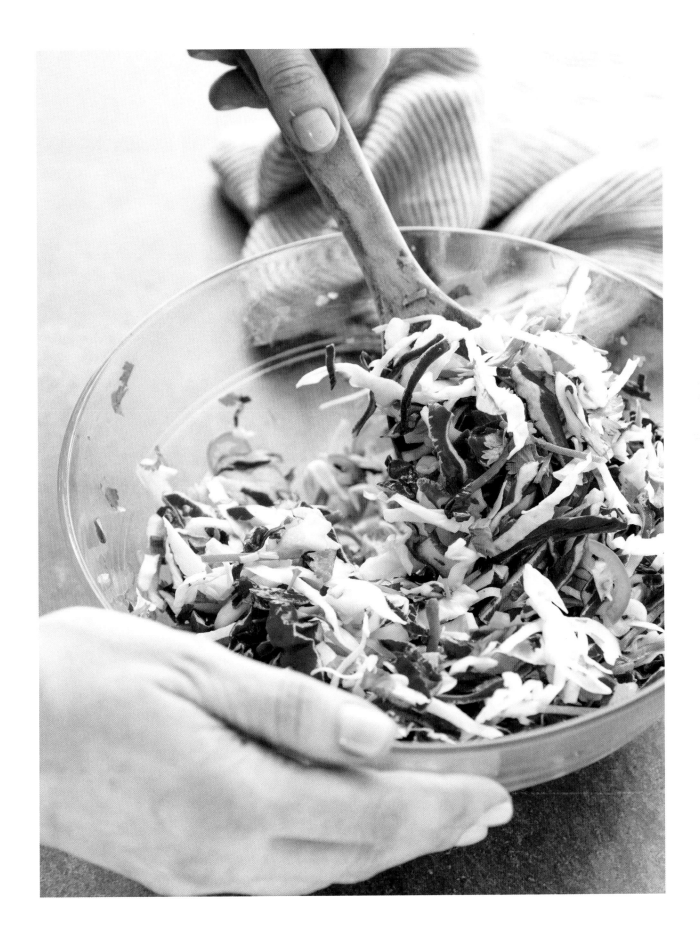

NUTS | EGGS | NIGHTSHADES | **FODMAPS** | DAIRY | **21DSD-FRIENDLY**

Cilantro Cauli-Rice

PREP TIME: **15 minutes** | COOK TIME: **5 minutes** | YIELD: **4 servings**

When you don't know what side to pair with a meal, a basic cauliflower rice is the perfect go-to. It works well as a rice replacement in any cuisine, or top it with red sauce as a replacement for pasta. It cooks quickly whether the cauliflower is fresh or frozen, so you can have it on the table in a flash!

1 medium head cauliflower, cut into florets

1 tablespoon cooking fat of choice

Sea salt and ground black pepper

1/4 cup finely chopped fresh cilantro leaves

Cilantro sprig, for garnish (optional)

Shred the cauliflower using a box grater or food processor into pieces the size of grains of rice.

In a large skillet over medium heat, melt the cooking fat. Add the shredded cauliflower and season with salt and pepper. Sauté for about 5 minutes, or until the cauliflower begins to become translucent, stirring gently to ensure that it cooks through.

Transfer the cooked cauliflower to a serving bowl and toss with the chopped cilantro. Garnish with a sprig of cilantro if desired.

TIP

To save time, buy packaged fresh or frozen riced cauliflower. If you use frozen for this recipe, it may take an additional 5 minutes to heat and cook through.

CALORIES: **65** | FAT: **4 g** | PROTEIN: **3 g** | CARBS: **8 g** | FIBER: **4 g** | NET CARBS: **4 g**

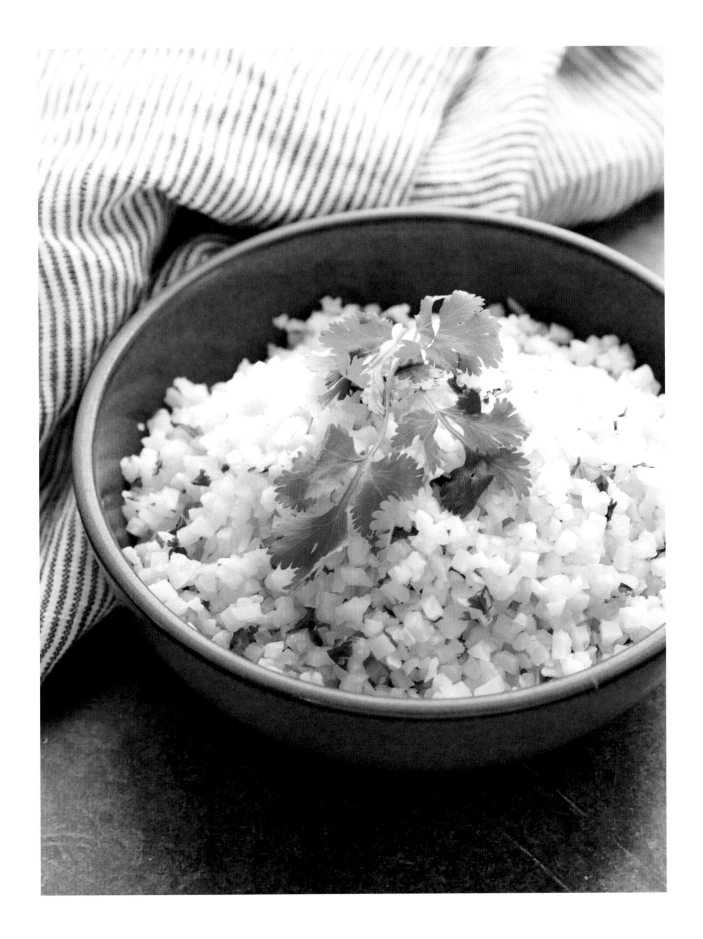

Creamy Cauliflower Purée

PREP TIME: 10 minutes | COOK TIME: 15 minutes | YIELD: 4 servings

To replace the creamy, silky texture of mashed potatoes, you can't beat cauliflower purée! The key to a perfectly smooth texture is steaming the cauliflower until it's practically falling apart. You can even use this as a base for a simple soup: just add some cooked onions and garlic and some broth (page 220).

1 medium head cauliflower, roughly chopped into 2- to 3-inch pieces (about 4 cups)

1/4 cup butter or ghee (page 336)

Sea salt and ground black pepper

Fill a large pot with 2 inches of water and place a steamer basket in the pot. Cover and bring to a boil over high heat. Add the cauliflower pieces to the basket and steam until fork-tender, about 15 minutes.

Place the cauliflower in a food processor. Add the butter and a few pinches of salt and pepper to taste. Puree until smooth and creamy.

> **TIP**
>
> If you don't have a food processor, you can use an immersion blender, a hand mixer, or a stand mixer, or mash the cauliflower by hand with a potato masher.

CALORIES: **136** | FAT: **12 g** | PROTEIN: **3 g** | CARBS: **8 g** | FIBER: **4 g** | NET CARBS: **4 g**

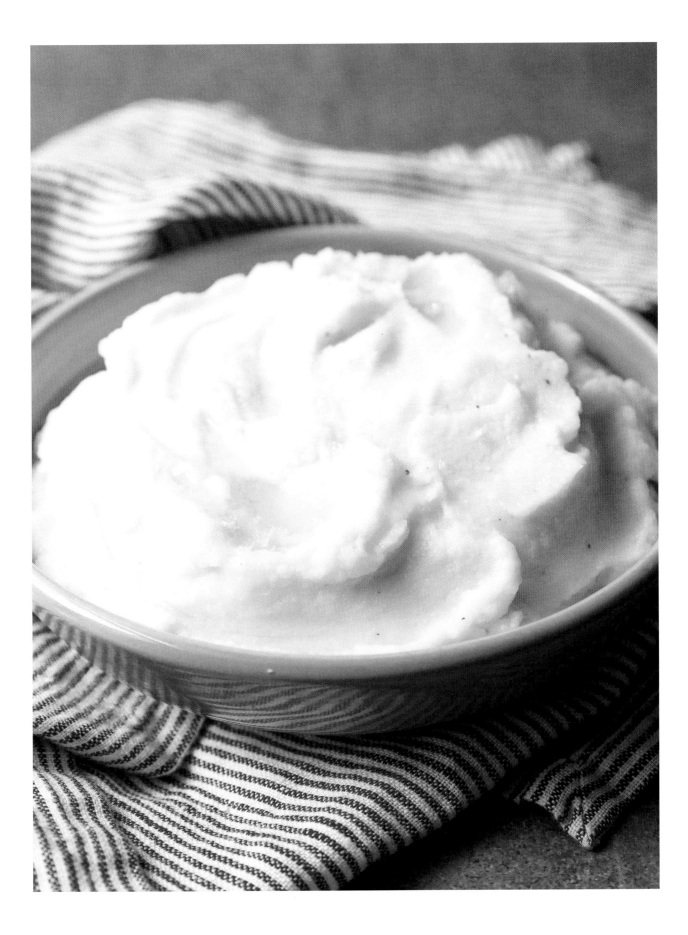

Mediterranean Roasted Cauliflower

PREP TIME: 10 minutes | COOK TIME: **40 minutes** | YIELD: **8 servings**

Roasted cauliflower is a perfect base for a lot of flavors—this time, Mediterranean! Pair it with Weeknight Roasted Chicken (page 212) or Mediterranean Meatloaf (page 232) for an exciting meal for the family. You can also finely chop this cauliflower and add it to a frittata with some feta cheese!

2 medium heads cauliflower, cut into florets

1/2 cup sliced pepperoncini, plus extra for garnish

1/4 cup capers

1/4 cup extra-virgin olive oil, melted ghee (page 336), or melted butter

4 ounces pancetta, diced (about 1/4 cup)

2 large cloves garlic, thinly sliced

1/2 teaspoon ground cumin

Sea salt and ground black pepper

Juice of 1 lemon

Preheat the oven to 375°F.

Place the cauliflower on a rimmed baking sheet along with the pepperoncini, capers, olive oil, pancetta, and garlic, then season generously with the cumin, salt, and pepper. Toss everything together to evenly distribute the oil and seasoning.

Bake for 35 to 40 minutes, until the cauliflower is golden brown, stirring once halfway through cooking.

Pour the lemon juice over the top before serving.

NIGHTSHADE-FREE?
Omit the pepperoncini.

TURN DOWN THE HEAT
If your family doesn't like hot peppers, leave out the pepperoncini or replace them with roasted bell peppers.

CALORIES: **156** | FAT: **12 g** | PROTEIN: **5 g** | CARBS: **10 g** | FIBER: **4 g** | NET CARBS: **6 g**

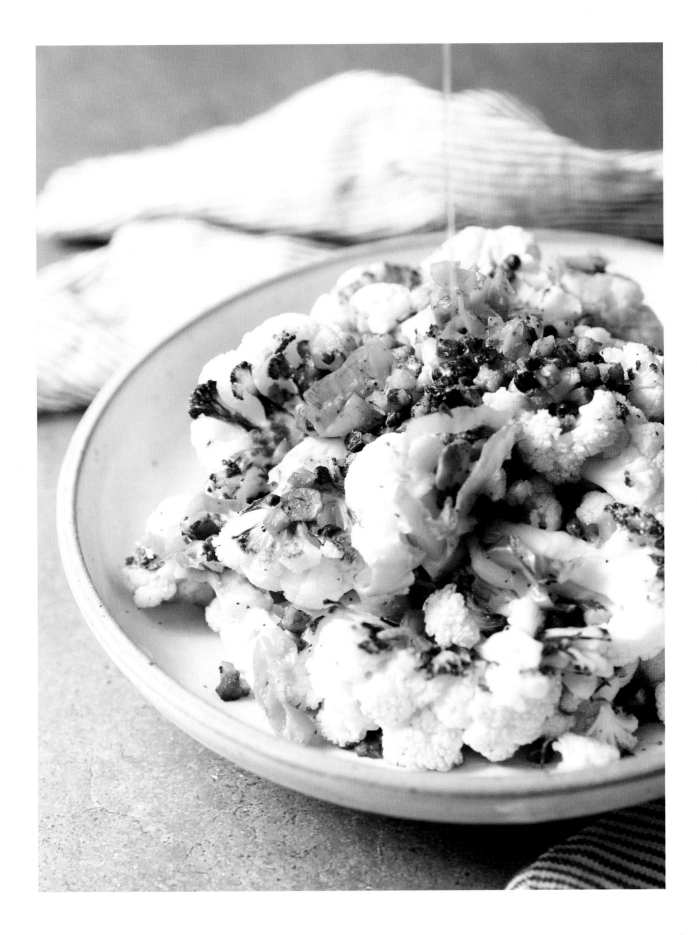

Blistered Shishito Peppers

PREP TIME: — | COOK TIME: **5 minutes** | YIELD: **4 servings**

Bell peppers can be a bit ho-hum as a side dish, so try this easy preparation for shishito peppers! About one in ten of these peppers may have a spicy kick, but most of them are mild, and they make a great side dish or even a snack. Dip them in Ranch Dressing (page 347) or Keto Hummus (page 302), or enjoy them plain with coarse sea salt!

2 teaspoons cooking fat of choice

12 ounces shishito peppers

Pinch of sea salt

Coarse sea salt, for garnish

Heat the cooking fat in a large skillet over high heat. Add the peppers, season lightly with salt, and sauté until charred, 4 to 5 minutes. Finish with coarse sea salt before serving.

CALORIES: **42** | FAT: **3 g** | PROTEIN: **1 g** | CARBS: **5 g** | FIBER: **3 g** | NET CARBS: **2 g**

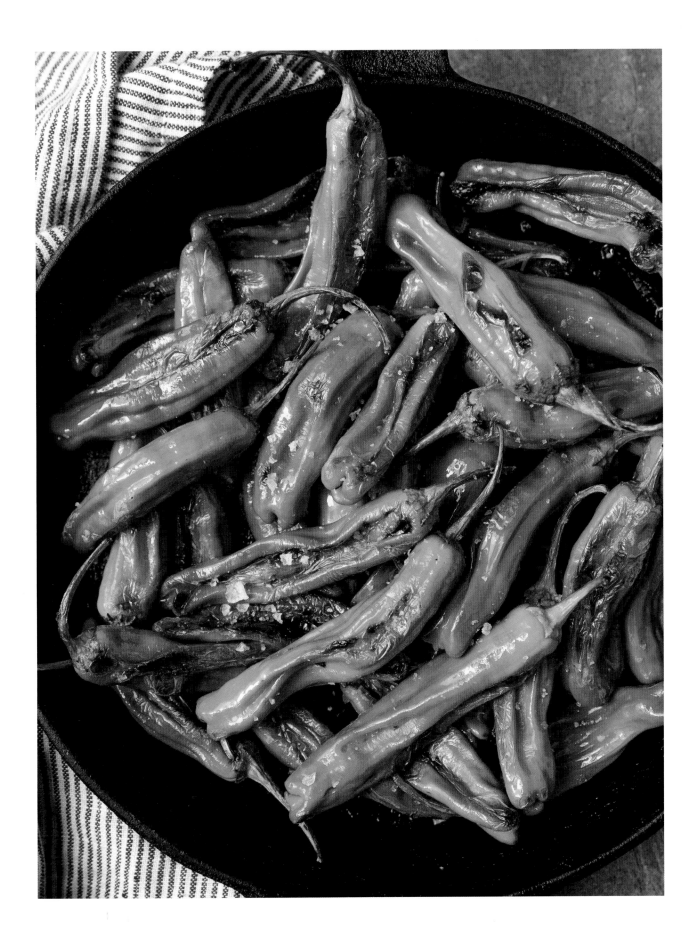

Marinated Onions

PREP TIME: 10 minutes, plus time to marinate the onions | YIELD: about 2 cups (1/2 cup per serving)

While pickled onions typically include sugar, these have no sugar at all and are a keto-friendly way to add some tangy flavor to lots of dishes. Enjoy these on burgers, in tuna salad, in tacos, or as a salad topper (they're used in several Easy Keto Meal Ideas on pages 154 and 155). Keep a batch of these on hand at all times; you'll be glad you have them!

1/3 cup red wine vinegar

1 teaspoon coarse or flake sea salt, or 1/2 teaspoon fine sea salt

1 teaspoon dried oregano leaves or dried chives

1/2 teaspoon garlic powder

1/4 teaspoon ground black pepper

2 medium red onions, cut in 1/4-inch-thick half moons

In a medium-sized mixing bowl, mix together the oil, vinegar, salt, and spices. Add the onions, stir to coat well, cover, and marinate overnight in the refrigerator.

The onions will keep in an airtight container in the refrigerator for 1 to 2 weeks.

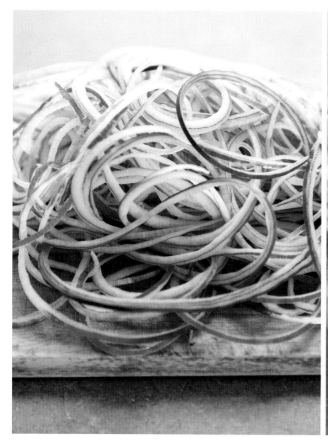 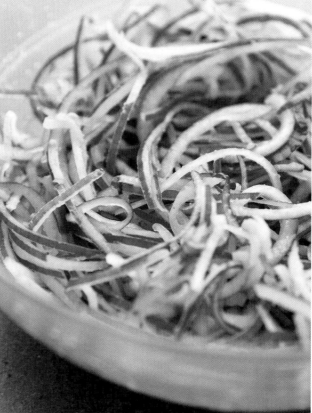

CALORIES: **26** | FAT: **0 g** | PROTEIN: **1 g** | CARBS: **5 g** | FIBER: **1 g** | NET CARBS: **4 g**

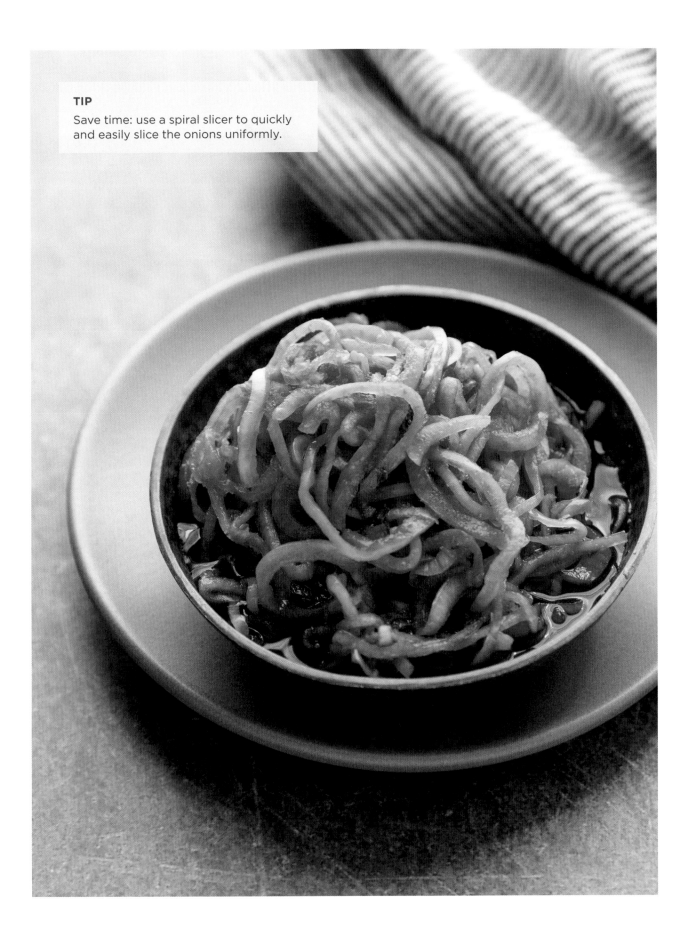

TIP
Save time: use a spiral slicer to quickly and easily slice the onions uniformly.

Spicy Roasted Asparagus with Lemon

PREP TIME: **5 minutes** | COOK TIME: **15 minutes** | YIELD: **4 servings**

Asparagus is a great low-carb veggie option, and this is one easy preparation! You can grill asparagus, too, but this roasting method is quick and easy, and it packs in way more flavor than steaming or boiling would. Eat these hot or prep them ahead to chop and put on a salad for lunch the next day.

1 pound asparagus, trimmed and rinsed

1 tablespoon cooking fat of choice, melted

1/2 teaspoon granulated garlic

Sea salt and ground black pepper

1 tablespoon extra-virgin olive oil

Juice of 1/2 lemon

1/4 cup shaved Parmesan cheese (optional)

Grated zest of 1 lemon

1 teaspoon red pepper flakes

Preheat the oven to 375°F.

Place the asparagus on a rimmed baking sheet and toss with the melted cooking fat. Sprinkle it with the granulated garlic and lightly season with salt and pepper. Roast for 10 to 15 minutes, until bright green and fork-tender. You'll need less time for very thin asparagus, more time for very thick asparagus.

Remove the asparagus from the oven and drizzle it with the olive oil and lemon juice, then top with the cheese (if using), lemon zest, and red pepper flakes.

NIGHTSHADE-FREE?
Omit the red pepper flakes.

DAIRY-FREE?
Omit the cheese.

TIP
Use the remaining lemon half to make a quick spritzer by squeezing the juice into a glass of sparkling water.

CALORIES: **83** | FAT: **7 g** | PROTEIN: **3 g** | CARBS: **5 g** | FIBER: **2 g** | NET CARBS: **3 g**

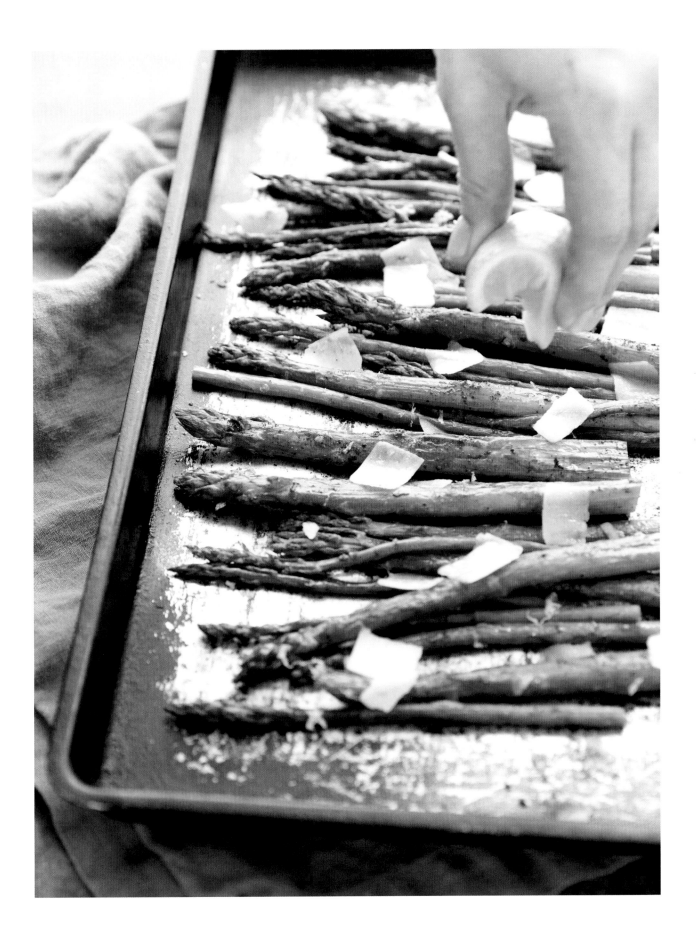

Bacon-y Caramelized Onions

PREP TIME: 10 minutes | COOK TIME: **45 minutes** | YIELD: **about 1 cup (1/4 cup per serving)**

Caramelized onions make the perfect burger topping and help to naturally sweeten my BBQ Sauce (page 341), which is delicious on ribs (see page 254) or as a dip for Keto Chicken Tenders (page 206). They do take time, but the deep flavor of these onions is worth the wait. Mix a small amount into some mayonnaise for a delicious spread. A little goes a long way with these!

2 tablespoons bacon fat (see Tip)

4 small yellow onions, thinly sliced

1/2 teaspoon sea salt

1/2 teaspoon dried rosemary leaves or thyme leaves (optional)

In a large sauté pan or skillet over medium heat, melt the bacon fat, then add the onions. Cook for 8 to 10 minutes, until the onions begin to become translucent. Add the salt and dried rosemary (if using).

Turn the heat down to medium-low and slowly cook the onions, stirring occasionally, for 45 minutes, allowing them to brown just slightly before stirring each time. If you find that the onions are browning too quickly or are sticking too much, reduce the heat slightly, add 1 to 2 tablespoons of warm water at a time to the pan, and stir it into the onions to keep them cooking evenly.

As they cook, the onions will become more and more browned and softened, and eventually they will look as they do in the photo. They will be rich-tasting and richly colored at the end of cooking. This process requires low, slow heat; faster, hotter heat will not yield the same results.

TIP
If you don't have bacon fat, you can use any cooking fat.

SERVING SUGGESTION
Enjoy these onions as a topping for burgers, sausages, or grass-fed hot dogs, or mix them into meatloaf or omelets.

CALORIES: **85** | FAT: **6 g** | PROTEIN: **1 g** | CARBS: **7 g** | FIBER: **1 g** | NET CARBS: **6 g**

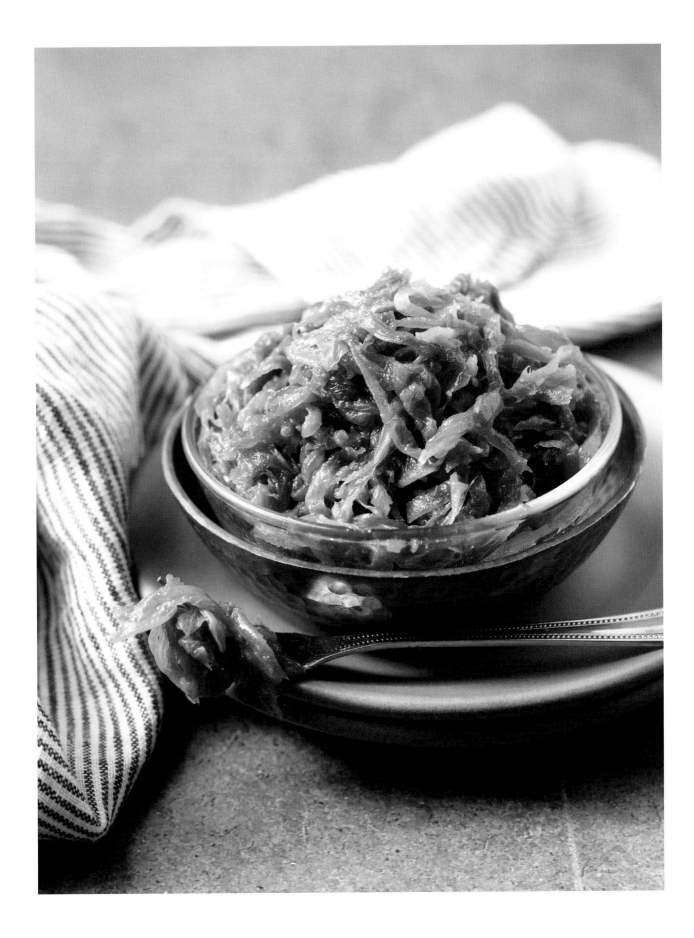

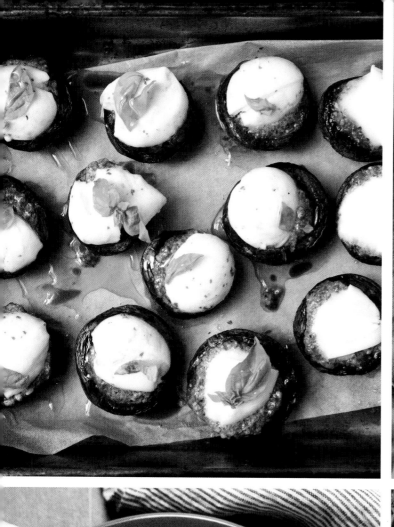

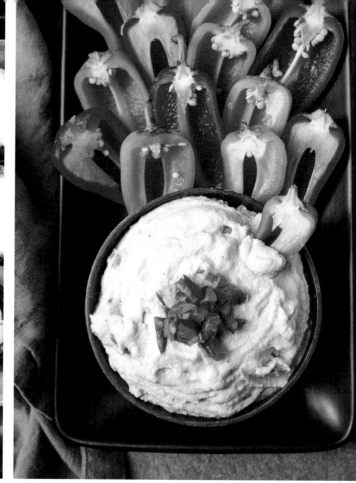

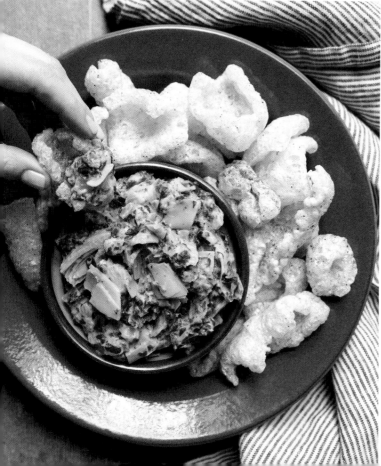

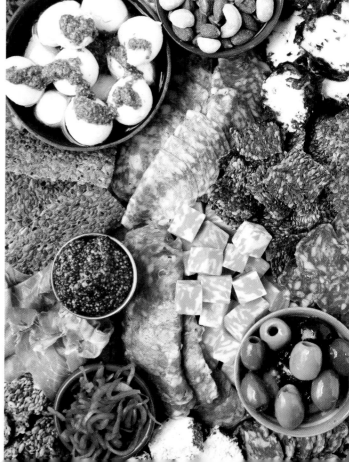

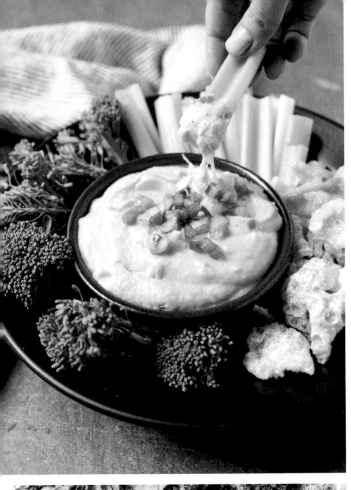

Snacks
& Dips

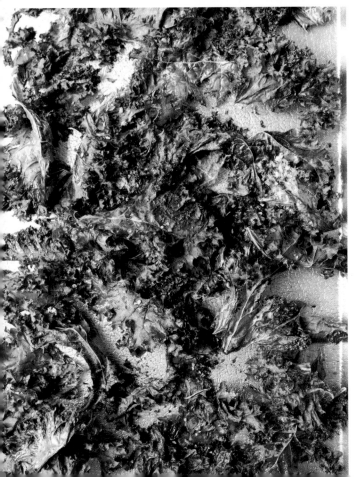

Herbed Cashew Cheese

PREP TIME: 10 minutes, plus time to soak the cashews | YIELD: 1 1/2 cups (1/4 cup per serving)

If you can't eat dairy and want a replacement for a soft, spreadable cheese (like cream cheese), try this! For a milder flavor, omit the raw garlic, or for a sweet version, season the plain base with a pinch of salt, cinnamon, and a few drops of stevia. The dairy-free base is a blank canvas for your creative ideas!

1 cup raw cashews

1 cup warm water

1/4 cup extra-virgin olive oil

1/4 cup water

2 tablespoons fresh lemon juice

1 clove garlic, minced or grated

2 tablespoons minced fresh chives

Sea salt and ground black pepper

Place the cashews in a small container and add the warm water. (If it doesn't cover the cashews completely, just add more warm water.) Soak for 1 to 4 hours unrefrigerated or up to overnight in the refrigerator.

Drain and rinse the cashews, then place them in a blender or food processor. Add the olive oil, the 1/4 cup water, the lemon juice, and the garlic. Process until smooth and creamy, stopping occasionally to scrape down the sides of the processor, about 5 minutes total. Mix in the chives and add salt and pepper to taste.

If you'd like a lighter texture, add warm water, 1 tablespoon at a time, until you achieve the desired consistency.

CALORIES: **288** | FAT: **25 g** | PROTEIN: **7 g** | CARBS: **13 g** | FIBER: **1 g** | NET CARBS: **12 g**

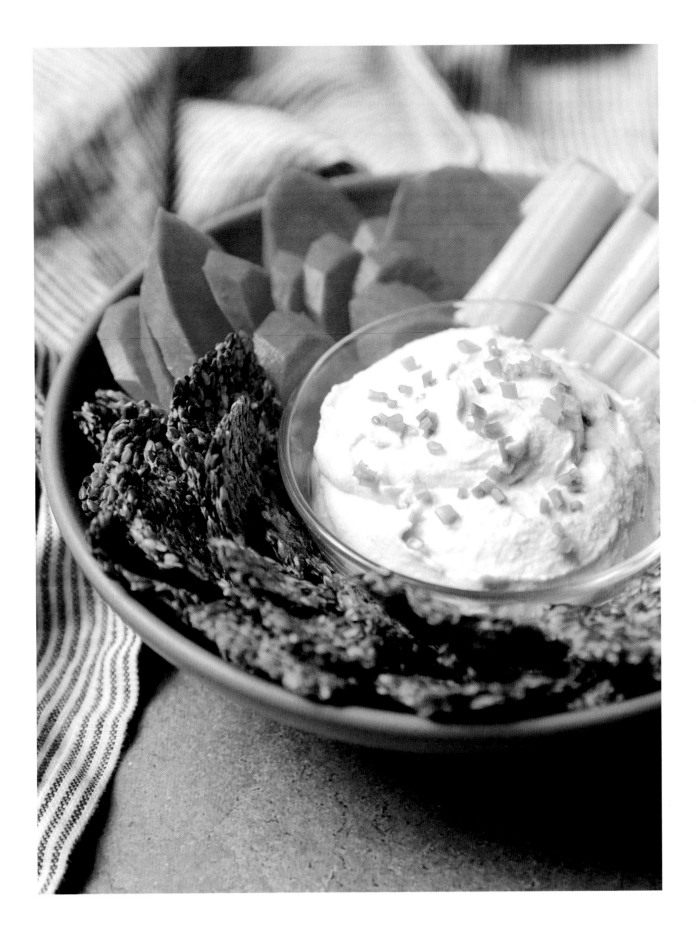

Bacon Jalapeño Poppers

PREP TIME: **10 minutes** | COOK TIME: **30 minutes** | YIELD: **16 poppers (4 per serving)**

These poppers make a great snack or game-day bite. They're a perfect balance of a little heat, some creamy filling, and smoky, salty bacon. I recommend using smaller jalapeños so that they're bite-sized and the bacon wraps easily.

8 jalapeños, halved lengthwise and seeded

1/2 cup Herbed Cashew Cheese (page 298)

8 slices bacon, cut in half

Ranch Dressing (page 347), for serving (optional)

Preheat the oven to 375°F. Line a rimmed baking sheet with foil, then place a wire baking rack on it.

Stuff the jalapeños with the herb cheese, then wrap a piece of bacon around each one.

Bake for 25 to 30 minutes, until the bacon is crispy.

Let cool slightly, then serve with ranch dressing on the side if desired.

TIP

You can use toothpicks to hold the bacon to the jalapeños—it has a tendency to shrink when baked.

CALORIES: **358** | FAT: **33 g** | PROTEIN: **10 g** | CARBS: **7 g** | FIBER: **1 g** | NET CARBS: **6 g**

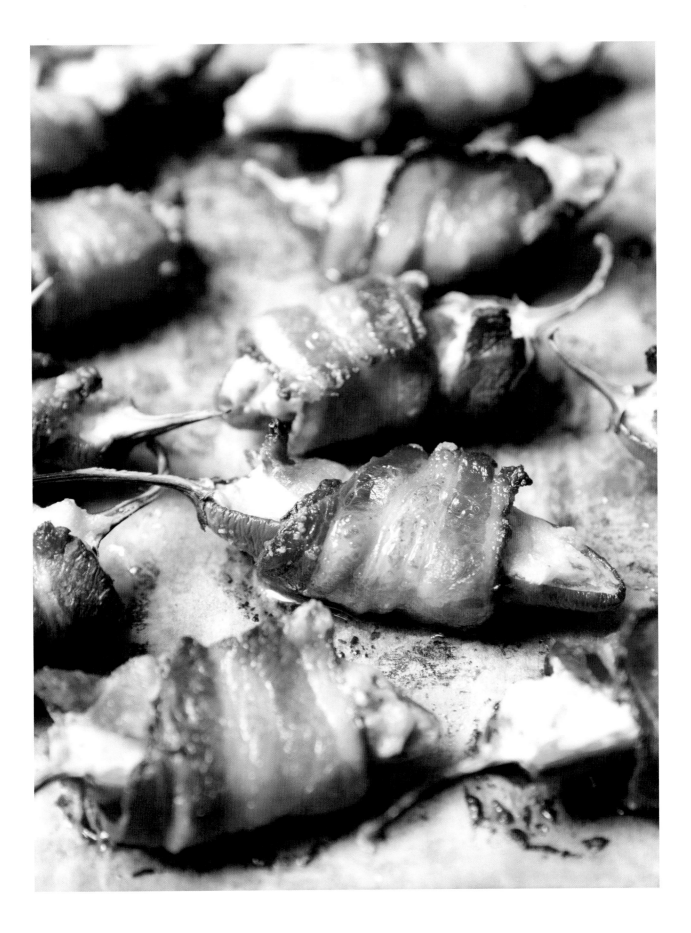

Keto Hummus

PREP TIME: 15 minutes | COOK TIME: 15 minutes | YIELD: about 2 cups (1/4 cup per serving)

A perfect snack or dip for a gathering, hummus is always a crowd-pleaser. This low-carb version will fool even the biggest hummus fans. Serve it as a dip for veggies or as a dippable side with lamb chops or meatballs seasoned with Mediterranean spices.

4 cups cauliflower florets

1/4 cup plus 1 tablespoon extra-virgin olive oil, divided

2 tablespoons raw or roasted tahini

Juice of 1 lemon (reserve the zest for garnish)

Pinch of ground cumin

Sea salt and ground black pepper

Pinch of paprika, for garnish (optional)

FOR SERVING

Olives

Sliced vegetables

Fill a large pot with 2 inches of water and place a steamer basket in the pot. Cover and bring to a boil over high heat. Add the cauliflower and steam for 15 minutes, until fork-tender.

In a food processor, combine the steamed cauliflower, 1/4 cup of the olive oil, the tahini, lemon juice, and cumin and process until smooth. Add salt and pepper to taste, along with more tahini or olive oil if you like.

Scoop the hummus into a serving dish and garnish with the lemon zest, remaining tablespoon of olive oil, and paprika (if using). Serve with sliced vegetables and olives.

Store in an airtight container in the refrigerator for up to 5 days.

NIGHTSHADE-FREE?
Omit the paprika.

NOTE
If you spot an orange cauliflower in your local market, use it instead of the white variety for a deeper-colored dip that looks even more like traditional hummus made from garbanzo beans.

TIP
When adding raw garlic to a dressing, sauce, or dip that will remain uncooked, more is not always better! The potency of raw garlic intensifies as it sits, so don't let this recipe be one where you read "1 clove" and translate it to "4 cloves," as garlic lovers often do when cooking!

CHANGE IT UP
Substitute zucchini for the cauliflower, but shred and strain it to remove most of its water content before adding it to the food processor.

CALORIES: **110** | FAT: **10 g** | PROTEIN: **2 g** | CARBS: **4 g** | FIBER: **2 g** | NET CARBS: **2 g**

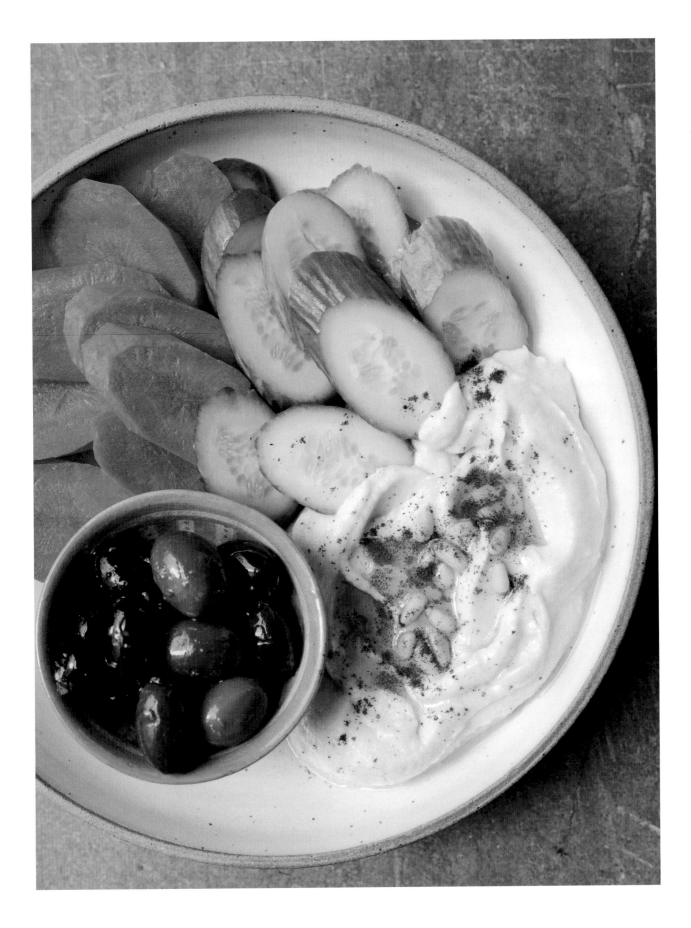

Quick Guacamole

PREP TIME: 15 minutes | YIELD: 2 cups (1/4 cup per serving)

Grab a few avocados at the grocery store and this guacamole comes together quickly, with just a few additions! My best tip for perfectly ripe avocados: leave them on the countertop, then, once they feel a bit soft when you press on them, either use or refrigerate them. They'll last a few more days this way!

4 ripe medium avocados, peeled, halved, and pitted

Juice of 2 limes

1 medium shallot, minced

1/4 cup chopped fresh cilantro leaves

Sea salt and ground black pepper

1 small jalapeño, minced (optional)

Sliced vegetables, for serving

In a large mixing bowl, mash the avocado with a fork. Stir in the lime juice. Add the shallot, cilantro, salt, and pepper and stir until well combined. If you like spicy guacamole, add the jalapeño and stir to combine.

Serve chilled or at room temperature with sliced vegetables.

Store in an airtight container, keeping the pit from one avocado inside the container to help it keep from browning. Keep in the refrigerator for up to 3 days.

NIGHTSHADE-FREE?
Omit the jalapeño.

CALORIES: **120** | FAT: **11 g** | PROTEIN: **2 g** | CARBS: **8 g** | FIBER: **5 g** | NET CARBS: **3 g**

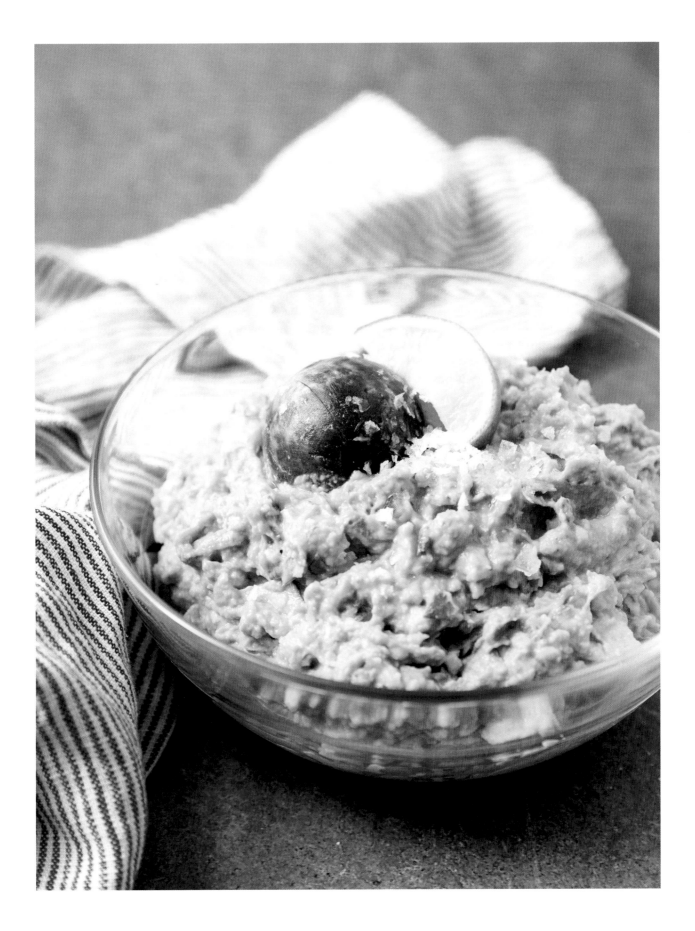

Quick Salsa

PREP TIME: 5 minutes | YIELD: **about 3 cups (1/4 cup per serving)**

Many store-bought salsas contain added sugar or other ingredients you don't need or want. While you can often find fresh pico de gallo that's healthy, salsa is very quick and easy to make at a fraction of the cost! Using a food processor will yield a smoother texture than pictured, but it is faster than chopping by hand!

1/4 cup fresh cilantro, stems and leaves, finely chopped

1 small red onion, finely chopped

8 roma tomatoes or other small to medium tomatoes, finely chopped

1 small jalapeño pepper, minced, seeded if desired for less heat (optional)

Juice of 1 to 2 limes

Sea salt and ground black pepper

Toss together all the ingredients in a large mixing bowl. Alternatively, place all the ingredients in a food processor and pulse until the desired consistency is reached.

Season with salt and pepper to taste.

Store in an airtight container in the refrigerator for up to 5 days.

CALORIES: **12** | FAT: **3 g** | PROTEIN: **1 g** | CARBS: **3 g** | FIBER: **1 g** | NET CARBS: **2 g**

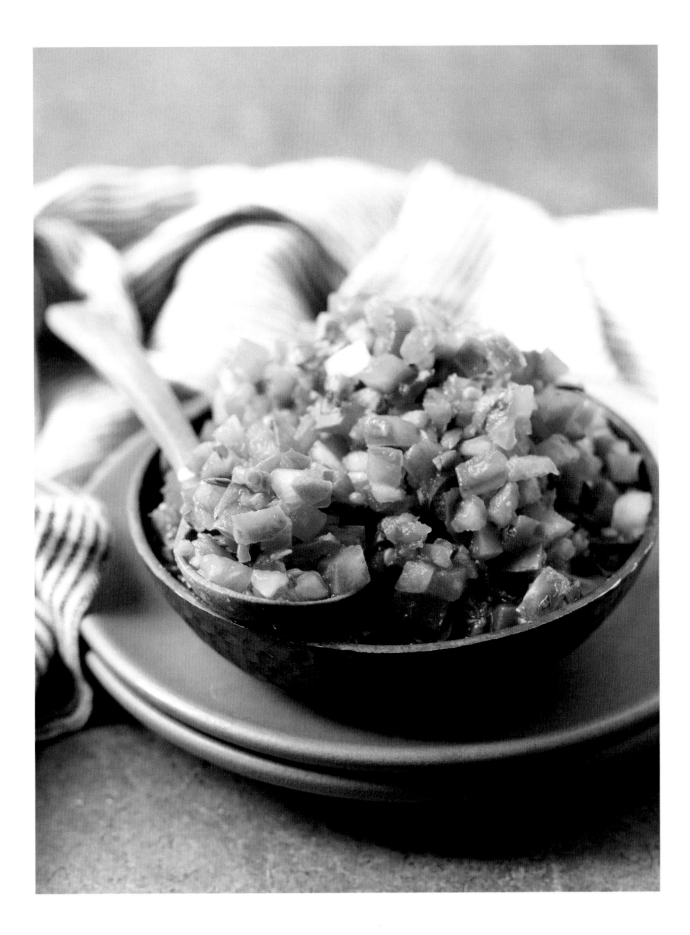

Baked Cheese Crisps

PREP TIME: **5 minutes** | COOK TIME: **10 minutes** | YIELD: **4 servings**

These couldn't be easier to make and are highly customizable. Add any spice blend you like to vary the flavor; just watch out for salt in the spice blends, as an already salty Parmesan cheese can get a bit over-the-top if you add more salt to it! I love chives, but adding some garlic or onion would also be great. These are perfect as a salad topper!

1 cup finely shredded Parmigiano-Reggiano cheese

1 tablespoon dried chives

TIP

If you have a silicone baking sheet liner, I highly recommend using it in place of parchment paper for this recipe; it will make the crisps easier to remove.

Preheat the oven to 375°F. Line a rimmed baking sheet with parchment paper.

Place heaping tablespoons of the cheese 1 inch apart on the prepared baking sheet, press down on them to flatten slightly, then sprinkle them with the chives.

Bake for 5 to 10 minutes, until browned and crispy. Keep an eye on the crisps during baking, as they can burn quickly.

Remove the crisps from the oven and cool completely before serving.

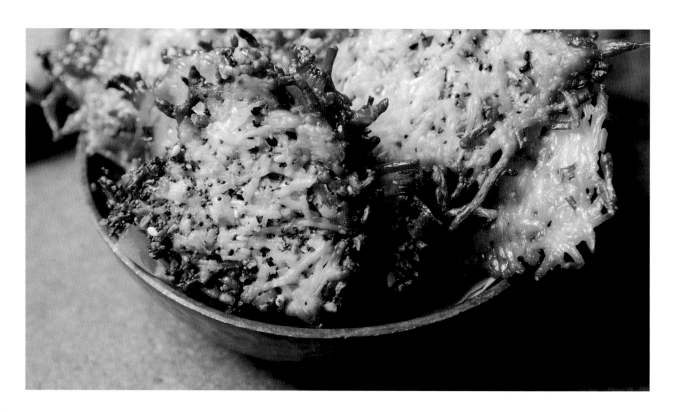

CALORIES: **219** | FAT: **15 g** | PROTEIN: **20 g** | CARBS: **2 g** | FIBER: **0 g** | NET CARBS: **2 g**

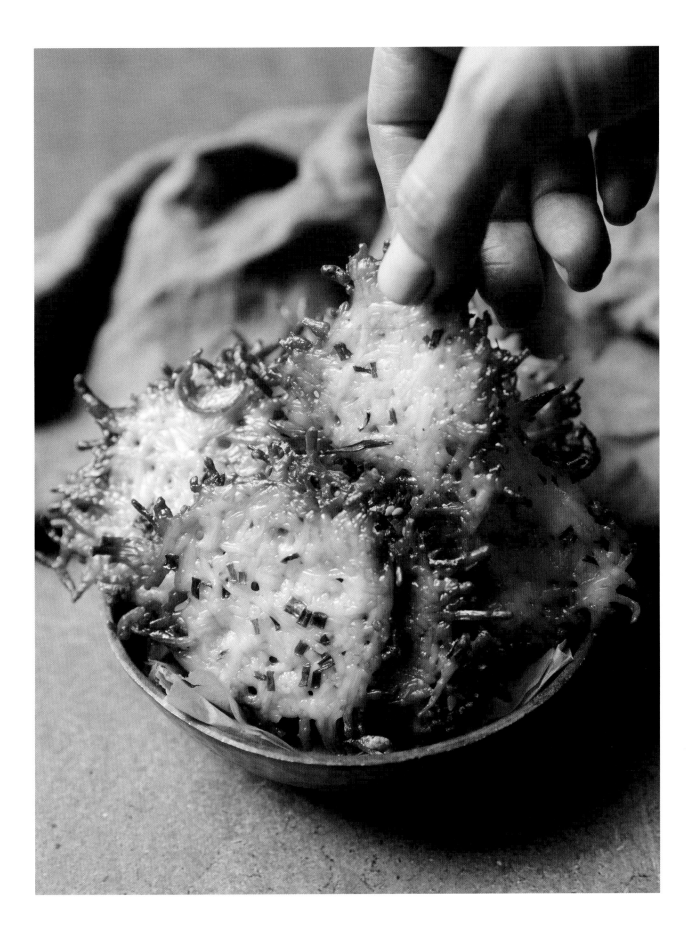

Pesto-Stuffed Mushrooms

PREP TIME: 20 minutes | **COOK TIME: 20 minutes** | **YIELD: 1 dozen mushrooms (3 per serving)**

My grandmother was known for her stuffed mushrooms appetizer, which we enjoyed at every holiday she hosted. These are a nod to her signature dish, without the carb-heavy breadcrumbs. You can use the pesto on page 343 or get a store-bought one (just watch out for junky oils). Top with fresh or shredded cheese and enjoy!

1 dozen baby bella mushroom caps, cleaned

8 ounces fresh mozzarella

1/2 cup Pesto (page 343)

Sea salt and ground black pepper

DAIRY-FREE?

Use my Herbed Cashew Cheese (page 298) instead of fresh mozzarella.

Preheat the oven to 350°F.

Place the mushrooms on a rimmed baking sheet cup side down and bake for 10 minutes, or until some of the moisture is released.

While the mushrooms are baking, slice the mozzarella into small pieces, approximately the size of the mushrooms.

Turn the mushrooms cup side up and fill each one with a spoonful of pesto and 1 or 2 pieces of mozzarella. Return the mushrooms to the oven and bake for about 10 minutes, until golden brown on top.

Sprinkle with salt and pepper before serving.

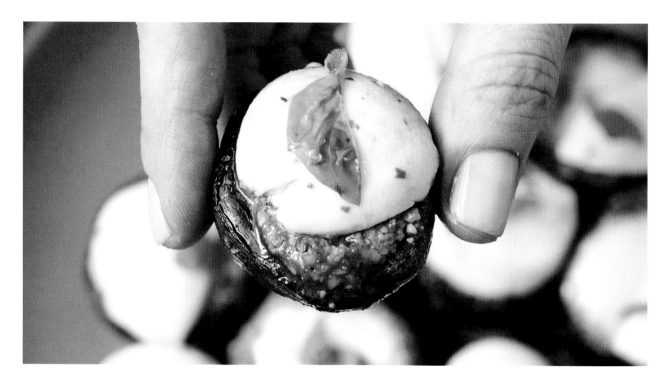

CALORIES: **132** | FAT: **11 g** | PROTEIN: **4 g** | CARBS: **5 g** | FIBER: **1 g** | NET CARBS: **4 g**

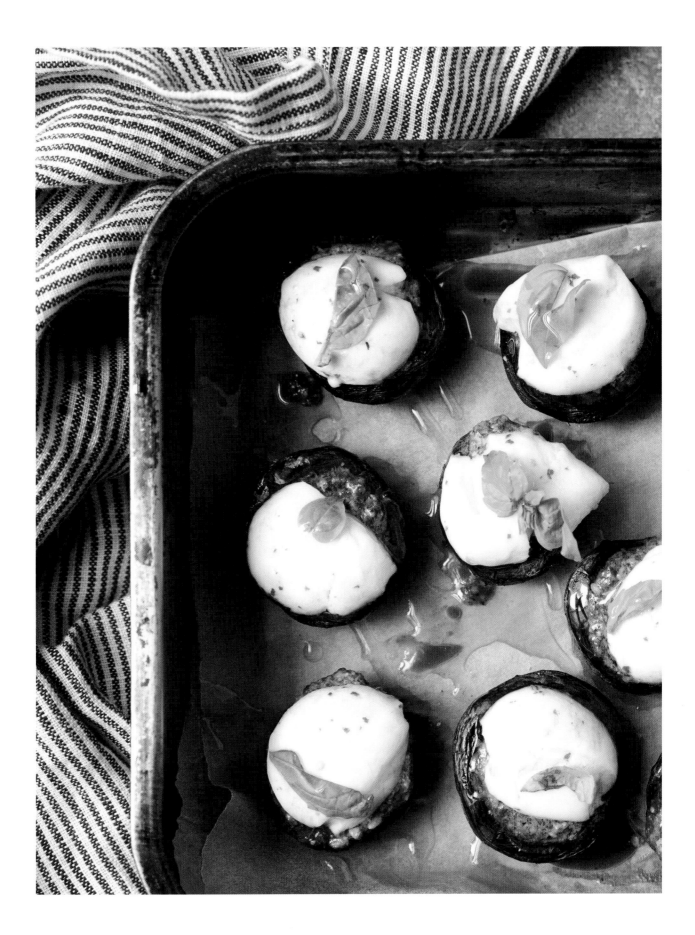

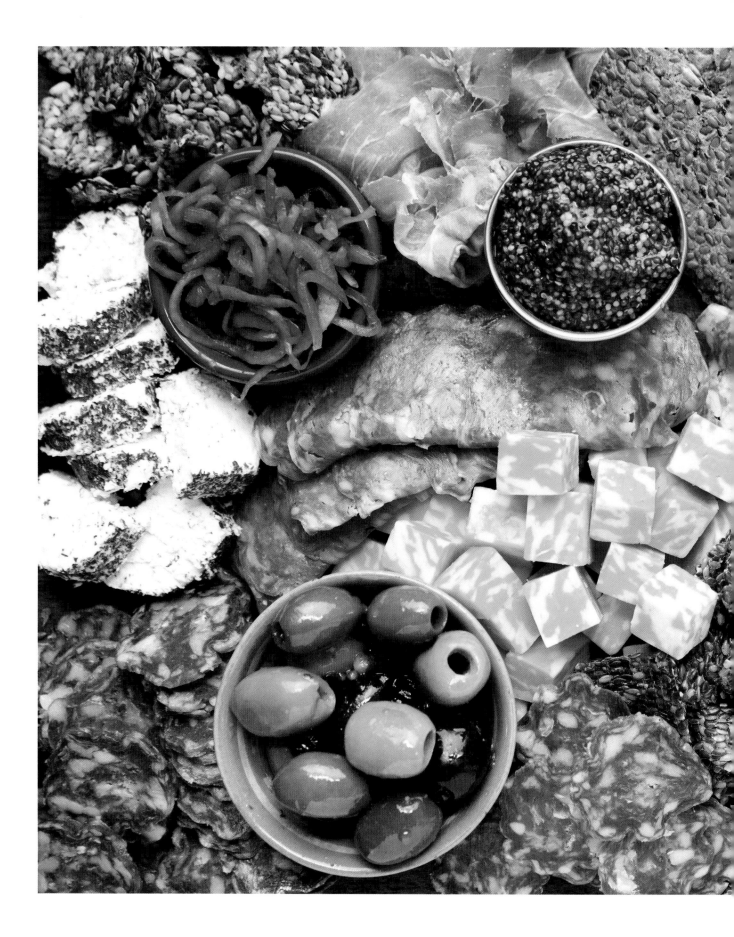

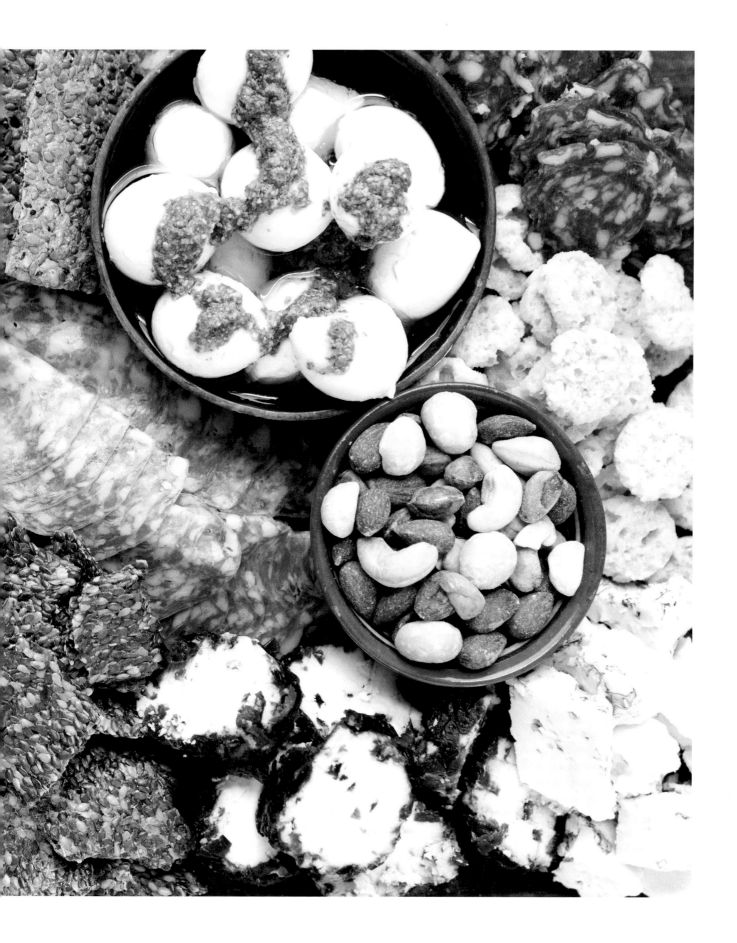

Keto Charcuterie Board

Charcuterie boards—spreads of meats, cheeses, nuts, and other savory finger foods—are perfect for special occasions and perfectly keto-friendly! Adding labels for everything on the board is a nice touch for parties, and folks who are gluten-free or have other dietary restrictions will particularly appreciate the information.

CHEESES

Choose a combination of hard and soft cheeses, and include one with a flavor mixed in (like a honey or olive chèvre, for example) if you like. I recommend using a small label to identify each cheese, so that your guests aren't unpleasantly surprised by the flavor if it's not their favorite. Labels are especially helpful for flavored and spicy cheeses (like a pepper jack, for example).

Some of my favorite hard cheeses for a charcuterie board are:

- Goat Gouda
- Cheddar
- Manchego

Some of my favorite soft cheeses for a charcuterie board are:

- Chèvre—plain, honey, fig, olive, or truffle
- Goat Brie

MEATS

Choose a combination of fresh and cured meats such as:

- Prosciutto, salami, chorizo, and coppa
- Turkey breast
- Roast beef
- Head cheese
- Pastrami
- Corned beef

SAVORY AND/OR FERMENTED ITEMS

I love including savory items like roasted veggies, nuts, cheese crisps, pickles, and other fermented goodies on a board. Even a small container of sauerkraut can go perfectly with meats, cheeses, and some mustard!

Some of my favorite savory and/or fermented items for a charcuterie board are:

- Pickles
- Marinated Onions (page 290)
- Sauerkraut
- Olives. Some of my favorites are oil cured, Castelvetrano, and Kalamata. I prefer using pitted olives because they're less messy, but some with pits really have great flavor.
- Roasted vegetables, like carrots, peppers, or potatoes
- Grilled vegetables, like zucchini, peppers, or eggplant
- Baked Cheese Crisps (page 308)
- Raw or roasted nuts, spiced, salted, or plain
- Hard- or soft-boiled eggs (or even some leftover frittata cut up into pieces)

SAVORY SPREADS & MUSTARDS

To add some punch to the combination of meat, cheese, and crunchy crackers or crispy toast, add a creamy spread. It can provide a lot of flavor and break up the fattiness of the bites.

Some of my favorite savory spreads and mustards for a charcuterie board are:

- Brown mustard
- Whole-grain mustard (the kind where it's mostly whole mustard seeds—this is especially awesome on a charcuterie board)
- Dijon mustard
- Onion jam (no sugar added)
- Bacon jam (no sugar added)

TIPS & HACKS TO OPTIMIZE THE LOOK OF YOUR BOARD

1. **Use a great board.** The backdrop for your food doesn't matter as much as the food itself, but it can make for a much more impressive presentation.

2. **Pick foods you love.** If you choose a few things you love and others you don't, you'll end up avoiding the things you don't love.

3. **Balance the foods.** Pick some sweeter foods and some that are more salty, sour, and pungent. Then, select some spicy meats and some mild ones. Next, pick some cured meats and some fresh (if you can!). Lastly, choose some fresh or fermented veggies and some that have been grilled or roasted.

4. **Slice carefully.** When you prepare the cheeses and meats, slice them evenly and thinly. You want to give your guests as many bites as possible to enjoy, so keep each piece on the small side. And even slices make for a more beautiful presentation.

5. **Be creative with the presentation.** One of the best-kept secrets about assembling charcuterie boards is this: you can throw together something really impressive looking with just scraps and almost-finished items from your fridge. The trick is to make it look lovely! Arrange the cheeses in staggered or zig-zag shapes, and select at least two or three options but no more than four or five. Break up the white and yellow cheeses with more brightly colored items, like meats and pickles. You can place everything right on the board, but think about using small bowls or dishes for items like sauces or olives. It helps keep the foods contained and the board clean, but using small dishes also adds some visual interest to the board.

Ranch Kale Chips

Kale chips bake up crispy and delicious and provide an often-missed texture in your keto diet. Season these chips with any of the spice blends you like on pages 330 and 331, or just use sea salt to keep them more basic. For the best texture, I recommend enjoying these immediately rather than storing them for later.

2 bunches curly kale or other variety

1 tablespoon olive oil or coconut oil, melted

1 teaspoon Ranch Spice Blend (page 331)

Preheat the oven to 350°F.

Rinse the kale leaves under cold water and pat them dry with a towel. Pull the leaves from the stalk by holding tightly onto the end of the stalk and running your hand up the sides. You can also just cut the stalks out. Discard the stalks or save them for juicing.

Roughly chop the kale into large pieces and place it in a large mixing bowl. Pour the oil over the kale and gently massage it in, spreading the oil evenly over all of the kale.

Arrange the kale in a single layer on 2 rimmed baking sheets and sprinkle both sides with the spice blend.

Bake for 10 minutes, then turn off the oven and leave the kale in the oven for an additional 10 minutes as the oven cools.

FODMAP-FREE?
Omit the Ranch Spice Blend and season with salt and pepper instead.

NOTE
Keep a close eye on the kale as it bakes. It can burn quite quickly if you're not paying attention.

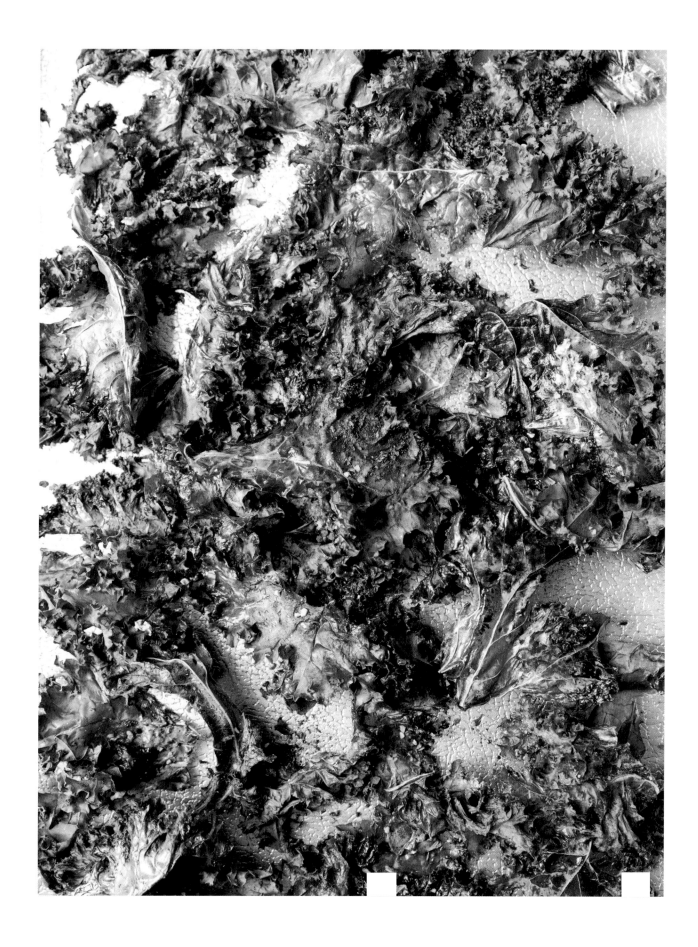

Cauliflower Queso Dip

PREP TIME: **10 minutes** | COOK TIME: **15 minutes** | YIELD: **1 1/2 cups (1/4 cup per serving)**

A keto diet can be extremely cheese-heavy, and while cheese is keto-friendly, I love the idea of powering it up with some veggies. This queso dip is the perfect way to enjoy that cheesy, melty texture while adding more nutrition. I recommend serving this warm so it remains soft and smooth!

1 1/2 cups chopped cauliflower

1/4 cup boiling water

6 ounces cheddar cheese, shredded (about 3/4 cup)

1/2 teaspoon granulated onion

2 or 3 pinches of sea salt

2 or 3 pinches of ground black pepper

1/2 cup Quick Salsa (page 306)

Fill a large pot with 2 inches of water and place a steamer basket in the pot. Cover and bring to a boil over high heat. Add the cauliflower and steam for 15 minutes, until fork-tender.

Transfer the cauliflower to a blender or food processor and add the boiling water, cheese, granulated onion, salt, and pepper. Blend until smooth. If the sauce is too thick, add water 1 tablespoon at a time until the desired consistency is reached. Taste and adjust the seasonings as desired.

Transfer the dip to a serving bowl, stir in the salsa, and serve.

Store in an airtight container in the fridge for up to 5 days or in a freezer-safe bag in the freezer until ready to use. After defrosting, stir to restore the texture.

NIGHTSHADE-FREE?
Omit the salsa.

   CALORIES: **130** | FAT: **10 g** | PROTEIN: **8 g** | CARBS: **3 g** | FIBER: **1 g** | NET CARBS: **2 g**

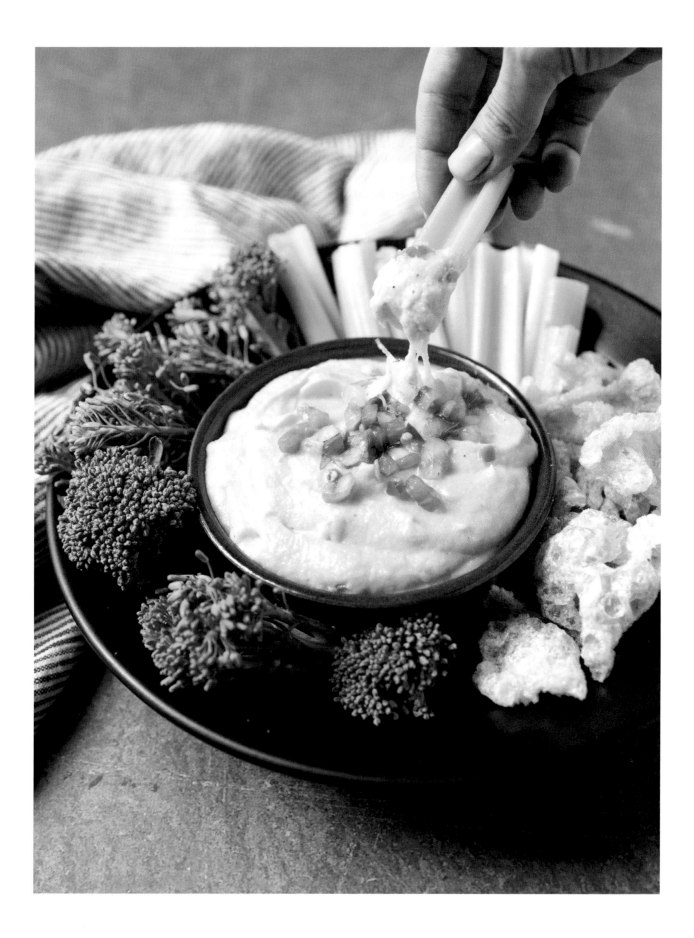

NUTS | EGGS | NIGHTSHADES | FODMAPS | DAIRY | 21DSD-FRIENDLY

Dairy-Free Cashew Queso Dip

PREP TIME: **10 minutes, plus time to soak the cashews** | COOK TIME: **15 minutes** |
YIELD: **1 1/2 cups (1/4 cup per serving)**

A dairy-free twist on a classic cheese dip, this version is perfect if dairy isn't a part of your diet. Use this as a base for other recipes or enjoy it straight-up! It's also great as a side dish with Creamy Cauliflower Purée (page 284).

FOR THE CASHEWS

1/2 cup raw cashews

1/2 cup warm water

1 cup chopped cauliflower

1/4 cup warm water

1/4 cup nutritional yeast

1/4 teaspoon granulated onion

2 or 3 pinches of sea salt

2 or 3 pinches of ground black pepper

1/2 cup Quick Salsa (page 306)

Place the cashews in a small container and add the warm water. (If it doesn't cover the cashews completely, just add more warm water.) Soak for 1 to 4 hours unrefrigerated or up to overnight in the refrigerator.

Fill a large pot with 2 inches of water and place a steamer basket in the pot. Cover and bring to a boil over high heat. Add the cauliflower and steam for 15 minutes, until fork-tender.

Transfer the cauliflower to a blender or food processor. Drain the cashews, then add them to the blender or food processor. Add the 1/4 cup warm water, nutritional yeast, granulated onion, salt, and pepper. Blend until smooth. If the sauce is too thick, add water a tablespoon at a time until the desired consistency is reached. Taste and adjust the seasonings as desired.

Transfer the dip to a serving bowl, stir in the salsa, and serve.

Store in an airtight container in the fridge for up to 5 days or in a freezer-safe bag in the freezer until ready to use. After defrosting, stir to restore the texture.

NIGHTSHADE-FREE?
Omit the salsa.

CALORIES: **80** | FAT: **5 g** | PROTEIN: **5 g** | CARBS: **7 g** | FIBER: **2 g** | NET CARBS: **5 g**

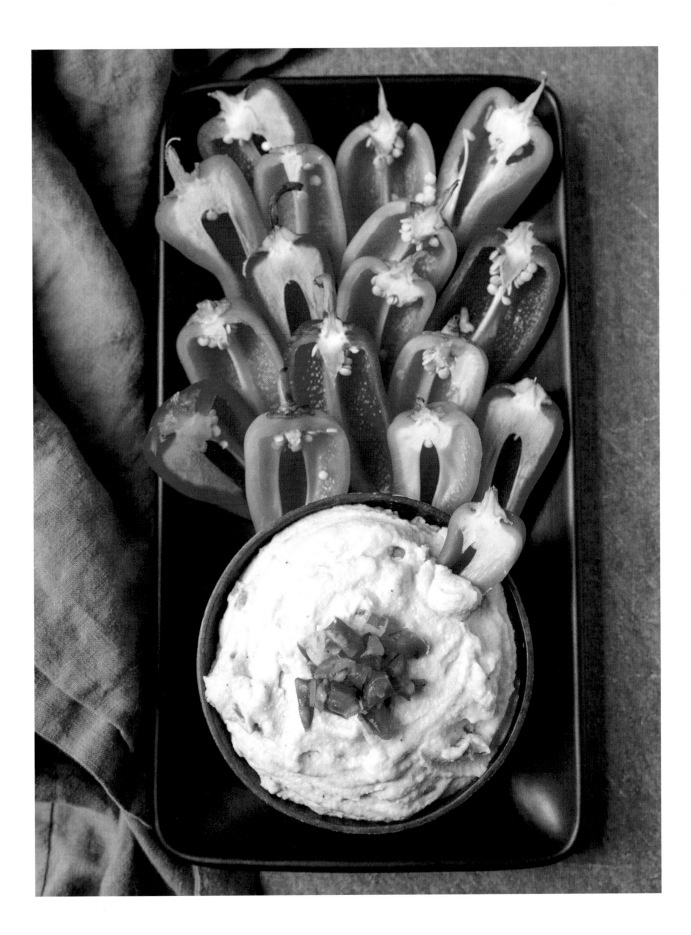

Spinach Artichoke Dip

PREP TIME: **15 minutes** | COOK TIME: **20 minutes** | YIELD: **2 cups (1/4 cup per serving)**

A game-day favorite that can be made and enjoyed anytime! This dip can be eaten with veggies or crackers, added to a Keto Charcuterie Board (page 314), or even used to stuff chicken before baking it. Make this for your next gathering—the whole crowd will love it, keto or not!

2 tablespoons extra-virgin olive oil, divided

1 medium yellow onion, finely chopped

2 large cloves garlic, grated or minced

Sea salt and ground black pepper

1/2 pound frozen chopped spinach, thawed, with the water squeezed out

4 ounces artichoke hearts, finely chopped

1 1/2 cups Cauliflower Queso Dip (page 318) or Dairy-Free Cashew Queso Dip (page 320, omit the salsa)

Chicharrones, for serving (optional)

Heat 1 tablespoon of the olive oil in a medium-sized saucepan over medium heat. Add the onion, season lightly with salt and pepper, and cook for 8 to 10 minutes, until translucent. Add the garlic and cook for an additional 2 to 3 minutes, until the garlic browns slightly.

Make a well in the center of the onion mixture and add the remaining tablespoon of olive oil. Add the spinach and artichoke hearts, lightly season with salt and pepper, and cook, stirring every minute or so, for 5 minutes, or until the spinach has wilted and the artichoke hearts have softened.

Remove the pan from the heat and add the cauliflower queso. Stir to combine and taste; add salt and pepper to taste if needed. Serve with chicharrones if desired.

This dip can be made up to a few days in advance for a party and served warm or at room temperature. Store leftovers in an airtight glass container in the fridge for up to a week. Reheat in a preheated 350°F oven for 10 minutes.

CALORIES: **146** | FAT: **11 g** | PROTEIN: **8 g** | CARBS: **7 g** | FIBER: **3 g** | NET CARBS: **4 g**

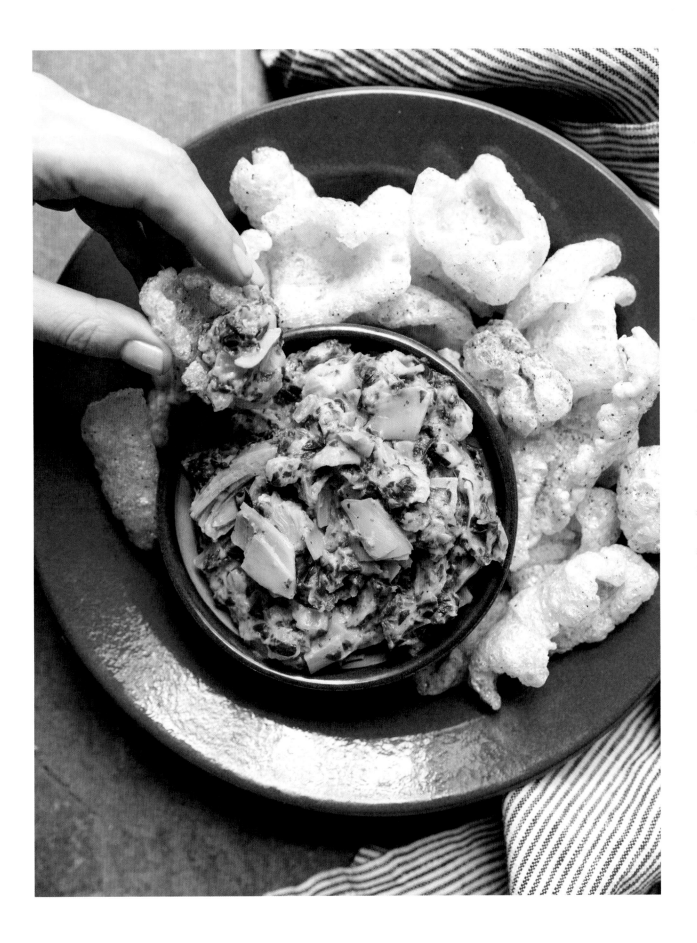

Simple Keto Romesco

PREP TIME: 15 minutes, plus time to soak the cashews | COOK TIME: 15 minutes | YIELD: 2 cups (1/4 cup per serving)

This bold roasted red pepper dip traditionally includes bread, but I've replaced it with a bit of our favorite low-carb veggie: cauliflower! This can be served as a dip or used as a sauce for grilled chicken, pork, or steak. You can even mix it with olive oil and lemon juice for a delicious salad dressing.

1/4 cup raw cashews

1/2 cup warm water

1 cup chopped cauliflower

1 (12-ounce) jar roasted red peppers, drained

1 small clove garlic, minced or grated

2 tablespoons extra-virgin olive oil

Grated zest of 1 lemon

Juice of 1 lemon

2 tablespoons chopped fresh cilantro leaves or parsley

1/4 teaspoon smoked paprika, plus extra for garnish

Pinch of cumin

Sea salt and ground black pepper

Baked Cheese Crisps (page 308), for serving (optional)

Place the cashews in a small container and add the warm water. (If it doesn't cover the cashews completely, just add more warm water.) Soak for 1 to 4 hours unrefrigerated or up to overnight in the refrigerator.

Fill a large pot with 2 inches of water and place a steamer basket in the pot. Cover and bring to a boil over high heat. Add the cauliflower and steam for 15 minutes, until fork-tender.

Transfer the cauliflower to a food processor. Drain the cashews, then add them to the food processor. Add the red peppers, garlic, olive oil, zest, lemon juice, cilantro, paprika, and cumin. Process until smooth. Add salt and pepper to taste.

Scoop the romesco into a serving dish and garnish with a pinch of smoked paprika. Serve with Baked Cheese Crisps, if desired.

CALORIES: **119** | FAT: **10 g** | PROTEIN: **3 g** | CARBS: **8 g** | FIBER: **1 g** | NET CARBS: **7 g**

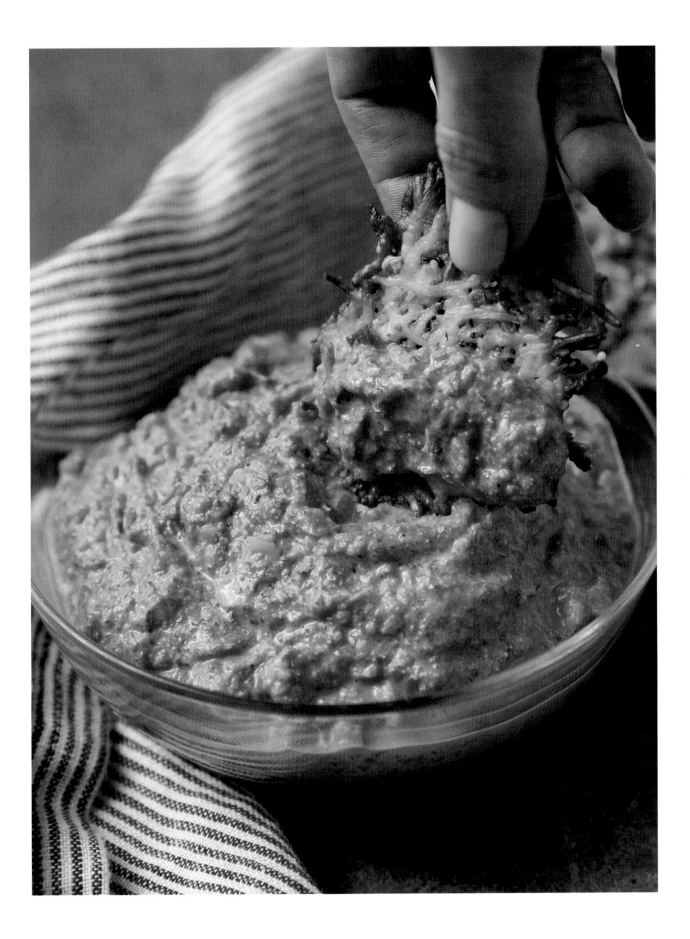

Caponata Dip

PREP TIME: 15 minutes | COOK TIME: 35 minutes | YIELD: about 2 cups (1/4 cup per serving)

Eggplant is a great low-carb vegetable that can be enjoyed as a main dish (see page 238) or made into this hearty dip. Try spreading it on a slice of deli turkey with some olives and eating it as a roll-up, or enjoy it spread on low-carb flax crackers or grilled chicken.

1 large eggplant (about 1 1/4 pounds), cut into 1/2-inch pieces

1 large yellow onion, cut into 1/2-inch pieces

4 large cloves garlic, peeled and smashed with the side of a knife

4 tablespoons extra-virgin olive oil, divided, plus extra for garnish

1/2 teaspoon sea salt

1/4 teaspoon ground black pepper

1/4 teaspoon ground cumin

1 medium tomato, chopped into 1-inch chunks

Juice of 1 lemon

2 tablespoons chopped fresh cilantro leaves

FOR GARNISH

Extra-virgin olive oil

Fresh cilantro leaves

Pinch of paprika (optional)

Pine nuts (optional)

FOR SERVING (OPTIONAL)

Low-carb flax crackers

Sliced vegetables

Preheat the oven to 375°F.

Place the eggplant, onion, garlic, 2 tablespoons of the olive oil, salt, pepper, and cumin in a large bowl and toss to combine.

Spread the mixture out on a rimmed baking sheet and bake for 30 to 35 minutes, until the eggplant is softened and browned, tossing halfway through.

Remove the eggplant mixture from the oven and transfer it to a food processor. Add the tomato, lemon juice, cilantro, and remaining 2 tablespoons of olive oil. Pulse until the mixture is just slightly chunky. Add salt and pepper to taste.

Scoop the dip into a serving dish and garnish with additional olive oil, cilantro, paprika (if desired), and pine nuts (optional). Serve with low-carb crackers and sliced vegetables, if desired.

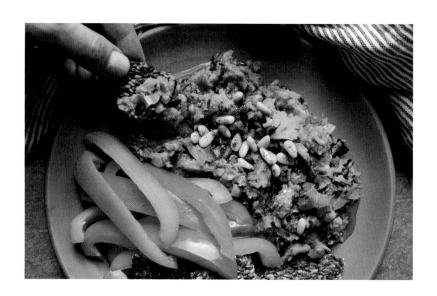

CALORIES: **90** | FAT: **7 g** | PROTEIN: **1 g** | CARBS: **7 g** | FIBER: **3 g** | NET CARBS: **4 g**

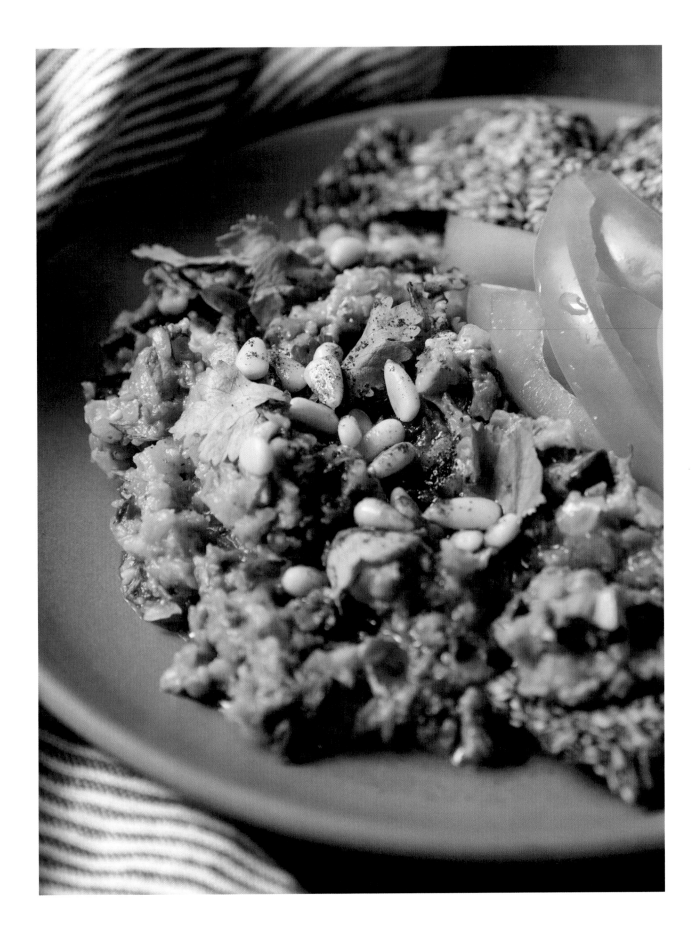

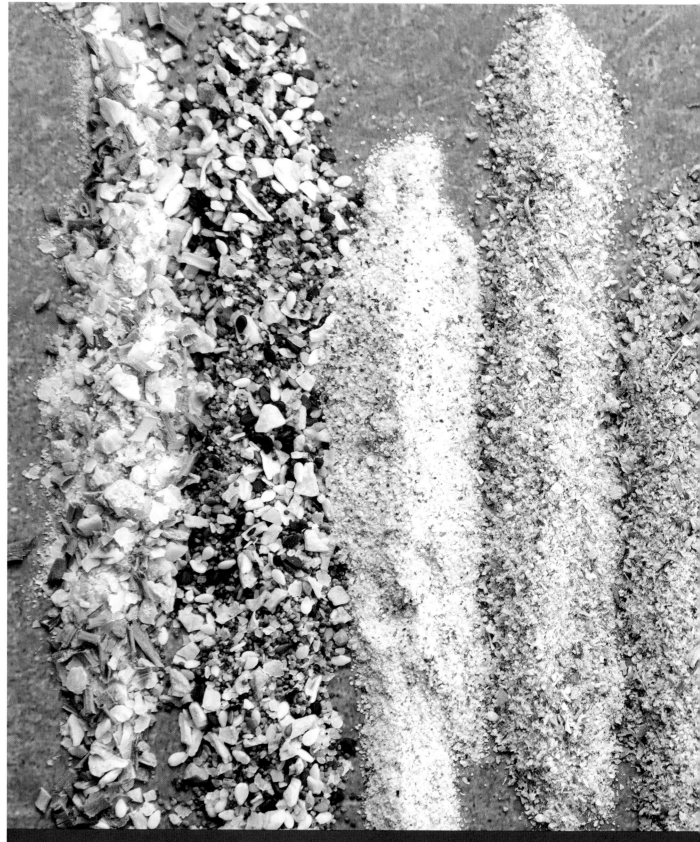

SUPER GARLIC   BAGEL   TRIFECTA   ITALIAN   GREEK

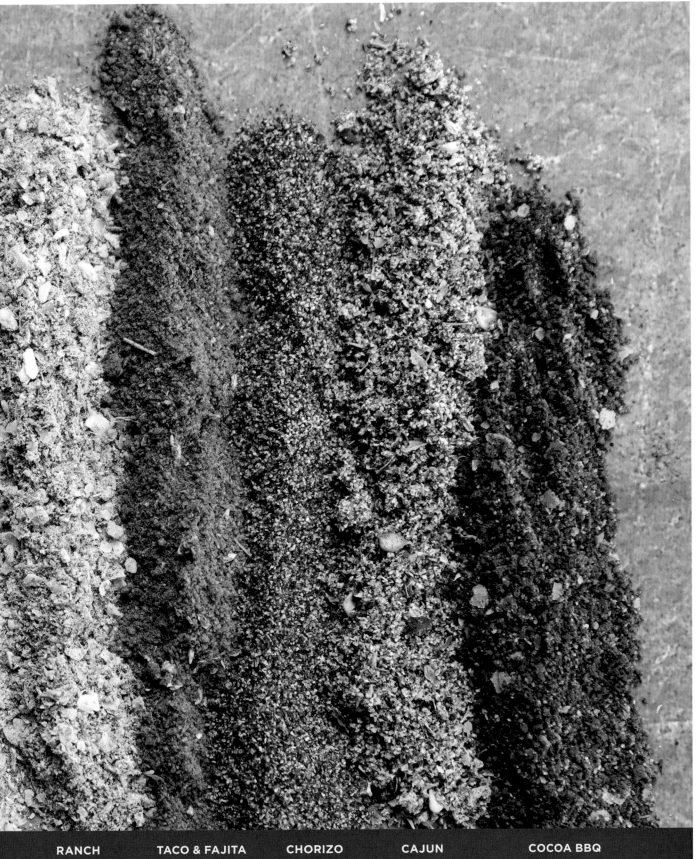

RANCH   TACO & FAJITA   CHORIZO   CAJUN   COCOA BBQ

Spice Blends

For each blend, combine all of the ingredients in a small bowl. Store in a small airtight container in a cool, dark place for up to a year. Use these blends as they appear in recipes throughout the book—or anytime!

SUPER GARLIC SPICE BLEND

NIGHTSHADES | **FODMAPS**

1/4 cup plus 1 teaspoon dried garlic flakes

2 tablespoons dried chives

1 tablespoon granulated garlic

2 teaspoons sea salt

BAGEL SPICE BLEND

NIGHTSHADES | **FODMAPS**

2 1/2 tablespoons dried garlic flakes

1 2/3 tablespoons poppy seeds

1 2/3 tablespoons dried onion flakes

1 1/2 tablespoons sesame seeds

1/2 tablespoon coarse sea salt

TRIFECTA SPICE BLEND

NIGHTSHADES | **FODMAPS**

1/4 cup plus 1 tablespoon granulated garlic

2 tablespoons plus 2 teaspoons sea salt

1 tablespoon ground black pepper

ITALIAN SPICE BLEND

NIGHTSHADES | **FODMAPS**

2 1/2 tablespoons dried parsley

1 1/2 tablespoons granulated garlic

1 1/2 tablespoons granulated onion

1 tablespoon dried ground sage

1 tablespoon ground fennel seeds

1 teaspoon sea salt

1 teaspoon ground black pepper, or 1/4 teaspoon white pepper

GREEK SPICE BLEND

NIGHTSHADES | **FODMAPS**

3 tablespoons dried lemon peel

3 tablespoons dried oregano leaves

2 tablespoons granulated garlic

1 tablespoon sea salt

2 teaspoons ground black pepper

RANCH SPICE BLEND

NIGHTSHADES | FODMAPS

2 tablespoons plus 2 teaspoons dried garlic flakes

1 tablespoon plus 1 teaspoon dried chives

1 tablespoon plus 1 teaspoon dried dill weed

1 tablespoon plus 1 teaspoon dried parsley

1 1/2 teaspoons sea salt

1 teaspoon celery powder or dried celery flakes

1 teaspoon dried lemon peel

1 teaspoon ground mustard

TACO & FAJITA SPICE BLEND

NIGHTSHADES | FODMAPS

2 tablespoons chili powder

1 1/2 tablespoons granulated garlic

1 1/2 tablespoons granulated onion

1 tablespoon ground coriander

2 teaspoons ground cumin

2 teaspoons smoked paprika

1 teaspoon sea salt

1 teaspoon ground black pepper

CHORIZO SPICE BLEND

NIGHTSHADES | FODMAPS

2 tablespoons chipotle powder

2 tablespoons smoked paprika

1 1/2 tablespoons granulated onion

1 1/2 tablespoons granulated garlic

1 1/2 teaspoons sea salt

1 teaspoon ground black pepper

CAJUN SPICE BLEND

NIGHTSHADES | FODMAPS

2 tablespoons dried oregano leaves

2 tablespoons paprika

1 1/2 tablespoons granulated garlic

1 1/2 tablespoons granulated onion

1 1/2 teaspoons sea salt

1 1/2 teaspoons ground black pepper

1 teaspoon dried thyme leaves

1/2 teaspoon cayenne pepper (you can add more if you like it hot)

COCOA BBQ SPICE BLEND

NIGHTSHADES | FODMAPS

2 tablespoons finely ground coffee beans

1 1/2 tablespoons sea salt

1 tablespoon paprika

1 tablespoon ancho chili powder

1 teaspoon granulated garlic

1 teaspoon granulated onion

1 teaspoon ground black pepper

1 teaspoon unsweetened cocoa powder

To order organic versions of these blends (and more) ready-made, visit balancedbites.com/spices.

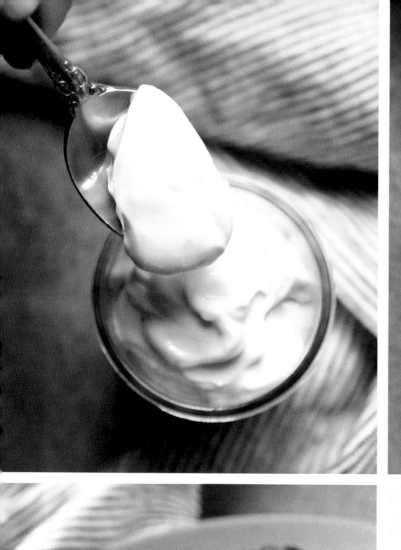
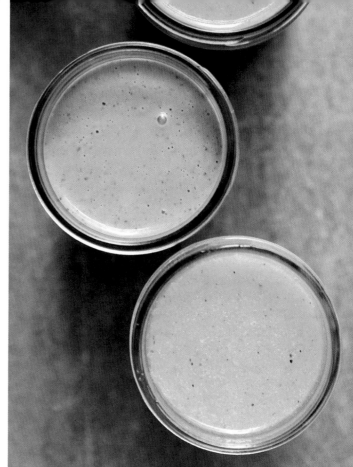
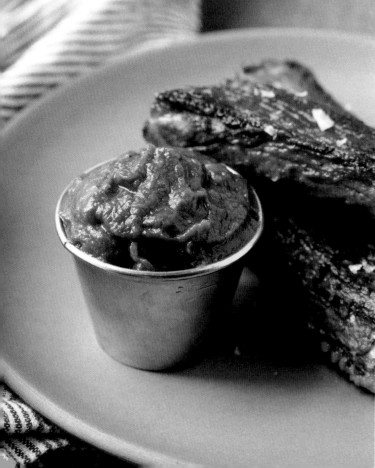
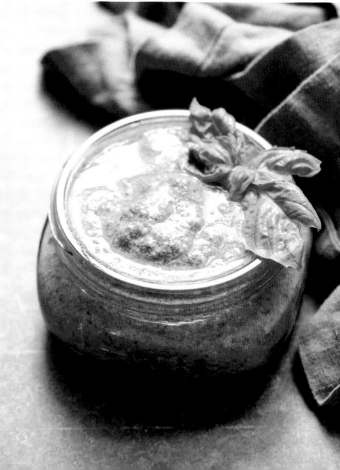

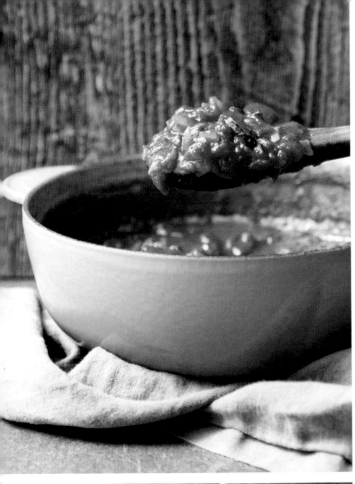

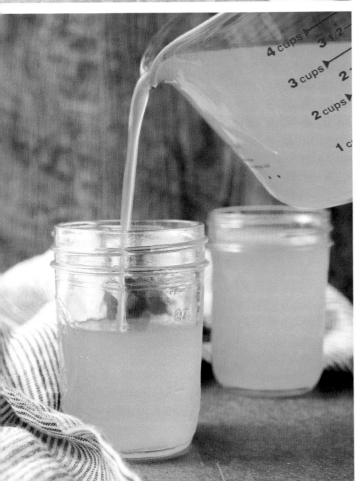

Condiments, Sauces & Dressings

Hollandaise Sauce

PREP TIME: **5 minutes** | COOK TIME: **10 minutes** | YIELD: **1 cup (2 tablespoons per serving)**

Take your eggs to the next level in the morning—maybe for a Sunday brunch—with rich hollandaise sauce! It can take a bit of practice, but this versatile sauce is a wonderful addition to your cooking repertoire.

3 large egg yolks

1 1/2 tablespoons fresh lemon juice

3/4 cup ghee (page 336) or butter, divided

Sea salt and ground black pepper

In a small saucepan, whisk together the egg yolks and lemon juice. Add half of the ghee. Cook over low heat, stirring constantly, for 1 to 2 minutes, until the ghee has melted.

Slowly add the remaining ghee and whisk for about 3 minutes, until the ghee has melted and the sauce has thickened. Add salt and pepper to taste.

Store in an airtight container in the refrigerator for up to 2 days. Reheat in a small saucepan over low heat and whisk in a teaspoon of water.

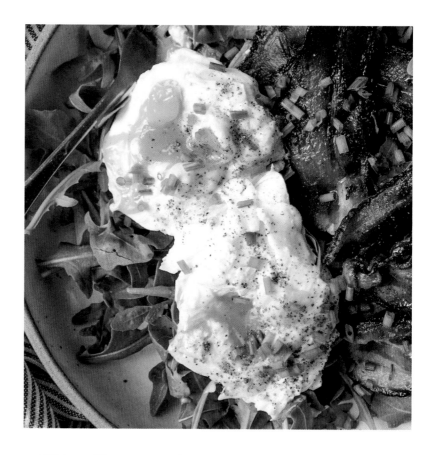

CALORIES: **174** | FAT: **19 g** | PROTEIN: **1 g** | CARBS: **1 g** | FIBER: **0 g** | NET CARBS: **1 g**

Healthy Homemade Mayonnaise

PREP TIME: 15 minutes | YIELD: **3/4 cup (1 tablespoon per serving)**

There are a few healthy brands of mayonnaise available in stores these days, but if you find yourself without any on hand or it's hard to find in your area, it's easy to make! You can add other flavors, like Pesto (page 343), to this mayo for a delicious spread for meats and vegetables.

2 large egg yolks

1 tablespoon fresh lemon juice

1 teaspoon gluten-free Dijon mustard

3/4 cup avocado oil, olive oil, or a blend of the two

In a medium-sized mixing bowl, whisk together the egg yolks, lemon juice, and mustard until blended and bright yellow, about 30 seconds.

Add 1/4 cup of the oil to the yolk mixture a few drops at a time, whisking constantly. Gradually add the remaining oil in slow, thin streams, whisking constantly, until the mayonnaise is thick and lighter in color.

Store in the refrigerator for up to a week.

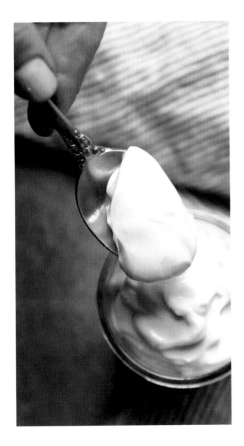

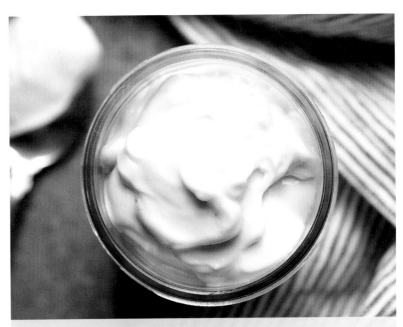

TIP

You can also make this recipe using a handheld immersion blender or a small blender. If using a regular-sized blender, double the recipe to make blending easier. Use the opening at the top of your blender to slowly drizzle in the oil.

CALORIES: **172** | FAT: **19 g** | PROTEIN: **1 g** | CARBS: **0 g** | FIBER: **0 g** | NET CARBS: **0 g**

Clarified Butter & Ghee

PREP TIME: **5 minutes** | COOK TIME: **30 minutes for clarified butter, 45 minutes for ghee**
YIELD: **4 cups (1 ounce per serving)**

It couldn't be easier to make your own clarified butter or ghee; all you need is a way to strain it and you're good to go. Ghee is my favorite cooking fat, but I find that I can tolerate it only if there are no dairy solids left behind, so I place a cheesecloth over a fine-mesh strainer for an ultra-strained version.

2 pounds unsalted butter

SPECIAL EQUIPMENT
Cheesecloth

TO MAKE CLARIFIED BUTTER:

Slowly melt the butter in a medium-sized heavy-bottomed saucepan over low heat. As the butter comes to a simmer, the milk solids will float to the top and become foamy while the separated oil will become very clear. Skim off the milk solids and remove the butter from the heat. Pour it through cheesecloth to strain out any remaining milk solids. Store the strained liquid in a glass jar.

TO MAKE GHEE:

Follow the instructions for making clarified butter, but allow the milk solids to continue to cook slowly until they become browned and begin to sink to the bottom of the pan. When there are no longer any solids floating at the top, the ghee is finished. Pour it through cheesecloth to strain out the browned milk solids. Store the strained liquid in a glass jar.

Clarified butter and ghee are shelf-stable and will last indefinitely in the pantry. However, if some milk solids remain and the temperature in your home becomes very warm, they may go off. To prevent this, store them in the refrigerator—just be aware that they'll become solid when chilled.

CALORIES: **257** | FAT: **29 g** | PROTEIN: **0 g** | CARBS: **0 g** | FIBER: **0 g** | NET CARBS: **0 g**

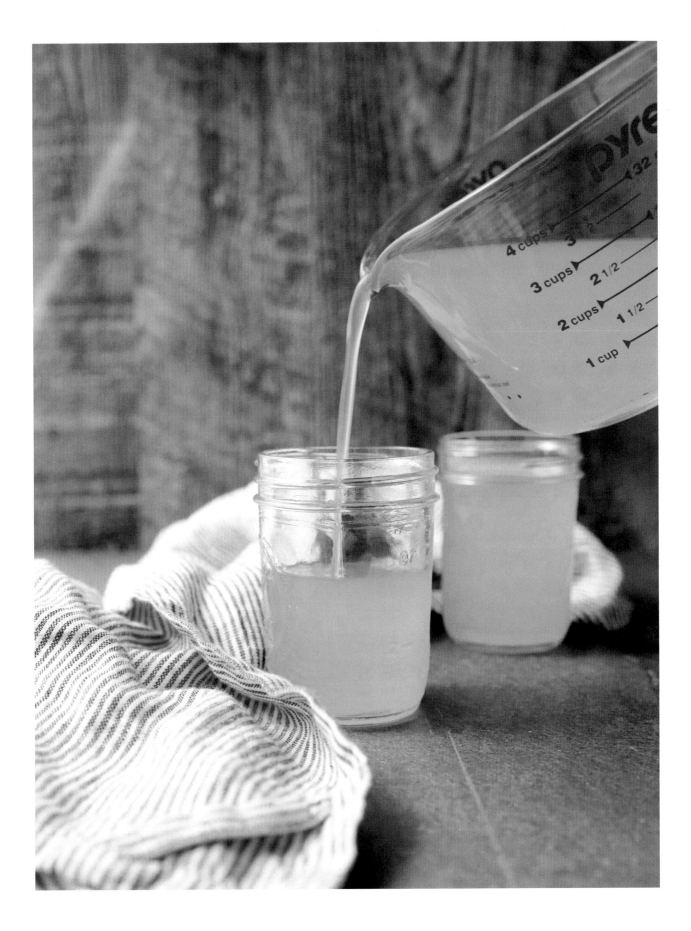

Simple Marinara

PREP TIME: 10 minutes | COOK TIME: **30 minutes** | YIELD: **3 cups (1/2 cup per serving)**

Finding clean-ingredient pasta sauce is much easier these days than it used to be, but if you're stuck without a jar on hand and you've got some canned diced or crushed tomatoes, you can whip up your own marinara in just a few minutes with this easy recipe. Try it the next time you're in a pinch!

2 tablespoons extra-virgin olive oil

1/2 cup diced yellow onions (about 1 small onion)

Sea salt and ground black pepper

2 or 3 cloves garlic, grated or minced

1 (28-ounce) can diced tomatoes, with juices

1 tablespoon chopped fresh basil leaves

In a saucepan, melt the olive oil over medium heat. Add the onion and cook until translucent, about 5 minutes. Season with salt and pepper.

Add the garlic and cook for about 1 minute, until lightly browned. Add the tomatoes, season with additional salt and pepper, and stir to combine.

Turn the heat down to low and simmer, stirring occasionally, for 15 to 20 minutes. Add the basil and simmer for 5 minutes more, then remove from the heat.

SERVING SUGGESTION

Serve over zucchini noodles or roasted spaghetti squash. Finish with a drizzle of extra-virgin olive oil for added flavor and richness.

CALORIES: **127** | FAT: **9 g** | PROTEIN: **2 g** | CARBS: **11 g** | FIBER: **3 g** | NET CARBS: **8 g**

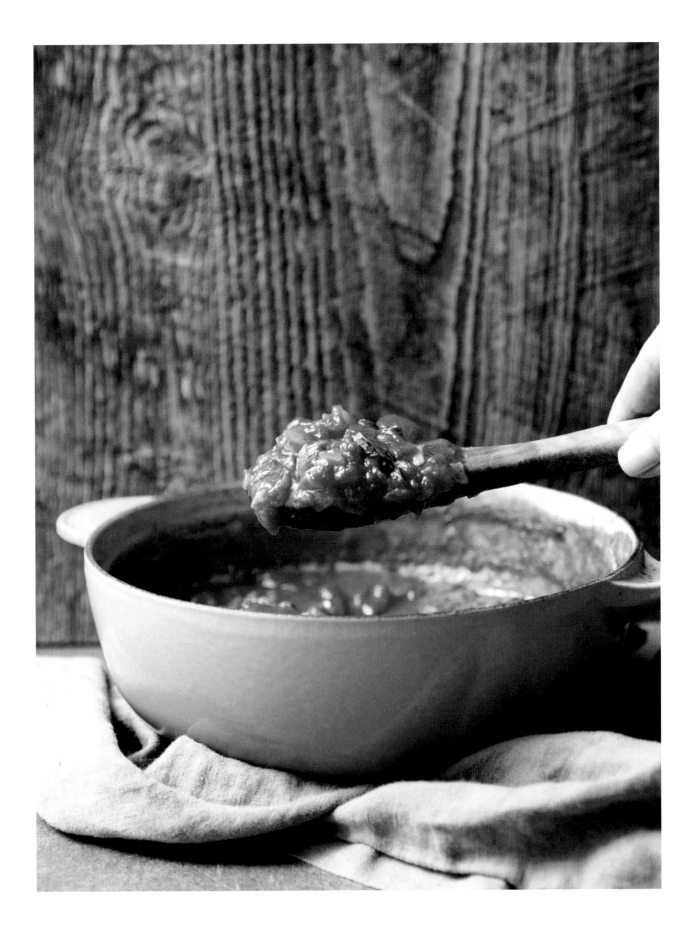

Sweetener-Free Ketchup

PREP TIME: **10 minutes** | COOK TIME: **45 minutes (stovetop), 4 hours (slow cooker)** |
YIELD: **1 1/2 cups (2 tablespoons per serving)**

Ketchup is often loaded with corn syrup or other added sugars, but this one has only real ingredients, and it tastes amazing! It's simple to make, and you can use a slow cooker or even an Instant Pot (use the same method as the slow cooker, then simmer it with the lid off for a few minutes). You'll love it!

1 small yellow onion, diced

2 medium apples, peeled and diced (green, Honeycrisp, or Gala)

2 cloves garlic, minced

1/4 cup water

2 tablespoons apple cider vinegar

1/2 teaspoon sea salt

1/4 teaspoon allspice

1/4 teaspoon ginger powder

1/4 teaspoon ground cinnamon

2 pinches of ground cloves

6 ounces tomato paste

TIP
Honeycrisp apples work especially well in this recipe, but only green apples are 21DSD-friendly

TO MAKE THIS ON THE STOVETOP:

Place all the ingredients in a small saucepan over medium heat and simmer, stirring regularly, for 15 minutes. Turn the heat down to low and continue to simmer for another 30 minutes as the sauce reduces, stirring occasionally to be sure it's not burning or sticking to the pan.

TO MAKE THIS IN A SLOW COOKER:

Place all the ingredients in a slow cooker and stir to combine. Set the slow cooker to low and cook for 4 hours.

Allow the mixture to cool slightly, then pour it into a food processor or high-speed blender and blend until smooth.

Once blended, place the ketchup in glass containers and allow it to come to room temperature before refrigerating.

Store in airtight containers in the refrigerator for several weeks or more. If you notice a change in color or smell or see any mold growth, toss it and make a new batch.

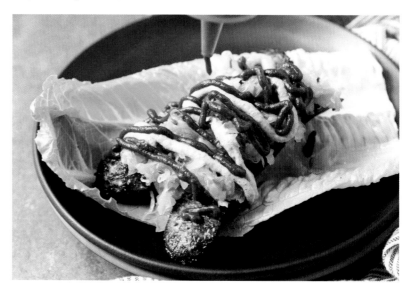

CALORIES: **28** | FAT: **0 g** | PROTEIN: **1 g** | CARBS: **7 g** | FIBER: **1 g** | NET CARBS: **6 g**

BBQ Sauce

PREP TIME: 10 minutes | YIELD: **2 cups (2 tablespoons per serving)**

Using homemade ketchup as a base and combining it with naturally sweet caramelized onions and some spices make this BBQ sauce rich in flavor and packed with nutrition. Enjoy it brushed on ribs; a little bit goes a long way!

2 cups Sweetener-Free Ketchup (page 340)

1/2 cup Bacon-y Caramelized Onions (page 294)

1/4 cup apple cider vinegar

1 teaspoon dry mustard

1/2 to 1 teaspoon chipotle powder, plus more if desired

1/2 teaspoon paprika

1/2 teaspoon sea salt

1/4 to 1/2 cup water (optional)

Combine all the ingredients except the water in a blender and blend on high for 2 to 3 minutes, until well combined.

If you prefer a thinner consistency, start by adding 1/4 cup water and blend for 1 more minute, then add another 1/4 cup water if desired. Taste and add more chipotle powder if desired for more heat.

Store in a glass jar in the refrigerator for up to 5 days.

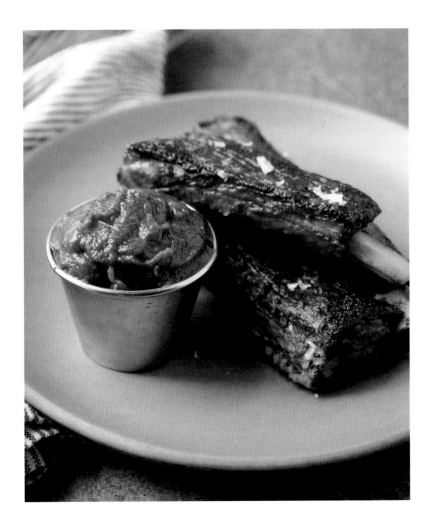

CALORIES: **32** | FAT: **1 g** | PROTEIN: **1 g** | CARBS: **6 g** | FIBER: **1 g** | NET CARBS: **5 g**

Avocado Crema

PREP TIME: **10 minutes** | YIELD: **3/4 cup (2 tablespoons per serving)**

Missing some of the ingredients for guacamole? Want to make a creamy avocado sauce without onions or garlic? This avocado crema is perfect. It's great over simple grilled fish or chicken, and it's especially tasty on tacos of any kind!

1 medium avocado, peeled, pitted, and halved

1/3 cup full-fat coconut milk

1/4 teaspoon ground cumin

1/4 teaspoon sea salt

Juice from 1 lime

1/8 teaspoon cayenne pepper (optional)

Place all of the ingredients in a food processor or blender and blend until smooth.

Store in an airtight glass container in the refrigerator for up to 3 days.

NIGHTSHADE-FREE?
Omit the cayenne pepper.

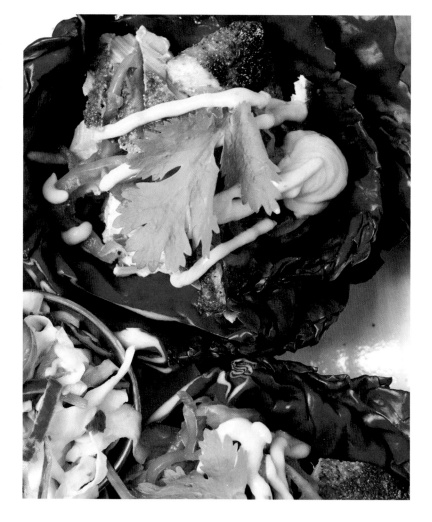

CONDIMENTS, SAUCES & DRESSINGS   CALORIES: **65** | FAT: **6 g** | PROTEIN: **1 g** | CARBS: **3 g** | FIBER: **2 g** | NET CARBS: **1 g**

Pesto

PREP TIME: 10 minutes | YIELD: 1 1/2 cups (1/4 cup per serving)

A classic Italian favorite, pesto is great on almost everything, from meat to eggs to salads, and even mixed into soups and other dishes, like Skillet Chicken Cacciatore (page 210). Try mixing pesto with a bit of Healthy Homemade Mayonnaise (page 335) for a delicious spread for turkey, chicken, and more.

2 tightly packed cups fresh basil leaves (from a 4-ounce clamshell pack)

2 large cloves garlic, peeled

1/4 cup pine nuts, or 1/2 cup walnut halves

1/4 cup shredded hard cheese, such as Parmigiano-Reggiano or Pecorino Romano

Grated zest and juice of 1 lemon

1/4 teaspoon sea salt

1/4 teaspoon ground black pepper

1/2 cup extra-virgin olive oil

Place the basil, garlic, nuts, cheese, lemon zest and juice, salt, and pepper in a food processor and pulse until the mixture comes together into a pastelike consistency. Add the olive oil and process until smooth. Taste and add more salt and pepper if desired.

Store in an airtight container in the fridge for up to 2 weeks.

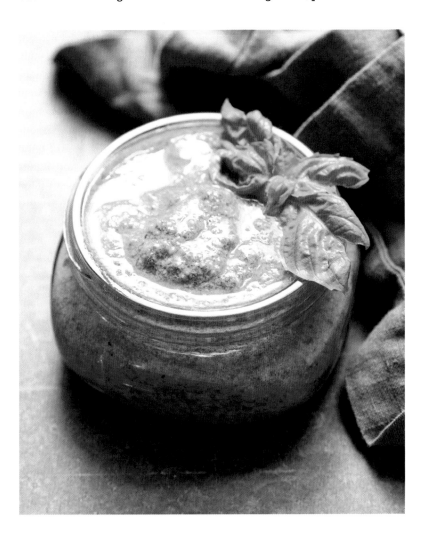

DAIRY-FREE?

Use 1/4 cup nutritional yeast instead of the cheese.

TIP

When adding raw garlic to a dressing, sauce, or dip that will remain uncooked, more is not always better! The potency of raw garlic intensifies as it sits, so don't let this recipe be one where you read "1 clove" and translate it to "4 cloves," as garlic lovers often do when cooking!

CALORIES: **241** | FAT: **24 g** | PROTEIN: **5 g** | CARBS: **3 g** | FIBER: **1 g** | NET CARBS: **2 g**

Salad Dressings

YIELD: 1 cup (1 tablespoon per serving)

FOR ALL DRESSINGS:

Place all of the ingredients, except the salt and pepper, in a blender and blend on low for 10 to 20 seconds. You can also whisk the ingredients together, but the dressing will not be as smooth. Taste the dressing, add salt and pepper to taste, and adjust the other seasonings to your liking. Add more oil, vinegar, and/or citrus juice as desired.

Store in an airtight glass container in the refrigerator for up to 3 weeks.

Basil Shallot Vinaigrette

2/3 cup extra-virgin olive oil

1/3 cup red wine vinegar

1/2 tightly packed cup fresh basil leaves

1 medium shallot (about 1 1/2 inches long), peeled (see Note)

1 teaspoon honey (optional)

Sea salt and ground black pepper

> **NOTE**
> If you wish to make this dressing in a bowl, mince the shallot before adding it to the bowl along with the other ingredients, then whisk to combine.

CALORIES: **84** | FAT: **9 g** | PROTEIN: **0 g** | CARBS: **1 g** | FIBER: **0 g** | NET CARBS: **1 g**

Balsamic Vinaigrette

2/3 cup extra-virgin olive oil

1/3 cup balsamic vinegar

1 teaspoon gluten-free Dijon mustard

1/2 teaspoon anchovy paste

Sea salt and ground black pepper

CALORIES: **86** | FAT: **9 g** | PROTEIN: **0 g** | CARBS: **1 g** | FIBER: **0 g** | NET CARBS: **1 g**

Lemon Herb Dressing

2/3 cup extra-virgin olive oil

1/3 cup fresh lemon juice

1 teaspoon gluten-free Dijon mustard

1/2 teaspoon minced shallots

1/2 teaspoon minced fresh cilantro leaves or basil (optional)

Sea salt and ground black pepper

CALORIES: **82** | FAT: **9 g** | PROTEIN: **0 g** | CARBS: **1 g** | FIBER: **0 g** | NET CARBS: **1 g**

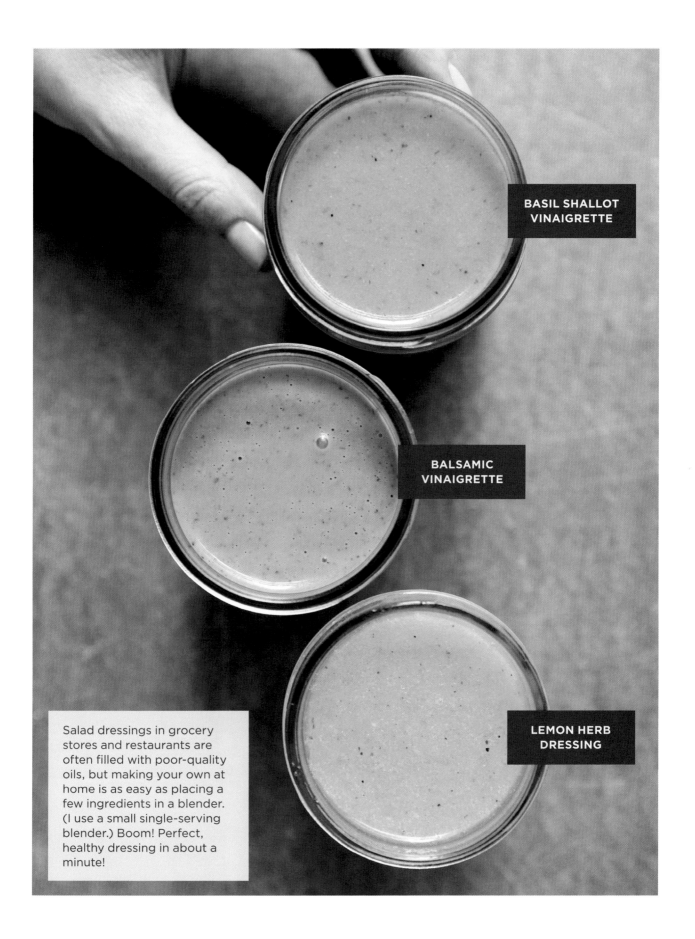

BASIL SHALLOT VINAIGRETTE

BALSAMIC VINAIGRETTE

LEMON HERB DRESSING

Salad dressings in grocery stores and restaurants are often filled with poor-quality oils, but making your own at home is as easy as placing a few ingredients in a blender. (I use a small single-serving blender.) Boom! Perfect, healthy dressing in about a minute!

Caesar Dressing

PREP TIME: **10 minutes** | YIELD: **1 cup (1/4 cup per serving)**

This extra-lemony take on Caesar dressing is perfect with baby kale (see page 202), but it's also great on a more classic romaine lettuce Caesar salad—or any kind of salad. Try this dressing with simple grilled chicken and roasted vegetables to turn the flavor way up!

2/3 cup extra-virgin olive oil

1/3 cup fresh lemon juice (about 2 lemons)

2 tablespoons grated hard cheese, such as Parmigiano-Reggiano or Pecorino Romano

1 teaspoon grated or minced garlic (1 to 2 cloves)

1 to 2 anchovy fillets, minced, or 1 to 2 teaspoons anchovy paste (see Note)

1/2 teaspoon gluten-free Dijon mustard

Sea salt and ground black pepper

Place all of the ingredients in a blender and blend on low for 10 to 20 seconds, until smooth. Taste the dressing and adjust the seasoning to taste with salt, pepper, and/or more oil or lemon juice.

Store the dressing in an airtight glass container in the refrigerator for up to 3 weeks.

DAIRY-FREE?

Use 2 tablespoons of nutritional yeast instead of the cheese.

NOTE

If you prefer a saltier dressing, use 2 anchovy fillets or 2 teaspoons of anchovy paste.

TIP

When adding raw garlic to a dressing, sauce, or dip that will remain uncooked, more is not always better! The potency of raw garlic intensifies as it sits, so don't let this recipe be one where you read "1 clove" and translate it to "4 cloves," as garlic lovers often do when cooking!

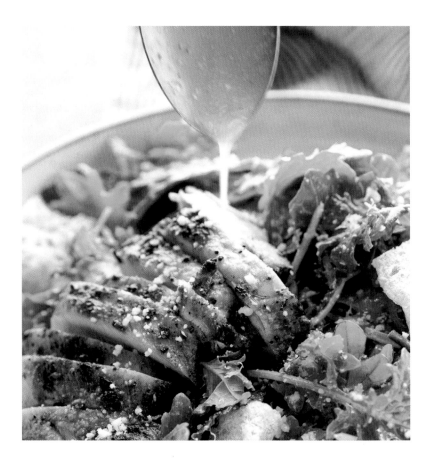

CALORIES: **390** | FAT: **40 g** | PROTEIN: **7 g** | CARBS: **3 g** | FIBER: **0 g** | NET CARBS: **3 g**

Ranch Dressing

PREP TIME: 5 minutes | YIELD: 1 cup (2 tablespoons per serving)

A classic favorite, this dressing can be used as a dip as well as on a salad. Store-bought versions contain junky oils, sugar, and lots of preservatives, and you can make an even better-tasting version at home. The spice blend here is key. (Don't forget, you can get my Ranch Spice Blend—and the other blends in this book!—premade and all organic at balancedbites.com/spices.)

1 cup full-fat sour cream

3 tablespoons fresh lemon juice
(1 large lemon)

1 tablespoon Ranch Spice Blend
(page 331)

2 tablespoons extra-virgin olive oil

1 heaping tablespoon chopped fresh
chives (optional)

1/2 teaspoon minced or grated
garlic (about 1 clove) (see Tips)

1/2 teaspoon red pepper flakes
(optional)

In a small mixing bowl, whisk together all the ingredients until well mixed.

If you prefer a thicker dressing, chill it in the refrigerator before serving.

Store in an airtight container in the fridge for up to a week.

NIGHTSHADE-FREE?
Omit the red pepper flakes.

DAIRY-FREE?
Use 1 cup plain coconut yogurt in place of the sour cream and add 1 tablespoon more of lemon juice for a total of 1/4 cup. You may need 2 lemons instead of 1 in this case.

TIPS

If the dressing is too firm after refrigerating, whisk in 1 tablespoon of warm water. You can use lemon juice instead if you like it more tart.

When adding raw garlic to a dressing, sauce, or dip that will remain uncooked, more is not always better! The potency of raw garlic intensifies as it sits, so don't let this recipe be one where you read "1 clove" and translate it to "4 cloves," as garlic lovers often do when cooking!

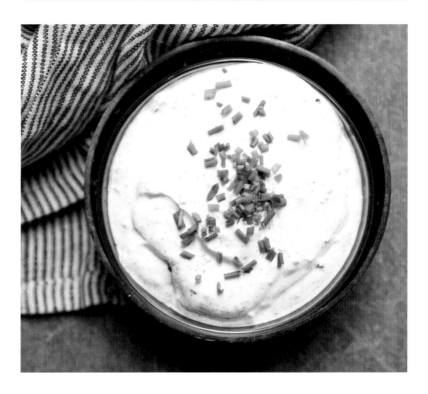

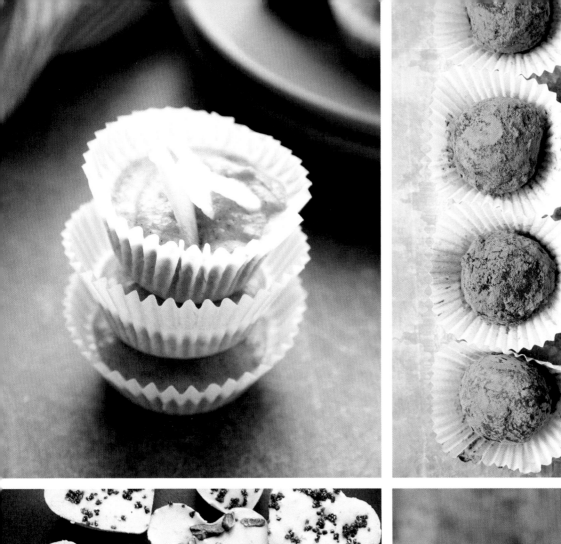

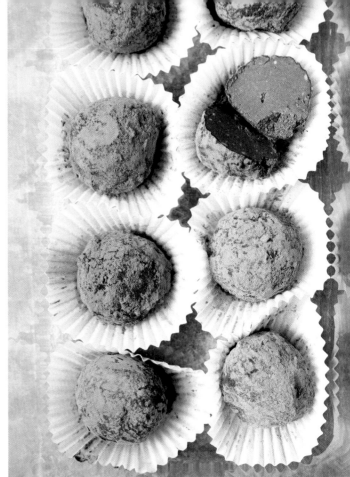

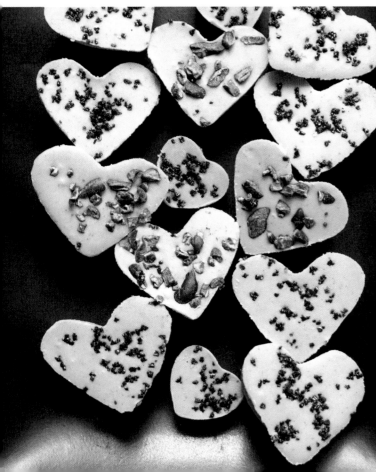

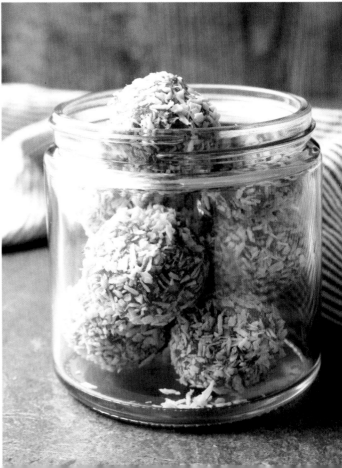

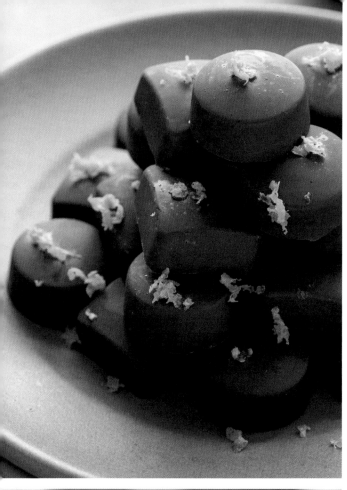

Treats

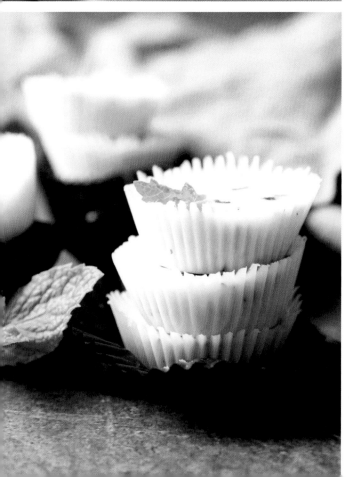

Ginger Fizz Mocktail

PREP TIME: **10 minutes** | YIELD: **4 servings**

This low-carb fizzy drink is a great way to enjoy summer fruit without lots of sugar. Using just about one-quarter of a peach per drink keeps the carbs low, but the flavor is amazing! If you own a juicer and can use fresh ginger juice, great; otherwise, a store-bought one will work.

1 fresh peach, peeled, pitted, and puréed (see Tips)

Juice of 2 lemons

1 teaspoon premade ginger juice, or 1 (2-inch) piece fresh ginger, peeled and juiced (see Tips)

Sparkling water

Sprig of mint, for garnish (optional)

In a pitcher, mix together the puréed peach, lemon juice, and ginger juice. Stir well to combine.

Add sparkling water to taste (depending on how diluted you want it to be) and serve with a slice of fresh peach.

> **TIPS**
>
> If peaches aren't in season, use frozen peaches instead: thaw about 8 slices to be the equivalent of 1 peach. Or, alternatively, use 4 ounces of fresh or frozen raspberries plus 2 tablespoons of water and follow the steps for creating and straining a raspberry purée on page 360.
>
> Ginger People is one great brand of bottled ginger juice, or you may find fresh ginger juice or "shots" locally in smaller juice shops.

CALORIES: **23** | FAT: **0 g** | PROTEIN: **0 g** | CARBS: **6 g** | FIBER: **1 g** | NET CARBS: **5 g**

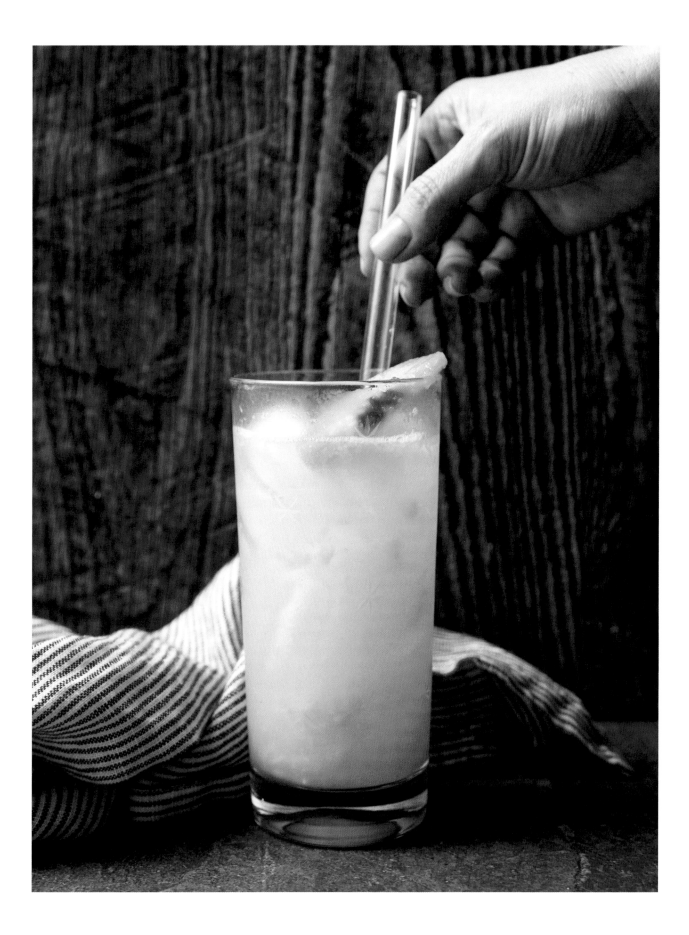

Dark Chocolate Orange Fudge

PREP TIME: 15 minutes, plus time to chill | YIELD: **2 dozen pieces (1 per serving)**

For an indulgent, chocolaty bite, not much is better than fudge! These sugar-free, stevia-sweetened morsels will satisfy that chocolate craving while delivering antioxidants, all without the high carb count.

3 tablespoons coconut butter, softened (see Notes)

2 tablespoons coconut oil, melted

4 ounces 100% dark chocolate, melted (see Notes)

1 teaspoon maple syrup

10 drops stevia extract

1/4 teaspoon pure vanilla extract

1/2 teaspoon orange extract (optional)

Grated zest of 1 orange (reserve 1 teaspoon for garnish)

SPECIAL EQUIPMENT (OPTIONAL)

Silicone candy mold(s) with about 1-inch wells

Place all of the ingredients in a large mixing bowl and stir until smooth. Taste and add up to 10 drops more stevia if desired.

Lay the silicone molds (if using) on a flat plate or small tray that will fit into your refrigerator. (I used small molds whose wells each hold about 1 teaspoon of the fudge mixture.) Using a teaspoon, spoon the mixture evenly into the molds.

Alternatively, portion the fudge into an ice cube tray or a parchment paper–lined mini muffin tin, filling each well completely. These containers will likely make 1 dozen pieces rather than 2 dozen, so each piece will be 2 servings.

Place the molds in the freezer for about 10 minutes, until the fudge is firm enough to pop out of the molds. Garnish with the reserved orange zest and serve cold. This fudge will melt at room temperature.

Store in an airtight container in the refrigerator or freezer for up to 6 weeks.

NOTES

To soften coconut butter, if the jar is microwave-safe (no metal), heat it in the microwave in 30-second increments, stirring between rounds, until it's liquid. Alternatively, place the jar in a saucepan and fill with water that reaches three-quarters of the way up the jar. Simmer on the stovetop over medium-low heat until the coconut butter softens enough to stir easily.

Using a high-quality chocolate is ideal. I love and recommend Pascha brand 100% dark chocolate chips. Note that with lower-quality 100% dark chocolate, you may need to add more stevia to make it a bit more palatable.

SPICE IT UP
Add a pinch of cayenne pepper to give this fudge a kick!

CALORIES: **59** | FAT: **6 g** | PROTEIN: **2 g** | CARBS: **3 g** | FIBER: **1 g** | NET CARBS: **2 g**

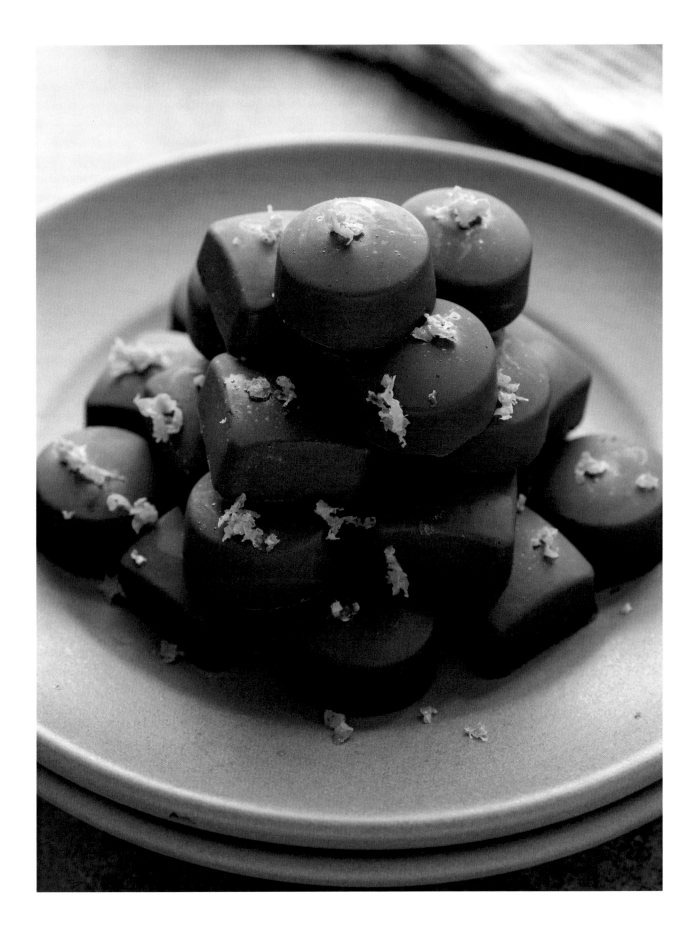

Salted PB Bites

PREP TIME: **20 minutes, plus time to chill** | COOK TIME: **10 minutes** | YIELD: **14 bites (1 per serving)**

Peanut butter and cacao butter combine in these treats for a creamy texture that's extra special. The collagen in these makes them a bit of a power treat, and they're great for kids and adults alike. If you like more texture, use crunchy peanut butter instead of creamy!

1/2 cup unsweetened peanut butter or other nut or seed butter

1/4 cup cacao butter, melted (see Note)

2 scoops grass-fed collagen peptides

1/4 teaspoon pure vanilla extract

2 pinches of ground cinnamon

2 pinches of sea salt

10 drops stevia extract

2 tablespoons cacao nibs

SPECIAL EQUIPMENT (OPTIONAL)

Silicone candy mold with at least 14 (3/4-ounce) cavities

In a medium-sized mixing bowl, whisk together all the ingredients except the cacao nibs until well combined. Taste and add more stevia if desired.

Pour the mixture evenly into the molds or an ice cube tray and sprinkle with the cacao nibs. Place in the refrigerator until completely chilled and set, about 30 minutes.

Release the bites from the molds or ice cube trays by inverting and twisting the tray to pop them out. If they aren't releasing as expected, set the bottoms of the containers in warm water, then invert the trays to release.

Store in an airtight container in the refrigerator or freezer for up to 6 weeks.

IN A RUSH?

Chill in the freezer for about 10 minutes, until set, rather than in the refrigerator.

NOTE

To melt cacao butter, place it in a small saucepan over low heat and stir constantly until it's fully melted. Alternatively, place it in a microwave-safe bowl and microwave on high in 30-second increments until fully melted.

TIP

It's fancy, but if you can find coffee salt, it makes a perfect topping for these bites in addition to the cacao nibs (as shown in the picture).

You could also use a mini muffin tin with paper liners instead of silicone molds.

CALORIES: **83** | FAT: **7 g** | PROTEIN: **4 g** | CARBS: **3 g** | FIBER: **2 g** | NET CARBS: **1 g**

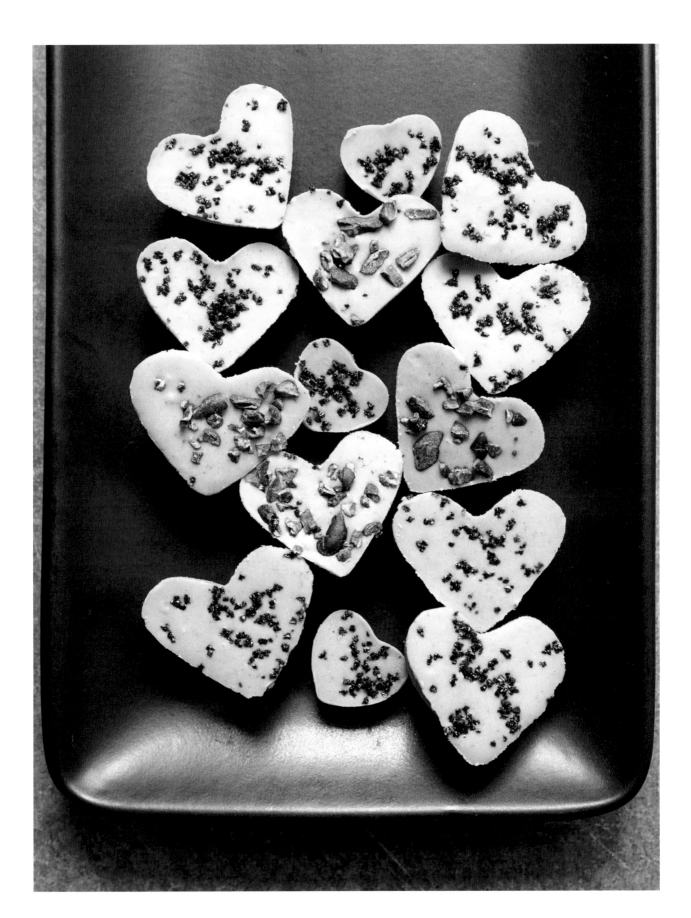

Creamy Raspberry Vanilla Treats

PREP TIME: **15 minutes, plus time to chill** | YIELD: **20 pieces (1 per serving)**

A great low-carb fruit option, raspberries give these treats a slightly sweet, slightly tangy bite. Coconut butter makes them creamy and naturally sweet, but adding a bit of stevia can make them as sweet as you like. Try adding cacao nibs for a "chocolate chip" effect and some crunch!

3/4 cup raspberries, fresh or thawed from frozen (one 6-ounce clamshell pack)

2 tablespoons water

1/2 cup coconut butter, softened (see Notes, page 352)

1/2 cup coconut oil, melted

5 drops stevia extract

Seeds from 1 vanilla bean pod, or 1/2 teaspoon pure vanilla extract (see Tip)

2 tablespoons unsweetened coconut flakes, for garnish (optional)

SPECIAL EQUIPMENT

24-well mini muffin tin

Line 20 wells of a 24-well mini muffin tin with mini parchment-paper liners.

Place the raspberries and water in a blender and pulse until smooth. Strain the mixture through a fine-mesh strainer or cheesecloth to remove the raspberry seeds. (You can use the back of a spoon to help push the mixture through the strainer.)

In a small mixing bowl, whisk together the raspberry purée, coconut butter, coconut oil, stevia, and vanilla bean seeds until well combined. Taste and add more stevia if you like.

Using a tablespoon, distribute the mixture evenly among the parchment-lined wells of the muffin tin. Top with the coconut flakes (if using). Place the muffin tin in the freezer for about 20 minutes, until firm. Serve cold; these treats will melt at room temperature.

Store in an airtight container in the refrigerator or freezer for up to 6 weeks.

TIP

To remove vanilla bean seeds, slice the bean lengthwise down the center, then run the back of your knife along the inside of the pod to scrape out the seeds.

CALORIES: **87** | FAT: **9 g** | PROTEIN: **1 g** | CARBS: **2 g** | FIBER: **1 g** | NET CARBS: **1 g**

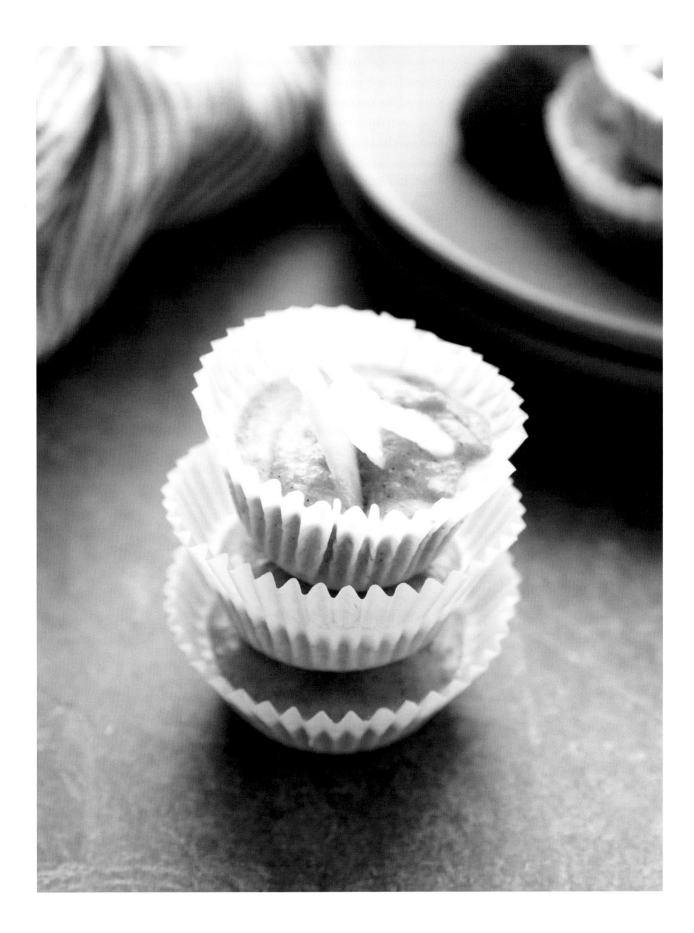

Mint Chip Cups

PREP TIME: **15 minutes, plus time to chill** | YIELD: **16 pieces (1 per serving)**

For an after-dinner or anytime treat, these mint cups are a delight! The minty flavor makes them refreshing, and the creamy coconut butter makes them satisfying. The cacao nibs are great no-sugar "chips" that add texture, but make these without cacao nibs if you prefer a smooth treat.

1/2 cup coconut butter, softened (see Notes, page 352)

1/4 cup cacao butter, melted (see Note, page 354)

1/4 cup coconut oil

5 drops stevia extract

1 teaspoon mint extract

2 teaspoons minced fresh mint

3 tablespoons cacao nibs

SPECIAL EQUIPMENT (OPTIONAL)
Mini muffin tin

Line 12 wells of a mini muffin tin with mini parchment-paper liners.

In a small mixing bowl, whisk together all the ingredients. Taste and add more stevia if you like.

Using a tablespoon, distribute the mixture evenly among the parchment-lined wells of the muffin tin. Place the muffin tin in the freezer for about 20 minutes, until firm. Serve cold; these treats will melt at room temperature.

Store in an airtight container in the refrigerator or freezer for up to 6 weeks.

CALORIES: **109** | FAT: **10 g** | PROTEIN: **1 g** | CARBS: **3 g** | FIBER: **2 g** | NET CARBS: **1 g**

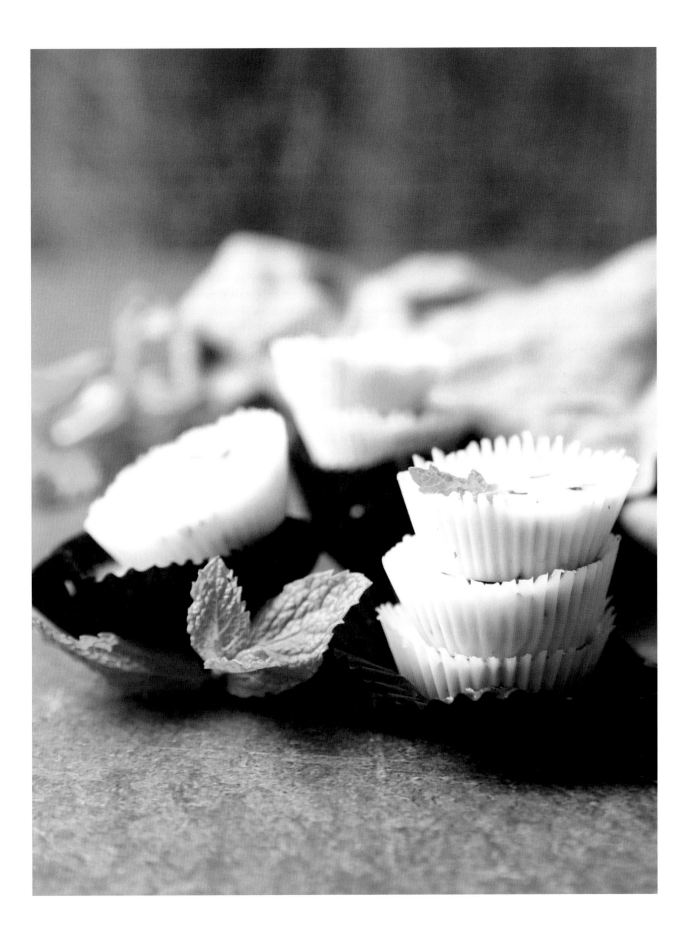

Raspberry Lemon Gummies

PREP TIME: 20 minutes, plus time to chill | COOK TIME: 10 minutes | YIELD: 24 gummies (2 per serving)

Feel like a kid again with these gummy treats (or serve them to your kids!). The tartness of the lemon with the sweetness of the raspberry and stevia makes them a healthy version of sour gummy candy.

1 cup fresh raspberries (one 6-ounce clamshell pack)

1/2 cup lemon juice (3 to 4 lemons)

1/2 cup water

1/4 cup unflavored grass-fed gelatin

10 drops stevia extract

SPECIAL EQUIPMENT (OPTIONAL)

Silicone gummy mold with at least 24 (3/4-ounce) cavities

Place the raspberries, lemon juice, and water in a blender and pulse until smooth. Strain the mixture through a fine-mesh strainer or cheesecloth to remove the raspberry seeds. (You can use the back of a spoon to help push the mixture through the strainer.)

Transfer half of the raspberry-lemon mixture to a small saucepan over medium-low heat.

While that half of the mixture warms, place the remaining half in a medium-sized mixing bowl and whisk in the gelatin, 1 tablespoon at a time. Whisk until the gelatin is well incorporated and the mixture is thick.

Pour the warm half of the mixture into the cool half and whisk thoroughly until smooth and well combined.

Add the stevia, taste, and then add more stevia if you like.

Pour the mixture into silicone gummy molds or a 6 by 9-inch glass or ceramic baking dish. Place in the refrigerator until completely chilled and set, about 30 minutes.

If you used a baking dish instead of gummy molds, use a small cookie cutter to cut out shapes or simply cut the gummies into squares or rectangles. To release the gummies from the molds or baking dish, set the bottoms of the containers in warm water.

NOTES

While whole raspberries are a high-fiber fruit, most of the fiber is found in the seeds. Since the seeds are removed for this recipe, the fiber has not been counted in the nutrition information below.

If you use a baking pan to make the gummies, keep in mind that the smaller the pan, the thicker the gummies will be.

CALORIES: **24** | FAT: **0 g** | PROTEIN: **4 g** | CARBS: **2 g** | FIBER: **0 g** | NET CARBS: **2 g**

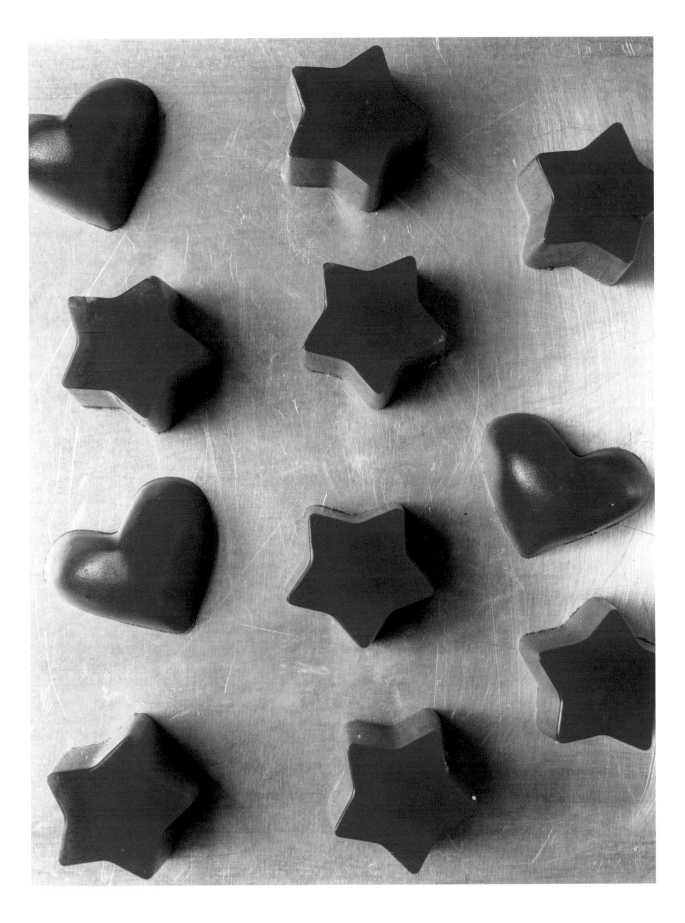

Sparkling Gummies

PREP TIME: 10 minutes, plus time to chill | COOK TIME: 10 minutes | YIELD: 16 gummies (2 per serving)

Looking for a way to enjoy flavored sparkling water beyond simply sipping on it? These gummies are a fun treat that you can make with any flavor you like. Alternatively, you can use plain sparkling water with some lemon or lime juice and stevia to get a more simple citrus flavor!

2 (12-ounce) cans naturally flavored sparkling water, divided

1/4 cup plus 2 tablespoons unflavored grass-fed gelatin

5 to 10 drops stevia extract

SPECIAL EQUIPMENT (OPTIONAL)

Silicone gummy mold with at least 16 (3/4-ounce) cavities

Heat 1 can of sparkling water in a small saucepan over medium-low heat.

While it warms, pour the remaining can of sparkling water into a medium-sized mixing bowl and whisk in the gelatin, 1 tablespoon at a time. Whisk until the gelatin is well incorporated and the mixture is thick.

Pour the warmed water into the bowl with the water and gelatin and whisk thoroughly until smooth and well combined.

Add the stevia, taste, and then add more stevia if you like.

Pour the mixture into gummy molds or a 9 by 9-inch glass or ceramic baking dish. Place in the refrigerator until completely chilled and set, about 30 minutes.

If you used a baking dish instead of molds, use a small cookie cutter to cut out different shapes or simply cut the gummies into squares or rectangles. To release the gummies from the molds or baking dish, set the bottoms of the containers in warm water.

NOTE
If you use a baking pan to make the gummies, keep in mind that the smaller the pan, the thicker your gummies will be.

CALORIES: **16** | FAT: **0 g** | PROTEIN: **4 g** | CARBS: **0 g** | FIBER: **0 g** | NET CARBS: **0 g**

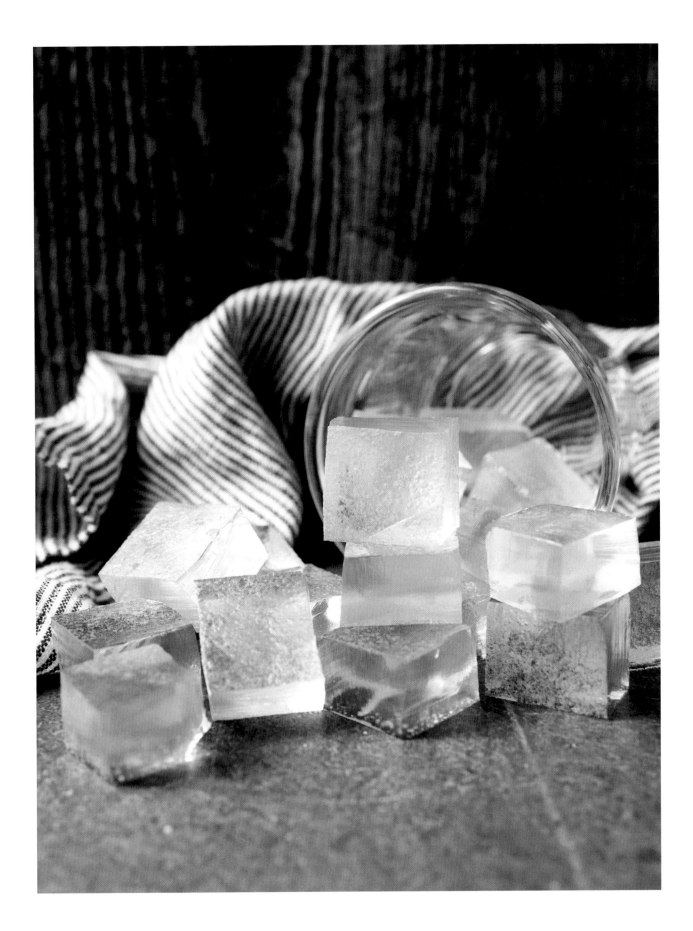

Chocolate Peanut Butter Truffles

PREP TIME: 15 minutes, plus time to chill | YIELD: 1 dozen truffles (1 per serving)

Chocolate and peanut butter is a classic flavor combination, and these truffles come together in just a few easy steps. They are great to keep on hand anytime, but they're especially nice for the holidays. You can also make these with cashew butter instead of peanut butter and add some mint extract for a chocolate mint truffle!

1/2 cup unsweetened creamy peanut butter

5 tablespoons cacao powder, divided

2 tablespoons cacao butter, melted (see Note, page 354)

1/2 teaspoon pure vanilla extract

10 drops stevia extract

Combine the peanut butter, 3 tablespoons of the cacao powder, the cacao butter, vanilla, and stevia in a medium-sized mixing bowl. Taste and add more stevia if desired. Refrigerate the mixture for about 10 minutes to firm up.

Place the remaining 2 tablespoons of cacao powder in a small bowl.

Once the peanut butter mixture is firm to the touch, form 1 tablespoon of the mixture into a ball and roll it in the cacao powder to coat. Place it in a mini muffin cup or on a pan or plate. Repeat with the remaining mixture.

Refrigerate for at least 20 minutes or up to overnight. Serve cold; these treats will melt at room temperature.

Store in an airtight container in the refrigerator or freezer for up to 6 weeks.

CALORIES: **76** | FAT: **6 g** | PROTEIN: **3 g** | CARBS: **4 g** | FIBER: **2 g** | NET CARBS: **2 g**

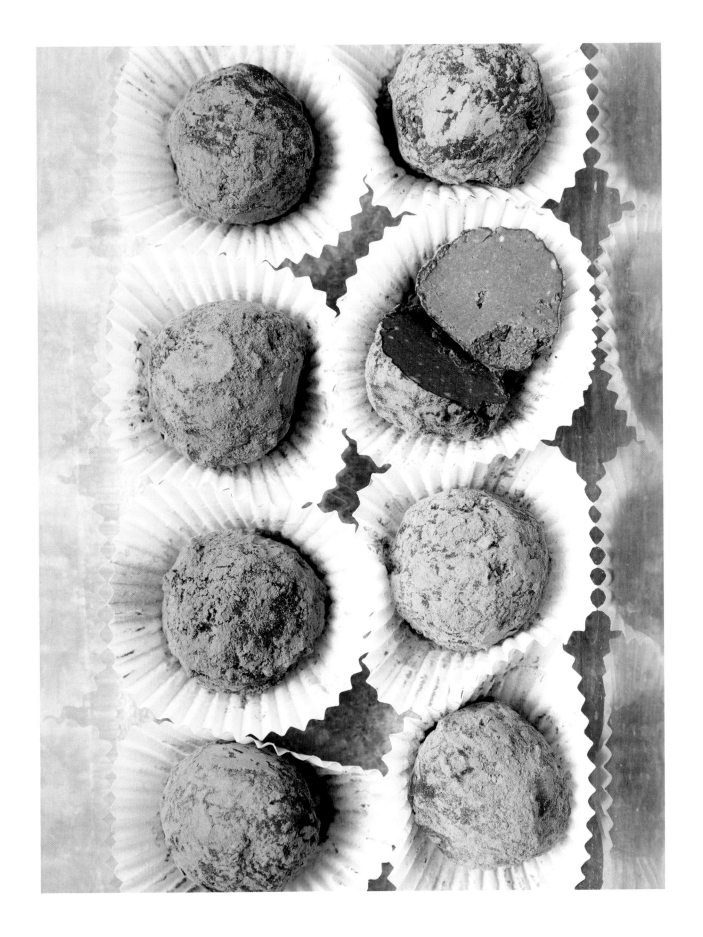

No-Bake Carrot Cake Bites

PREP TIME: **15 minutes** | YIELD: **1 dozen bites (1 per serving)**

Possibly my favorite treat in this book, these bites are delicious, and the cashew butter adds a natural sweetness—you may not want to add much stevia to these! These are also a great way to add more protein to your day; just up the collagen to two scoops if you like.

1 small carrot, peeled

1/2 cup unsweetened cashew, almond, or sunflower seed butter

1 scoop collagen peptides

1/4 teaspoon pumpkin pie spice

5 drops stevia extract

2 tablespoons chopped walnuts

1/2 cup unsweetened shredded coconut

Shred the carrot on a box grater, then finely mince the shreds. Alternatively, roughly chop the carrot and then process in a food processor until it's in very fine pieces. Place the carrot on a cheesecloth or a few layers of paper towels and squeeze out any excess water. Take care when completing this step, as the carrot juice may stain. You should have 5 or 6 tablespoons of minced carrot.

Combine 1/4 cup of the minced carrot (reserve the rest), the cashew butter, collagen peptides, pumpkin pie spice, and stevia in a medium-sized mixing bowl. Taste and add more stevia if desired. When the mixture is well combined, fold in the walnuts. Freeze the mixture for about 10 minutes to firm it up.

While the cashew butter mixture is in the freezer, combine the shredded coconut and 1 tablespoon of the minced carrot in a small bowl.

Once the cashew butter mixture is firm to the touch, form 1 tablespoon of the mixture into a ball and roll it in the coconut-and-carrot mixture to coat. Place it in a mini muffin cup or on a pan or plate. Repeat with the remaining mixture.

Refrigerate for at least 20 minutes or up to overnight. Serve cold; these treats will melt at room temperature.

Store in an airtight container in the refrigerator or freezer for up to 6 weeks.

CALORIES: **104** | FAT: **9 g** | PROTEIN: **3 g** | CARBS: **5 g** | FIBER: **1 g** | NET CARBS: **4 g**

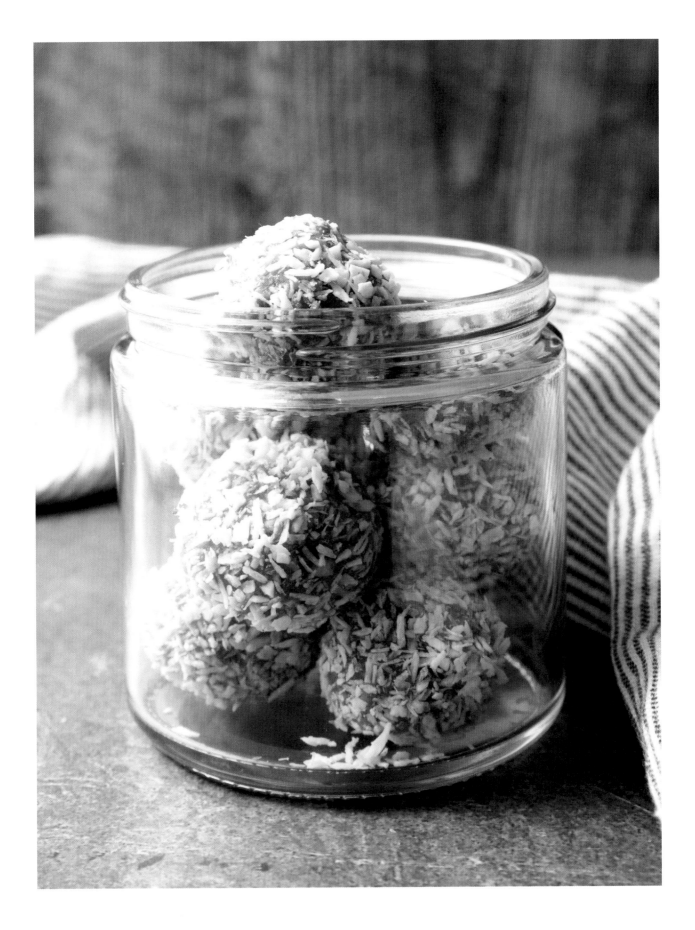

RECIPES	PG	NUTS	EGGS	NIGHT-SHADES	FODMAPS	DAIRY	21DSD-FRIENDLY
Chorizo Scramble Breakfast Tacos	168		M	●	●	M	●
Poachies Breakfast Salad with Hollandaise Sauce	170		●	●	●		●
Easy Soft-Boiled Eggs	172		●				●
Chunky Cobb-Style Egg Salad	174		●				●
Kale, Bacon & Goat Cheese Frittata	176		●		M	M	●
Italian Sausage, Peppers & Spinach Frittata	178		●	●	●	M	●
10-Minute Breakfast Hash	180			●	●	M	●
Matcha Chia N'Oatmeal	182				M		
Lemon Blueberry Keto Muffins	184	●	●		●	M	
Pumpkin Spice Keto Pancakes	186		●		●		
Chocolate Raspberry Smoothie	188				M		
Pumpkin Spice Smoothie	190				●		
Dreamy Matcha Latte	192				M		M
Creamy Keto Coffee	193				M		M
Chicken Salad Collard Wraps	196		M		●		●
Crispy Chicken Spinach Alfredo	198	●	●	●	●	●	●
Hidden Veggie Ranch Burgers	200			M	●		●
Baby Kale Caesar Salad with Grilled Chicken	202				●	M	●
The Best-Tasting Chicken	204				●		●
Keto Chicken Tenders	206		●	M	●		●
Cacio e Pepe Spaghetti Squash with Grilled Chicken Thighs	208					●	●
Skillet Chicken Cacciatore	210			●		M	●
Weeknight Roasted Chicken	212						
White Chicken Chili	214			M	●		●
Thai Red Curry Soup	216			●	●		●
Simple Shredded Chicken	218				M		●
Chicken Broth	220				M		●
Umami Steak & Arugula Salad	224				●	M	●
Beef Fajita Bowl	226			●	●		●
Power Bacon Cheeseburgers	228			●	●	M	●
Sloppy Joe Chili	230			●	●	M	●
Mediterranean Meatloaf	232		●	M	●		●
Beef Satay Skewers	234	●		M	●		●
Meat & Greens Bowl	236			●	●	M	●
Spiced Stuffed Eggplant	238			M	●	M	●
Simple Shredded Beef	240				M		●
Thai Meatballs	244			●	●		●
Tacos al Pastor	246			●	●		●
Super Garlic Stir-Fry Bowl	248			M	●		●
Spaghetti Bolognese Bake	250			M	●	M	M
Meatballs Marinara	252			●	●	M	●
Cocoa BBQ Ribs	254			●	●		●
Cajun Pork Tenderloin	256			M	●		●
Simple Shredded Pork	258				M		●
Blackened Fish Tacos	262			●	●		●
Shrimp Pad Thai	264	●			●		●
Lemon Caper Salmon	266				●	●	●
Sole Italiano	268			●	●		●
Glazed Salmon with Seared Bok Choy	270			●	●		●
Deli Tuna Salad	272		●	●	●		●
Niçoise Salad	274		●	●	●		●
Salmon Avocado Roll-Ups	276				●		●

● contains this allergen or is this type of recipe
M can be modified to be free of this allergen or to comply with this type of meal

RECIPES	PG	NUTS	EGGS	NIGHT-SHADES	FODMAPS	DAIRY	21DSD-FRIENDLY
Spicy Citrus Slaw	280			M	●		●
Cilantro Cauli-Rice	282				●		●
Creamy Cauliflower Purée	284				●		●
Mediterranean Roasted Cauliflower	286			M	●		
Blistered Shishito Peppers	288			●			●
Marinated Onions	290				●		●
Spicy Roasted Asparagus with Lemon	292			M	●	M	●
Bacon-y Caramelized Onions	294				●		●
Herbed Cashew Cheese	298	●			●		●
Bacon Jalapeño Poppers	300	●		●	●	●	●
Keto Hummus	302			M	●		●
Quick Guacamole	304			M	●		●
Quick Salsa	306			●	●		●
Baked Cheese Crisps	308					●	●
Pesto-Stuffed Mushrooms	310	●			●	M	●
Keto Charcuterie Board	314						
Ranch Kale Chips	316				M		●
Cauliflower Queso Dip	318			M	●	●	●
Dairy-Free Cashew Queso Dip	320	●		M	●		●
Spinach Artichoke Dip	322			●	●	●	●
Simple Keto Romesco	324	●		●	●		●
Caponata Dip	326	●		●	●		●
Super Garlic Spice Blend	330				●		
Bagel Spice Blend	330				●		
Trifecta Spice Blend	330				●		
Italian Spice Blend	330				●		
Greek Spice Blend	330				●		
Ranch Spice Blend	331				●		
Taco & Fajita Spice Blend	331			●	●		
Chorizo Spice Blend	331			●	●		
Cajun Spice Blend	331			●	●		
Cocoa BBQ Spice Blend	331			●	●		
Hollandaise Sauce	334		●				●
Healthy Homemade Mayonnaise	335		●				●
Clarified Butter & Ghee	336						●
Simple Marinara	338			●	●		●
Sweetener-Free Ketchup	340			●	●		M
BBQ Sauce	341			●	●		●
Avocado Crema	342			M	●		●
Pesto	343	●			●	M	●
Salad Dressings	344						
Caesar Dressing	346				●	M	●
Ranch Dressing	347			M	●	M	●
Ginger Fizz Mocktail	350				●		
Dark Chocolate Orange Fudge	352				●		
Salted PB Bites	354	●					
Creamy Raspberry Vanilla Treats	356				●		
Mint Chip Cups	358				●		
Raspberry Lemon Gummies	360						
Sparkling Gummies	362						
Chocolate Peanut Butter Truffles	364	●					
No-Bake Carrot Cake Bites	366	●			●		

RECIPE INDEX

Breakfast

168
Chorizo Scramble Breakfast Tacos

170
Poachies Breakfast Salad with Hollandaise Sauce

172
Easy Soft-Boiled Eggs

174
Chunky Cobb-Style Egg Salad

176
Kale, Bacon & Goat Cheese Frittata

178
Italian Sausage, Peppers & Spinach Frittata

180
10-Minute Breakfast Hash

182
Matcha Chia N'Oatmeal

184
Lemon Blueberry Keto Muffins

186
Pumpkin Spice Keto Pancakes

188
Chocolate Raspberry Smoothie

190
Pumpkin Spice Smoothie

192
Dreamy Matcha Latte

193
Creamy Keto Coffee

Main Dishes: Chicken

196
Chicken Salad Collard Wraps

198
Crispy Chicken Spinach Alfredo

200
Hidden Veggie Ranch Burgers

202
Baby Kale Caesar Salad with Grilled Chicken

204
The Best-Tasting Chicken

206
Keto Chicken Tenders

208
Cacio e Pepe Spaghetti Squash with Grilled Chicken Thighs

210
Skillet Chicken Cacciatore

212
Weeknight Roasted Chicken

214
White Chicken Chili

216
Thai Red Curry Soup

218
Simple Shredded Chicken

220
Chicken Broth

Main Dishes: Beef

224
Umami Steak &
Arugula Salad

226
Beef Fajita Bowl

228
Power Bacon
Cheeseburgers

230
Sloppy Joe Chili

232
Mediterranean
Meatloaf

234
Beef Satay
Skewers

236
Meat & Greens
Bowl

238
Spiced Stuffed
Eggplant

240
Simple Shredded
Beef

Main Dishes: Pork

244
Thai Meatballs

246
Tacos al Pastor

248
Super Garlic Stir-
Fry Bowl

250
Spaghetti
Bolognese Bake

252
Meatballs
Marinara

254
Cocoa BBQ Ribs

256
Cajun Pork
Tenderloin

258
Simple Shredded
Pork

Main Dishes: Seafood

262
Blackened Fish
Tacos

264
Shrimp Pad Thai

266
Lemon Caper
Salmon

268
Sole Italiano

270
Glazed Salmon
with Seared
Bok Choy

272
Deli Tuna Salad

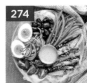
274
Niçoise Salad

276
Salmon Avocado
Roll-Ups

Sides

280 Spicy Citrus Slaw

282 Cilantro Cauli-Rice

284 Creamy Cauliflower Purée

286 Mediterranean Roasted Cauliflower

288 Blistered Shishito Peppers

290 Marinated Onions

292 Spicy Roasted Asparagus with Lemon

294 Bacon-y Caramelized Onions

Snacks & Dips

298 Herbed Cashew Cheese

300 Bacon Jalapeño Poppers

302 Keto Hummus

304 Quick Guacamole

306 Quick Salsa

308 Baked Cheese Crisps

310 Pesto-Stuffed Mushrooms

314 Keto Charcuterie Board

316 Ranch Kale Chips

318 Cauliflower Queso Dip

320 Dairy-Free Cashew Queso Dip

322 Spinach Artichoke Dip

324 Simple Keto Romesco

326 Caponata Dip

Spice Blends

330

Super Garlic Spice Blend
Bagel Spice Blend
Trifecta Spice Blend
Italian Spice Blend
Greek Spice Blend

Ranch Spice Blend
Taco & Fajita Spice Blend
Chorizo Spice Blend
Cajun Spice Blend
Cocoa BBQ Spice Blend

Condiments, Sauces & Dressings

334
Hollandaise Sauce

335
Healthy Homemade Mayonnaise

336
Clarified Butter & Ghee

338
Simple Marinara

340
Sweetener-Free Ketchup

341
BBQ Sauce

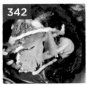
342
Avocado Crema

343
Pesto

344
Salad Dressings

346
Caesar Dressing

347
Ranch Dressing

Treats

350
Ginger Fizz Mocktail

352
Dark Chocolate Orange Fudge

354
Salted PB Bites

356
Creamy Raspberry Vanilla Treats

358
Mint Chip Cups

360
Raspberry Lemon Gummies

362
Sparkling Gummies

364
Chocolate Peanut Butter Truffles

366
No-Bake Carrot Cake Bites

GENERAL INDEX

ACKNOWLEDGMENTS

First and foremost, to you, my readers: That I am fortunate enough to share my advice, insights, wisdom, recommendations, and food with you is truly a blessing. I am grateful for this opportunity, and I don't take this responsibility lightly. I value your trust in me, and I hope to always deliver a balanced, sane, and health-focused approach in each of my books. I aim to be a "soft landing," to provide nondogmatic advice, and I want to say thank you for supporting my approach over the years and for your purchase of this book. I write these books for you—your presence matters.

To Team Balanced Bites—April, Holly, Moriah, Amanda, Niki, and Amy—a wonderful crew of women who have stood side by side with me through not only this book but many books before: You are the bedrock. Without you all keeping the lights on and the wheels turning in our entire operation, I honestly would not have the time and space I need to write these books. I value each of you for your individual input, ideas, creativity, and loyalty. You ladies are all so special to me.

To my friends and colleagues, Liz, Cassy, Mary, Caitlin, Jenny, Beth, and so many others who have told me I'm a trusted voice on this topic and that my voice was one you wanted to hear in this space: I appreciate your words so very much. Without your support and affirmations, this book may not have happened.

To many of my peers in the keto book space, Jimmy, Leanne, Kyndra, Tasha, Julie, Suzanne, and Jen: Thank you for the kind and warm welcome so many of you have extended via social media. I wasn't sure what to expect when writing a book on keto, but you've been awesome and I can't wait to meet and collaborate with so many of you.

To my publicist, Amanda: Thank you for being my number one (and perhaps most energetic) fan and cheerleader and for helping me to see my own potential. I've absolutely loved working with you.

To my editor, Erin: Thank you for being my copilot in getting my ideas organized. I'm fully aware that my words would just float on the page without your help to corral them into chapters that make sense. I so appreciate your support, encouragement, and shared love of humor in my dark moments from beginning to end.

To my publisher, Erich, and the whole Victory Belt team: Thank you for giving my ideas the opportunity to help so many people. I'll forever be grateful.

And to my husband, Scott: Thank you for always having my back while I'm writing books and feeling the stress of it on a daily basis with me. I appreciate your acts of service, not only in the mountains of dishes you washed as I cooked every recipe but also in your everyday presence. You are the best partner I could have asked for—you're my favorite.